SOCIAL THEORIES OF FERTILITY AND THE MALTHUSIAN DEBATE

SOCIAL THEORIES OF FERTILITY AND THE MALTHUSIAN DEBATE

BY

D. E. C. EVERSLEY

GREENWOOD PRESS, PUBLISHERS
WESTPORT, CONNECTICUT

Library of Congress Cataloging in Publication Data

Eversley, David Edward Charles.
Social theories of fertility and the Malthusian debate.

Reprint of the ed. published by the Clarendon Press, Oxford.
Bibliography: p.
1. Fertility, Human. 2. Demography. I. Title.
HB891.E85 1975 301.32'1 74-9219
ISBN 0-8371-7628-X

Originally published in 1959 by the Clarendon Press, Oxford

This reprint has been authorized by the Clarendon Press Oxford

Reprinted in 1975 by Greenwood Press, a division of Williamhouse-Regency Inc.

Library of Congress Catalog Card Number 74-9219

ISBN 0-8371-7628-X

Printed in the United States of America

PREFACE

THE study presented here arose out of an attempt to give a systematic account of recent trends in population movements, and theories associated with these, in lectures given to students in the University of Birmingham. Faced with an apparently chaotic mass of Malthusian and anti-Malthusian literature, I began to see something of a connecting thread only when H. L. Beales, to whom I had turned for advice, suggested that the key was to be found in the work of Richard Jones, Malthus's successor at Haileybury. In this way, another volume came to be added to the long list of those which might have been written by one who knows more about English social history than almost anyone else, but chooses to leave the credit for his ideas to accrue to his grateful pupils.

Professor D. V. Glass read and criticized the manuscript in its early stages and towards the end, and made many valuable suggestions in a field where he has unique knowledge. Dr. K. H. Connell contributed some Irish references. Mr. R. F. Willetts of this University, and my uncle, Dr. W. A. Morel, helped with classical sources, and Mrs. Margaret Hilton with French authors. Many other friends and colleagues placed their specialized knowledge and critical powers at my disposal. I am particularly grateful to Dr. Josephine Klein and Mr. Esra Bennathan for the detailed suggestions and help in systematization. My father, Dr. O. R. Eberstadt, read the proofs and saved me from a good many mistakes.

The subject of this book ranges over a number of fields outside my own, and the investigation did not follow the methods of any particular school of historical or sociological writing. These factors have inevitably led to defects in structure and in arbitrary judgements. I should like to make it clear that those who helped by discussion and criticism are not to be blamed for these faults.

The compilation of the manuscript would not have been possible without the help of a succession of skilful assistants. The excerpts from authors (and there were many more of these than found their way into text or footnotes) were transcribed by Miss Edna Davies and Mrs. Corinne Lovatt. The latter did most of the work on foreign and classical sources, and also typed a great part of the draft manuscript. Most of the final version was typed by Mlle Françoise Larregain. Mrs. Virginia McDonald and Miss Janet Blackman performed the laborious task of checking manuscript and footnotes, preparing the bibliography and index, and transforming an untidy mass into something at least partly conforming to the publishers' exacting standards. To all these, and the kind and patient publishers themselves, I owe warm thanks.

Finally, I would like to thank my own University for meeting the considerable expenses involved in the preparation and typing of the manuscript. If others lament the passing of the age of private patronage, I should only like to testify that its modern official counterpart is as generous, probably attaches fewer strings, and asks no questions if six years elapse between the first grant and the day of publication.

D. E. C. EVERSLEY

University of Birmingham
March, 1959

CONTENTS

I

INTRODUCTORY

The sociological approach to population

THE ghost of Parson Malthus is still abroad. Every year we hear fresh warnings of a threatened world famine. Population grows at an alarming rate. Yet for more than a hundred years the decline of fertility in many countries has been the principal subject of books about population. Today, there is a fair amount of unanimity concerning the general causes of this decline. In the words of the United Nations report:

> It is a striking feature of the literature on the decline of fertility that many explanations of the decline which appear different at first sight turn out upon closer inspection to be fairly similar. Most recent authors believe that the decline in fertility is due to a complex of inter-related causes, acting upon one another and jointly bringing about the decline. They generally agree that the decline in fertility is closely connected with the changes that have fundamentally transformed European society in the last two centuries, but attempts to associate the decline exclusively with a particular aspect of these changes, such as, for example, urbanization, have not proved satisfactory. Those writers who attribute the decline in fertility to 'civilization' as a whole have perhaps most clearly shown this to be true.[1]

In other words, most writers now agree that there is a good answer to Malthus's worst fears. The argument runs something like this: There is not so much danger of population outrunning subsistence, since there are factors at work in many societies which tend to diminish the rate of increase, and it is possible that these influences may increasingly operate in the countries where the growth is now fastest. They are: a rise in the standard of living, the adoption of 'Western civilized habits', and the progress of democratic institutions. To put forward these arguments is to record contemporary opinion. We are not here concerned with the question of whether they are in fact true, or indeed whether it is desirable that these countries should adopt 'Western civilized habits', or democratic institutions.

The object of this study is to investigate how these views came to be

[1] United Nations, Department of Social Affairs, Population Division, *The Determinants and Consequences of Population Trends* (New York, 1953), p. 77, para. 36.

held. To the historian of theory in the social sciences, it seems curious that demography should now be so firmly wedded to sociology. It did not begin in this way. Originally, the study of population movements was the most important part of what in England was called 'Political Arithmetic'. This subject, as it was treated by such writers as Graunt in the seventeenth century, later became 'Political Economy', and so population study came to be part of economics. So, in a sense, it has remained, and most books on economics have sections which describe both the effects of changes in economic organization on population size, and the effects of changes in the structure of population on economic activity. Some hold that population is merely a dependent variable, others give it a more important position.

For Malthus certainly, as for his classical contemporaries and the neo-classical economists of the age of Alfred Marshall, this subordination of population theory to economics was complete. But when we look more closely at the type of statement that was required to explain what actually occurred, it invariably means an observation on social behaviour or social medicine. This is so whether the mechanism of change in rates of growth relates to marriages, births or deaths, or migration.

Unfortunately, it is precisely on these points that the classical economists are weakest, partly perhaps because they were not particularly interested in behaviour, and partly because detailed discussions might have raised topics they considered indelicate. Yet as the arguments about the truth of the Malthusian propositions raged, it became increasingly clear that the question whether or not population would continue to grow rapidly depended not so much, as Malthus thought, on the availability of subsistence, but on the reaction of individuals to their environment. Availability of food and other necessaries, of course, is part of this environment, as is the employment which gives rise to wages wherewith to buy food, but increasingly the investigators saw the importance of other factors.

To study the history of population dogmas, then, is to trace the rise in the consciousness of writers in the social sciences of patterns in social organization and social behaviour. To this extent such an investigation is also an inquiry into the history of modern sociology. But it is not primarily conceived for this purpose. There are two more immediate reasons for undertaking this task. The history of theories, of *Dogmengeschichte* as Roscher and later Schumpeter called it, can add materially to our knowledge of any past period if we learn from it what men thought about various aspects of science, theology, or politics. Their ideas will have been derived, in many cases, from their own experience, and in that way books of theory become documentary sources of facts. The changing response to the impact of these experiences on ways of thinking and on policy also repays study.

Secondly, an analysis of past bodies of theory is of great help to the present student in almost every field. Every age produced its own ideological distortions, its prejudices and superstitions. By tracing the influences which gave rise to particular ideas, we are helped in our attempts to rid our own thinking of much of its inevitable bias. We need not be Marxists to acknowledge that the circumstances of our time obtrude themselves into our thought processes, even if we aim at producing social theories of general validity.

The field of population studies affords rich material for the student of ideas. This is due, no doubt, to the fact that the experiences which lead to ideas about population are at once the most common ones of everyday life, and connected with the deepest mysteries. Populations grow or shrink, because children are born, people sicken or die, get married or take monastic vows, because they eat well or starve, because there is a flood or an abundant harvest. Life itself, most ages have held, is God-given and God-taken. Growth and survival are the reward of virtue. Disease and death follow on wickedness. As these earlier ideas became refined the connexion between good behaviour and an increasing population became a physiological, rather than a theological, concern.

Although many authors have commented both on the need for a history of population theories, and the advantages to be derived for the general historian from such a history, a comprehensive account has not yet appeared. The task would be formidable. Since, at every turn, the factors affecting, and affected by, the growth and decline of population are the subject-matter of economics, politics, sociology, medicine, law, theology, and half a dozen other fields of study, those who have worked in them in the past have often devoted much thought to this matter. A list of works dealing exclusively with population would run into several thousand items. If we included those which devoted at any rate substantial sections to it, we should need to list tens of thousands. These would include most of the major classical works in the social sciences up to fairly recent times, when specialization set in. There are a great many general surveys and still more monographs on particular aspects, countries, and individual writers. Malthus alone is honoured by at least one new scholarly discussion every year, quite apart from the innumerable tracts and propagandist volumes which have been written about him since 1798. A list of some of the more important recent writings on the history of population theory and the Malthusian controversies will be found in the first Bibliographical Note at the end of this chapter.

The most comprehensive recent general outline of the development of population theories appeared at the beginning of a volume published in 1953 by the Department of Social Affairs (Population Division) of the United Nations Organization, *Determinants and Consequences of Population Trends*. There is still room, however, for a full analytical treatment fitting the major trends of thought into the framework of social and economic history.

On all these secondary sources the writer interested in old and scarce books must draw heavily, but it is not necessary to go again over the ground they cover. The difficulty is one of choice. The aim here has been to illustrate trends, not to make a complete list of authors who have advanced one sort of view. The writers quoted have been chosen because the ideas they put forward can be seen fairly clearly, not only as part of their own work in general, but also, and chiefly, as characteristic of their period. Naturally there are in this field, as in others, the inevitable Leonardos, the people who can see far beyond the horizon of their age. They may be mentioned as curiosities. But of all academic exercises, that of finding 'firsts' is probably the most futile, if it is done for the sake of the date alone. It is no doubt interesting if someone used the word 'unemployment' in the seventeenth century, but it is important to know that it came into current usage in the third quarter of the nineteenth. So it is here. The writers chosen, therefore, are for the most part those who translated the evidence they saw around them into generalizations about population. The basis for this choice is the belief that such an idea as that 'greater social mobility diminishes fertility' can really only emerge at a time, and in a country, where a change in the extent of social mobility took place. It is conceivable, of course, that such a statement is purely historical, that is to say, based on documentary evidence about a past age. The frequency with which writers cited in this book appeal to the evidence of the authors of Greece and Rome might suggest that this is quite usual. But closer analysis shows that, as we shall see, this appeal is merely a courtesy of a kind which is bestowed, in other types of literature within the moral sciences, on the Bible. In no case has this appeal been found to relate to a theory which was held to have been true only in classical times, or in contradiction to the investigator's contemporary experience. Seen in this way, the history of population theory becomes social history. But it is necessary to explain in some further detail the main features of the discussion through the ages, and the vocabulary which it uses.

Until the end of the eighteenth century, it was usual to regard a stationary population as normal and a growing population as desirable. A decline meant that there was something wrong—either there was a lack of subsistence, or pestilence, war, or vicious manners produced premature death and barrenness. It was the essence of good government to encourage growth by ensuring food, checking disease, and prohibiting luxury. Then, towards the end of the eighteenth century, the first voices were heard warning against over-population in a general sense. It is true that in particular countries at various periods there had been complaints that there was not enough land to support a growing population, usually in mountainous areas where settlement was confined to a few fertile valleys or mercantile seaboard cities. Such warnings were heard in ancient Greece, and led to demands for colonization. Rome saw its empire as an outlet for the unemployed talents of younger sons. The Vikings spread over northern Europe and to Scotland in search of land, and again in Elizabethan England colonists began a movement which, in time, added vast tracts of territories available for cultivation. But this sort of relative over-population, remediable by methods recognized as normal and efficient from Alexander to Hitler, these spasmodic searches for *Lebensraum*, did not give rise to any general theory of pressure. To Malthus we owe, if not the original idea, at any rate the spreading of the notion that population tended to increase faster than subsistence, and that only misery, or vice (the positive checks) or restraint (the preventive check), would ensure that people and food were in equilibrium. Part of what has been written since Malthus's day has been about the meaning of the word 'tendency'. Much more, however, has been published about the nature of this 'restraint' and the circumstances under which it was likely to operate.

Before discussing the various meanings that can be attached to Malthus's expressions, it should be clearly stated that what he, and his followers and adversaries, discussed was the *will* to have fewer children, or none, not the means to that end. If the means were late marriage, or a solitary life, allied with perfect chastity, then no further explanation is necessary. But if the means were a limitation of children in wedlock (a possibility Malthus hardly envisaged), then the question is inextricably bound up with abortion or contraception. Abortion falls outside the scope of the writings we are now considering—it was seldom advocated openly and the full extent to which it has contributed to the decline in the rate of population growth can never be measured. Contraception, to some extent, is in the same category: although it is widely advocated, not a great deal is so far known about the extent to which it has been effective. Most writers agree, however, that since the end of the nineteenth century, it has played a dominant role in Western Europe and North America in *translating into practice the desire to limit the family*. This much has to be clear: the first thing we look for is that desire—some reason why one should not go on to enlarge one's family. One very good reason, of course, may be the woman's wish not to undergo again the pains and difficulties of child-birth. Here again very little is so far known. In many families the desire to prevent further conceptions will be the result of complex ideas, in which all our standard of living arguments may well be mixed up with physical pain. The avoidance of pain and trouble in itself forms a constituent part of a higher standard of living and, as will be shown, the woman's ability to assert her right to limit her suffering is in itself also part of the progress of civilization.

There is some justification then for treating the question of the will to limit families quite apart from the means to that end. The means are part of technological progress. But the spur to that progress, and the breaking-down of the barriers which once prevented the dissemination of birth-control propaganda—these things are an integral part of the main stream of thought about population.

The term 'restraint' is then to be seen as a psychological one. The various sub-categories are related to its motivation. Admittedly, a good many of the theories to be discussed translate the effects of certain categories of influences into physiological consequences. Thus, some writers claim that luxurious living, or town dissipations, lead merely to an avoidance of marriage, or artificial means to prevent children after marriage; others again seek to prove that these modes of living actually reduce reproductive capacity in one way or another. A third category of writers does not draw such a hard-and-fast distinction between psychological and physiological effects, and merely observes that a given social or economic influence will produce the result indicated—lower fertility. Often the analysis will include such explanations as that of the nervous impotence of the intellectual (or rake, or whatever category is described)—thus obviating the need for any distinctions!

On the whole, however, the physiological explanations belong to an earlier age, and they will therefore figure in this account mainly as forerunners of later theories. But it should be noted that in recent years new explanations along similar lines have made their appearance, for instance those relating to the influence of high or low protein content in food on the fertility of nations.

The historical material

It has been shown that the views we must investigate are necessarily found in a very wide variety of publications. The subject has been commented on in all countries where the size of population caused concern, and since both under- and over-population were already known in the ancient world, the literature must be held to include writings on a large number of topics in every age and region. It is likely that the wish to restrict the size of one's family (or, in some areas, the number of daughters at least), began to be formed with civilization as such. As soon as man emerged from the cave-dwelling or hunting stage, into an ordered and more comfortable domestic life, there would arise in some families a point where the strength, skill, or prestige contributed by additional children would be less, in the opinion of the parents, than the trouble and expense of bringing them up. This assertion cannot of course be proved until we have the literary evidence of Greece and Rome, but this constitutes no reason for doubting the existence of such sentiments. The question rather is: who thought it their duty to record and describe this phenomenon, who wrote about the pattern of population movements? In the first place, one would answer, the historian, the writer describing contemporary fears of depopulation, or over-population. In the ancient world, however, the historian was most often also a philosopher, or at any rate a moralist, and thus, for instance, the evidence of Polybius should be read as a censorious comment on the manners of his time rather than a dispassionate account.

Secondly, the matter was of concern to theologians (a class hardly distinguishable in the ancient world from the philosophers). For them, too, the population problem was essentially a moral one: what was God's (or the Deity's) purpose? Was there, as many later claimed, a categorical imperative in the Old Testament: 'Be Fruitful and Multiply' —a command to be disobeyed at the parents' peril? Was excessive fear about the future, and hence caution, a failure to trust in God's goodness? Was the failure to produce a son an affront to the spirits of departed ancestors?

This analysis of the demographic situation, outdated as it may appear to us, is to be found in works on population until very recent times, and even now we know that in some countries population problems are very much the preoccupation of the priesthood. In the eighteenth century, as we shall see, the search for a natural, or God-given, order of population was prominent in the work of theologians.

Next to the philosophical and theological material the most important category of writings may be termed political. From about the seventeenth century onwards, the prevailing notions of politics emphasized a large (and healthy) population as the first prerequisite of a great power.[1] With the beginning of national wars, and an ever-increasing scarcity of readily available mercenaries in the open market, the number of a king's subjects assumed the utmost importance. In this way the seventeenth, and more particularly the eighteenth century, provide us with a rich harvest of works devoted to the analysis of the causes why in one place or another, the subjects fail to multiply. These inquiries gave rise to innumerable quaint speculations, but also to some of the first serious scientific work in the field, that done by the English 'Political Arithmeticians'.

It would have been well if this trend had continued. The raw material for demographic work, as opposed to theorizing in a vacuum, was available and could have been improved. In London and some other towns there were 'Bills of Mortality', summaries of deaths arranged by causes in the parishes where burial took place; there were the parish registers themselves, and there were many other sources at least of partial statistics. At the end of the seventeenth century Gregory King had made an estimate of the size and social structure of the population, mainly on the basis of the Hearth Tax returns of the reign of Charles II, the lists of households in each parish with the number of hearths they contained as assessed by the constables for the purposes of the tax levied. There were, in the reign of William and Mary, taxes on the parochial registrations. Hospitals kept records of admissions and deaths. Bishops made counts of the number of houses in their parishes. These multifarious sources were used by a great number of writers at the time, but unfortunately not very many of them appear to have had it as their primary objective to arrive at the truth about the movements of

[1] This thought also underlies the Augustan legislation.

population. Instead, as their titles often indicate, they used, or rather misused, the facts at their disposal to prove their assertions—whether about the incompetence of the government, the absence of morals in their age, or the goodness of the Divine Author. Others engaged in metaphysical speculation for its own sake. The eighteenth-century scientists were driven by a restless desire to establish the pattern of the 'natural order' in all matters. Everything had to conform to rules, and human beings were not excluded. It is not surprising that the 'laws' discovered by the eighteenth-century writers hardly stand up to examination. The factual material was extremely faulty, and their shortcomings were not even commented on by some of those who used them. Sometimes there were deliberate, often no doubt unintentional, falsifications of the original data. They all copied from each other. Classification of diseases, as causes of death, was very poor, smallpox being one of the few which are defined beyond doubt. The eighteenth-century controversies centred mainly on the question whether the population was growing or not, at least from about 1760 onwards. (A fuller account of this period will be found in the publications listed in the second Bibliographical Note at the end of this chapter.) Gregory King's estimate was then the only one available which could pretend to any sort of accuracy, but its value was not universally recognized. The first census was not taken until 1801. Various attempts had previously been made to have this necessary task performed earlier, but they failed against popular prejudices—there was a widespread fear of taxation, and militia service, and an idea that enumeration was contrary to divine law. In Parliament objections were based on the belief that the revelation of numbers might give comfort to the King's enemies.

This was the position in England. Abroad, only Sweden offered any factual material of higher quality than the British statistics. Austria and the other Scandinavian countries also could show attempts at enumeration, but there was really nothing anywhere on which serious analytical work could be based. But this was no bar to prolific writings, notably in France. Everywhere there was the conviction that more people were needed, and in France, where costly wars, epidemics, and famines had wrought havoc at the beginning of the eighteenth century, the fears of the politicians were not groundless. This welter of half-truths, metaphysics, moralizing, political and religious pamphleteering, and plagiarism would be at best only entertaining, and at worst, rather monotonous and bulky reading, if it were not for the fact that the attitudes revealed are useful mirrors of the societies in which their authors lived. Thus there is a great difference between the worlds of the high ecclesiastic dignitary, Johann Peter Suessmilch, in mid-eighteenth-century Berlin, that of the moral philosopher Ferguson in Edinburgh at the same time, of Dr. Thomas Short in London, and of the elder Mirabeau in Paris. Within the same country, differences over time are significant even though we may now consider all the attitudes which we compare to be of equal worthlessness. To do full justice to the authors concerned, one should not really quote rather isolated statements from their works without the context, or without at any rate summarizing their main teaching. This, however, would be a space-consuming undertaking, and for this reason only major works have here been accorded so much courtesy.

If the seventeenth and eighteenth centuries, then, have a somewhat unreal appearance in retrospect, the nineteenth century begins, on the whole, to wear a modern aspect. Malthus marks the change. On this point no one would disagree, though emphasis differs. Some see him still as the archmetaphysical speculator who happened to have put his finger on a point of some practical consequence, others hail him as the pioneer of the scientific approach. Again, most writers today say that the change in tone was due to Malthus himself, but some of his detractors give more credit to the changing circumstances of the time, of which he was but a shrewd commentator. We must reserve some evaluation of this problem for a later chapter. What we cannot doubt is that with him the language of population literature changes. The old, familiar assumption that a larger population was 'good' in every case, hardly ever challenged in the eighteenth century, was dropped in favour of an equally simple, but not so universally accepted view that a fast-growing population was a menace.

This general view coloured the terminology, and even the moralizing of our authors. Refinements of living which limited families were once classed with famines and wars as dreadful obstacles to a desired end. After Malthus, the same refinements were welcomed as suitable alternative checks to growth in the place of the 'positive' checks, which were the same as previously—vice and catastrophe.

After Malthus, then, though there were still a few who denied the existence of any problem, every writer became either a Malthusian, an anti-Malthusian, or a neo-Malthusian. Some of the literature was still purely polemic, and just as in previous times there had been political implications in attitudes to population, so now there was some tendency for the side which followed Malthus to regard itself as scientific and liberal, and their opponents as revolutionaries, just as these regarded themselves as progressives and the Malthusians as arch-reactionaries. Although these terms scarcely seem to have any meaning to us today, they were real enough in the period which Mr. Kenneth Smith has described in *The Malthusian Controversy*. In spite of these shortcomings, the books of the early nineteenth century are the most valuable from the point of view of this attempt to discover the origins of our modern population theories.[1]

With the second half of the nineteenth century, and more particularly in our own time, more level-headed investigations of causes and effects have gradually won the day. Since contraception began to be generally feasible, and the will to use it became widespread, the spectre of over-population receded and was, in two generations, replaced by the menace of an ageing or depopulated Western world. Eventually, Malthus re-emerged when the facts of the population increase of the Far East became known. But in most cases observations no longer aroused the passions of politicians, theologians, or philosophers, and the great bulk of this recent literature deals with statistical inquiries into the nature of the observed trends.

The language of population literature

Perhaps at this stage a word of explanation is first necessary about the terms used in this literature, since they have a habit of changing their meaning. The whole field is now known as population studies. The most important single discipline within this field is demography, the description of population movements, which primarily makes use of the techniques of applied statistics. 'Political Arithmetic' thus is properly speaking the ancestor of demography, since it was concerned with the counting of heads. Later on, there developed 'Vital Statistics', the measurement of births, deaths, and marriages, together with the study of causes of deaths, and epidemics. This subject in turn led to the study of public health and hygiene. Modern demography is still concerned with these matters, but primarily deals with the measurement of the growth and changes in composition and location of population. Under this heading come measurements of the expectation of life (which also forms part of actuarial science), of age structure, sex composition, emigration and internal migration, and other fundamental components of population structure. For our purposes, the most

[1] An evaluation of Malthus's position will be found at the end of this book.

important of these activities is the study of fecundity (potential fertility) and actual fertility, which is measurable. The term now applied to the phenomena described in this book is, usually, 'differential fertility', and this may mean differences between races, nations, classes, occupations, religions, regions and so on.

So far we have listed only descriptive writings, which were mostly of a statistical nature or at any rate based on field work and observation. The evaluation of this material is the task of population theory today. Most writers on this subject today, of course, base themselves on the material prepared by the demographers. But this was not always so. There is no clear-cut development of epochs, but broadly speaking the ancient world literally did not count at all, but theorized from general observation, and this state of things did not change until the seventeenth century. Even then it did not become usual to rely solely on observation, indeed the great majority of writers still gave their prejudices at least as much weight as either common sense or other people's statistics. Malthus stands out as a man who scorned all statistics, and never even made use of the four census reports which came out in his lifetime. But his contemporary John Rickman, who was responsible for these censuses, and Rickman's great successor, William Farr, finally brought demography into population studies. After their time, only the incorrigible cranks totally ignored the facts, and followed Malthus into the world of deductive reasoning applied to everyday life.

About the middle of the nineteenth century a fresh division took place. On one hand, the statisticians perfected the approach to fact-finding. On the other hand, the first modern sociologists began to be more interested in the mechanism of population changes, the response in attitudes, and ultimately in behaviour, of individuals and families in a changing environment. In France, this departure becomes notable with Le Play and his school (who investigated the changing structure of the family in post-Napoleonic France). In England, the outstanding figure was Herbert Spencer, a 'social biologist'. As sociology developed, notably in the twentieth century, it became ever more psychological in its approach to population. That is to say, writers took the facts of demography for granted, and concentrated on the processes that went on in people's minds. This, of course, was the final breach with economics. Words like instinct, needs, ambition, frustration, sublimation, status began to replace subsistence, employment, wages, and the poor laws. Yet they were all talking about the same thing.

More recently something of a reunion between these different approaches has again taken place. Although one still has, occasionally, approaches to population which are narrowly biological, or psychological, or economic, the majority of textbooks at least take all aspects into account. Monographs on particular aspects may, of course, be different. Statisticians write about methods of projecting population into the future in purely mathematical terms, whereas an economist might discuss prospects of employment in connexion with a possible effect on the marriage-rate, or a sociologist the probable response to a continued housing shortage.

This must necessarily be a very rough outline of what demography and population theory mean. But we must still draw attention to some linguistic or methodological difficulties which are peculiar to the field investigated here.

The diversity of the interests which prompted investigations into population complicates the analysis of ideas because of the constant need to disentangle the observed fact from the terms of abuse or praise with which it is recorded. Not only would the same phenomenon be a menace to one age and a boon to the next, but even contemporaries would disagree and thus make it more difficult to make judgements about events. The most obvious case is that of the refinements of civilization. To one age they were 'luxuries'; they were akin to debauch and whoredom. Feather beds, rich food daintily served, the daily bath —these were the adjuncts of decay. But no sooner had it been recognized that it was precisely those who knew nothing of these joys who bred the fastest, and threatened to overrun the world, than the commentators called these things adjuncts of genteel living. Soon it was taught that the promotion of these articles of equipment, or habits, from the category of luxuries, to that of decencies and even necessities, was a matter of vital moment to the civilized world.

Similarly, it was the fashion, both in the ancient world and in more recent times, to deplore the threatened extinction of ancient aristocracies and their replacement by crude upstarts. But when it was found that the very hope of rising in the world, and perhaps eventually taking one's place in the ranks of the nobility was, apparently, a sure way of engendering habits of prudence, the decay of the old orders and the recruitment of new leaders of society from below was hailed as one of Nature's most providential arrangements. So it was with women. Once indolence and vice had been said to lead them to resort to unnatural means of preventing pregnancy, but at the end of the nineteenth century fashion as well as philosophy began to praise those who would assert their 'right to their own body', or engage seriously in pursuits unconnected with home or family.

Towards the end of the nineteenth century, as the threat of depopulation began to overtake first France, and then other countries, the values of the earlier ages were revived, and once more the recent virtues found themselves condemned as vices. Selfishness, decadence, and even death of nations were the themes. Conversely, to bear children—whether for the glory of the country, or the *Führer*—was highly laudable, and encouraged by allowances not so different from the Speenhamland system. The old Poor Law and the French welfare state have this in common: that people are, in the view of the critics of the system, encouraged to have children which they could not afford unaided. Improvident, they serve the purposes of the state and the economy.

Closely connected with this changing description of practically identical processes is another trick of rhetoric: to take whatever specific you happen to advocate as a cure for all the world's evils, and make it do now one thing, now the opposite, according to what the world considers are the evils of the moment. Thus, for instance, the redistribution of land, diminishing large estates and creating a new class of smallholders, was, in the eighteenth century, considered an excellent means of increasing population. In the nineteenth, as if by magic, precisely the same process was held to be a sure cure for over-population.

The danger here for the historian is that he may be tempted into the position of a referee: tell me, the reader begs, which of these ideas was correct? To answer this question, however, is the task, say, of an agrarian historian. The recorder of theories must use the ideas in all their imperfections. When one finds writers using indiscriminately such terms as 'fertility' and 'fecundity', or 'fertility' and 'birth-rate', one wishes to correct the author. But it is best to leave the errors, and rather attempt to show how they arose than to give a correct version.

Similarly, we must beware of treating any of the influences which will be described as in any way scientifically proven merely because a great many authors happen to draw attention to them. In Germany, for instance, the idea that *Wohlstand und Kultur* were a sure remedy for over-population gained so much currency towards the end of the nineteenth century that those who wanted Germany to be a large and strong nation actually came to oppose further cultural advances lest they should weaken the nation.[1]

Method

As has already been pointed out, the literature of the subject is so large that one must necessarily be extremely selective. To choose a 'representative' view of an age, a place, or a school of thought is comparatively simple: to determine in what order these subdivisions should be arranged is very difficult. A neat division into epochs would reveal the gap in population literature between the later Roman Empire and the Reformation. National views, as such, in this field, count for little, except inasmuch as the experience of, for example, France or Ireland has been so peculiar as to produce its own literature. Again, as far as the usual great schools of philosophy are concerned, one could easily state what the utilitarians or the *encyclopédistes* thought about population, but this would tell us little about the things we are interested in: in other words, we should know more about how utilitarianism responds to a given problem, but less about the challenge the observed population movements presented to its adherents.

It has therefore been thought best to divide the complex argument as far as possible into its component parts, and to see what contributions various ages, places, and schools of thought have made to it, despite the fact that this does violence to time, that it ignores national achievement, and that it invariably fails to do justice to the authors concerned. J. S. Mill contributed more to knowledge than the theory of the prudent peasant proprietor, and Marx was not, primarily, a critic of Malthus. No attempt will be made to remedy this defect: the reader who wishes to know more about the general history of the time, or the work of a specific author, will have to look elsewhere.

It seems necessary to give reasons for introducing the ancient world into the history of a modern theory. First of all there are good precedents—almost every history of theory seems to begin with Greece. Secondly, ancient Greece provides us with the first recorded example of the fear of over-population.[2] Thirdly, many demographers still

[1] See K. Kautsky, *Vermehrung und Entwicklung in Natur und Gesellschaft* (Stuttgart, 1910), pp. 192 ff., where he warns against the claims of bourgeois thinkers that these factors were always anti-genitive: they were neither a sure remedy for over-population, nor, given the proper social framework, would they weaken the state.

[2] Cf. J. Beloch, *Die Bevölkerung der griechisch-römischen Welt* (Leipzig, 1886), pp. 491 ff., and U. Kahrstedt, 'Die Bevölkerung des Altertums', *Handwörterbuch der Staatswissenschaften* (4th ed., Jena, 1924), ii. 655 ff.

claim to find some of their best illustrative material in the ancient world.[1] Lastly, the Greek and Roman writers dominated Western thinking up to the eighteenth century to an extent which now seems incredible. Doctors could not write without constant reference to Hippocrates and Galen; Aristotle and Plato dominated much of philosophical and political literature. As late as 1830 an economist like Michael Sadler thought it necessary to bolster up his peculiar theories with (badly distorted) quotations from the classics. Their views, therefore, are essential to the understanding of later attitudes.

Such a division into categories is naturally somewhat arbitrary. The separation of arguments about education from those about intellectual activity is artificial, yet the two were put forward in different contexts and not always by the same authors. Similarly economic historians will be sceptical about the division of societies into those which were stationary in their economic organization, and those which were developing. Obviously no society is completely static for long, and there is no clear measurement of what constitutes rapid development. Yet there is a noticeable difference in the sort of assertions that are made about population movements in, say, mid-eighteenth-century France and mid-nineteenth-century Britain: in one case the observations made are held to be of general validity (towns are bad, aristocracies die out, the court is debilitating, and so on); in the other case the reference is continuously, and specifically, to the phenomena of change and of movement: urbanization, social promotion, cheapening of industrial products, increasing requirements of skill and education, and the like.

The development of the ideas in outline

The plan of this essay is as follows: First, we trace the origins of ideas which had significance already in pre-industrial societies. That is to say, we try to answer the question: given the fact that some people were less fertile than others, how was this explained by the societies of the ancient world, and in the early modern world? These explanations are sometimes complex, and include hypotheses which we now dismiss as mere superstitions. Thus, the classical moralists and naturalists are full of the effects of different phases of the moon, of the propitiation of the gods, and of the application of herbal infusions or spells. Although this sort of explanation is fascinating to the anthropo-

[1] See A. Landry, 'Quelques aperçus concernant la dépopulation dans l'antiquité gréco-romaine', *Revue historique* (1936), clxxvii. 1–33. He quotes a German, Zumpt, writing as early as 1841, whose main field was classical antiquity, and who yet was also amongst the first to predict the course of population development in his own time.

logist, it has here been ruled out, since it has no bearing on the development of modern population theory. But other types of theory are direct precursors of the present ideas on the subject.

The first of these concerns the effects of luxury. What this word meant, and how its meaning changed, from gross debauchery to running hot water and the confusion about physiological and psychological effects of indulgence, forms the substance of the first section. Luxury was associated on one hand with towns, and so we study views on the effects of urban living. On the other hand, the greatest opulence was to be found amongst the aristocracies, and their notorious infertility was noticed by a large number of writers.

In the next chapter the emphasis changes slightly. For the first time there is a recognition of important differences in economic status, and of social attitudes connected with status. Moreover, there is a consideration of the effect of movement from one social and economic class to another. This does not imply any recognition of a changing society, but merely the possibility of the movement of individuals within a society which is not noticeably altering its characteristics. The basis of this type of argument is the belief that those who are poor are heedless of the consequences of additions to the family. From the Roman concept of the proletariat, the offspring-yielding class, we advance to the modern description of the shiftless, and prolific, day-labourer of western Europe. The corollary to this proposition is that of the next section, namely that those who have in some way managed to obtain a foothold in an income (or status) group a little above the absolute minimum, will restrict their fertility in some way to preserve that achievement. A further extension of this thought comes in the last section of Chapter Three, where we see what happens if one applies this kind of foresight to one's children, and restricts numbers, either because their dowries or education make them particularly expensive, or because one feels that a family means not only lowering one's own prospects, but also denying the possibility of the maintenance of the standard of living for the children themselves.

We now proceed to a different sort of world, which was fully described only in post-Malthusian times. Chapter Four deals with the economic basis of voluntary restraint of fertility in a society which is rapidly transforming its economic basis and therefore the attitudes of its people. The first essential to the understanding of the origin of such attitudes is the recognition of the changing basis of meaning of the words 'necessities', 'decencies', and 'luxuries' (a division due to

Nassau Senior), a change which in itself implies movement, a dynamic situation in which individuals change their behaviour as they progress through society.

This progress, or the hope of it, forms the subject of the second section in this chapter, where we show how the prospect of rising in the social and economic scale was held to restrict fertility, and finally, in the third section, we summarize those authors who made the process of upward movement into a whole social system, of which infertility was an essential part.

In Chapter Five we move from the rather simple economic analysis of the effects of differences in income to rather more indirect influences on fertility. First amongst these is the process of acquiring property by wider sections of the community, and the general equalization, or rather closer approximation, of incomes. In the second section of Chapter Five this process is connected with political organization: the institutions of democracy and, in particular, civil liberty, which make this equalization possible, and guarantee the safety of property. This includes the removal of all artificial barriers to free promotion through society.

In the last two sections of this chapter we describe arguments relating to two particular social aspects—the role of education in shaping the ambitions and tastes of the population, and the results of according higher status to women; a process which, for social as well as possibly economic reasons, seems to have accompanied industrialization everywhere to some extent, as well as being characteristic of the higher levels of society.

In Chapter Six we have collected a number of theories which might be termed special variants of the general ideas put forward in the previous chapters. The first of these concerns food—the supposition that richer food, or more food, leads to infertility, or conversely, that starvation is actually favourable to fecundity. Secondly, there is the idea that intellectual or sedentary activity, as opposed to active manual labour, promotes barrenness, a persistent if unproven assertion. A good deal of controversy surrounds the third special category, the theories relating to the effect of religion. One occasionally comes across the idea that the movement away from religion, or 'enlightenment', acts as a check to fertility, either because this means that objections to birth-control are overruled, or because the ideal of the family is broken down. In either case, both friends and opponents of this movement connect it in some way with the progress of society.

In Chapter Seven we abandon the somewhat atomistic approach of the earlier sections, and begin to consider the ideas which place these various influences on the individual in their social context. The beginning is provided by the plunge into social biology, the grandiose attempt by Spencer (and others) to postulate conditions of equilibrium and compensating mechanisms which accorded with the idea of an orderly natural universe held in earlier times. Human beings are seen, even in their emergence into complex modern societies, as following, by means of a mechanism not always adequately explained, a social law ensuring their survival. From this we go on to discuss other equilibrium theories, all of which can be applied to explain a fall in fertility as numbers increase. Some of these are of a purely statistical nature. We end this chapter with references to theories derived from the observed tendency of birth-rates to fall as survival rates improve, especially those of newborn children, and as advances in general medicine and public health change the conditions of life of the people.

In Chapter Eight we draw together all these diverse theories into the kind of synthesis which became fashionable in western Europe in the later nineteenth century. A number of variants can be distinguished: first we deal with the theory that there is a form of general progress of civilization, which inculcates the higher wants, and therefore automatically restricts fertility. This idea already dates back to the time before Malthus, but we find, in the second and third sections, that after the *Essay on Population* it became something of an obsession with his opponents, and was proudly brandished as the answer to all fears, and finally made into a law of nature to fit in with the optimistic concepts of the age of the Great Exhibition.

But elsewhere, less sanguine interpretations of the progress of civilization were put forward. In France, the decline of fertility alarmed the nation, and stagnation and decadence rather than progress came to be associated with the changes in national life. In the final section of this chapter we give an account of the more elaborate cultural theories associated especially with German writers, and the grandiose ideas of the life-cycle of nations and the coming decline of Western civilization which culminated in Oswald Spengler's work.

Finally, in the ninth chapter, we try to place the development of the arguments in this book into their proper perspective. First of all, the principal characteristics of the writings are summarized and placed into two main categories: those that relate to the unchanging order of the preindustrial world, and those which find their expression chiefly against the background of rapidly changing conditions, especially in industrializing societies. In the second section we then attempt to place Malthus into the emerging pattern. It will be shown that most of the modern theories of fertility were foreshadowed by him, but that he could never bring himself to grant that they had the power to act as powerful antidotes to the dangers which he feared. Despite his obvious shortcomings, he emerges as the dominant figure in the history of population theory, forcing a change in the whole context and language of the subject.

In the third section of the last chapter, we come to face the question of the correct place for the arguments concerning the social determination of fertility in the general structure of population theory. For this purpose we need a definition of the requirements of such a theory. Since it emerges from the discussion of this topic that investigators have never been clear as to the proper home of population studies, an attempt is made to elucidate the position by examining two different views of the subject as part of economics: the neo-classical view as represented by Alfred Marshall, and a modern Marxist view put forward by Sydney Coontz. The last part of this section is concerned with a general description of the process of theorizing in this field and the difficulties which are apparently inherent in this. We end with a re-appraisal of the standard-of-living theories as useful pointers to the nature of social and economic change, rather than a significant part of modern population theory, despite the widespread acceptance which they have found amongst investigators.

The progress of theories from the simplest to the most elaborate does not conform to any rigid time-scale. When English writers argued from the experience of an industrial world where the power of landlords had already been much reduced, their counterparts on the continent of Europe still thought in terms of agrarian states with commercial urban centres. Scotland in the eighteenth century had a different economic and social life from England. For this reason, we can only broadly classify theories as belonging to preindustrial, industrializing, or fully industrialized societies. Of these, the second is the most interesting, for it is then that such concepts as the rising family, the property-acquiring family, and the changing standards of requirements have most meaning. The complex arguments of the last chapters belong to the stage of accomplishment, and even of incipient decline. The arrest of population growth in itself, of course, even if it can be traced to a higher standard of living, is sometimes taken as an indication of imminent decay.

A last word of caution is necessary. The fact that types or arguments can be identified, and assigned to epochs in history, does not mean that analogies go very far. The reasoning associated with recent Western history cannot be projected back into primitive societies, not only for want of facts, but because there is no basis for these complex relationships in an agrarian, bartering, and custom-bound society. This bars evidence from social anthropologists, and makes us cautious in our approach to Greece and Rome. Many writers have been tempted to use such words as 'decadence' and 'race-suicide' to give unitary explanations for apparently similar phenomena in widely different societies. It therefore seems advisable in this essay to relate the emergence of similar explanations of movements to the chronology of the stages of evolution only in similar societies. This procedure alone would caution us against simple fancies of the type which solves the Indian population problem by providing the Bengal peasant with roast beef and two vegetables for his Sunday dinner. It should be said, however, that such 'historicist' fancies, to use Karl Popper's term, are at least hallowed by tradition:

> The natives of Indostan being confined, by the laws of their religion, to the use of vegetable food, and requiring little except rice . . . are populous. . . . If any revolution, or what might be called perhaps refinement of manners, should generate in these people a taste for the flesh of animals . . . the population, from this single change, would suffer in a few years a great diminution.[1]

This was written in 1785 by Archdeacon William Paley, the author of the *Natural Theology, or Evidence of the Existence and Attributes of Deity collected from the Appearances of Nature.*

BIBLIOGRAPHICAL NOTES TO CHAPTER ONE

1. *Works on the history of population theory*

(a) *General works*

P. Aries, *Histoire des populations françaises et de leurs attitudes devant la vie depuis le XVIIIe siècle* (Paris, 1948).

J. Bonar, *Theories of Population from Raleigh to Arthur Young* (London, 1931).

L. Elster, Sub art. 'Bevölkerungswesen', *Handwörterbuch der Staatswissenschaften* (4th ed., Jena, 1924), Bd. II.

[1] W. Paley, *The Principles of Moral and Political Philosophy* (19th ed., London, 1793, 2 vols.), ii. 355.

J. A. Field, *Essays on Population and Other Papers* (H. F. Hohmann, ed. and comp., Chicago, 1931).
R. Gonnard, *Histoire des doctrines de la population* (Paris, 1923).
G. Mackenroth, *Bevölkerungslehre; Theorie, Soziologie und Statistik der Bevölkerung* (Enzyklopädie der Rechts- und Staatswissenschaft. Abteilung Staatswissenschaft, Berlin, 1953).
P. Mombert, *Bevölkerungslehre* (Jena, 1929).
J. J. Spengler, *France Faces Depopulation* (Durham, North Carolina, 1938).
—— *French Predecessors of Malthus* (ibid., 1942).
C. E. Stangeland, *Pre-Malthusian Doctrines of Population; a Study in the History of Economic Theory* (New York, 1904).

(b) *On the Malthusian controversy*

H. A. Boner, *Hungry Generations: The Nineteenth-Century Case against Malthusianism* (New York, 1955).
D. V. Glass (ed.), *Introduction to Malthus* (London, 1953).
R. L. Meek (ed.), *Marx and Engels on Malthus* (London, 1953).
K. Smith, *The Malthusian Controversy* (London, 1951).
J. Stassart, *Malthus et la population* (Liège, 1957).

2. *Works on the background to the population controversy in England before Malthus*

D. V. Glass, 'Gregory King's Estimate of the Population of England and Wales, 1695', *Population Studies* (1949–50), iii. 324 ff.
—— 'The Population Controversy in Eighteenth Century England. Part I: The Background', *Population Studies* (1952–3), vi. 69 ff.
—— 'Some Aspects of the Development of Demography', *Journal of the Royal Society of Arts* (1956), civ. 854 ff.
E. C. K. Gonner, 'The Population of England in the Eighteenth Century', *Journal of the Royal Statistical Society* (1912–13), lxxvi. 261 ff.
H. J. Habakkuk, 'English Population in the Eighteenth Century', *Economic History Review* (1953), vi, no. 2, 117 ff.

The books and articles listed above are only a few among the large number which may be consulted by readers wishing to provide themselves with more background information. The most recent publications contain extensive lists of further references. Unfortunately, no general bibliography of population literature exists, other than that printed by the United Nations, Department of Social Affairs, Population Division, in *The Determinants and Consequences of Population Trends* (New York, 1953).

II

SOME THEORIES CURRENT IN PREINDUSTRIAL SOCIETIES

I. LUXURY

'Sed iacet aurato vix ulla puerpera lecto.' (JUVENAL)[1]

What is luxury?

THE word luxury, as commonly employed, signifies the consumption of goods and services on an excessive scale. There is usually an element of censure in the use of the term. But the common observation of a large number of writers brands it as a singularly imprecise term. What reasonable measure of consumption is it that luxury is supposed to exceed? It is worth looking at the employment of the word at different times. In seventeenth-century France, as Spengler has shown, luxury production simply meant manufacture—i.e. the provision of goods not made at home or found in nature.[2] If it had been done without by an earlier age, it was unnecessary and therefore a luxury.

From the beginning, therefore, the branding of luxury as an enemy of fertility is associated with the diffusion of comforts amongst all classes as well as the obvious debauches of the rich. This would seem to suggest that this particular argument would normally emerge at times of considerable advances in the economic and social field. In fact, general luxury stood condemned in all ages, but the idea that the term is a relative one emerged with full clarity only in the middle of the eighteenth century. It is curious to note that it does so almost simultaneously in a number of countries. The clearest statement perhaps is that of Adam Ferguson, Professor of Philosophy in Edinburgh (1723–1816), and he is worth quoting in full:

> We are far from being agreed on the application of the term *luxury*, or on that degree of its meaning which is consistent with national prosperity, or with the moral rectitude of our nature. It is sometimes employed to signify

[1] Juvenal, *Satires*, 6, line 594.

[2] J. J. Spengler, *French Predecessors of Malthus* (Durham, North Carolina, 1942), p. 110.

a manner of life which we think necessary to civilization, and even to happiness. It is, in our panegyric of polished ages, the parent of arts, the support of commerce, and the minister of national greatness, and opulence. It is, in our censure of degenerate manners, the source of corruption, and the presage of national declension and ruin. It is admired, and it is blamed; it is treated as ornamental and useful, and it is proscribed as a vice.

With all this diversity in our judgements, we are generally uniform in employing the term to signify that complicated apparatus which mankind devise for the ease and convenience of life. Their building, furniture, equipage, cloathing, train of domestics, refinements of the table, and in general, all that assemblage which is rather intended to please the fancy, than obviate real wants, and which is rather ornamental than useful. . . .

We may propose to stop the advancement of arts at any stage of their progress, and still incur the censure of luxury from those who have not advanced so far. The house-builder and the carpenter at Sparta were limited to the use of the axe and the saw; but a Spartan cottage might have passed for a palace in Thrace; and if the dispute were to turn on the knowledge of what is physically necessary to the preservation of human life, as the standard of what is morally lawful, the faculties of physic, as well as of morality, would probably divide on the subject, and leave every individual, as at present, to find some rule for himself. The casuist, for the most part, considers the practice of his own age and condition as standard for mankind. . . . A censor born in a cottage, and accustomed to sleep upon straw, does not propose that men should return to the woods and caves for shelter; he admits the reasonableness and the utility of what is already familiar, and apprehends an excess and corruption, only in the newest refinement of the rising generation.[1]

Ferguson went on to condemn luxury in its extreme form, where it proved to be harmful to democratic government because it led to corruption—but he remained anxious to stress that unless there were these evident evil effects on the body politic, it could neither be defined nor condemned.

Contemporary with Ferguson in Scotland we have the economist Sir James Steuart of Coltness, who stressed that the production of luxuries within any given system was a matter for political, not moral judgement—that is, whether a given consumption of things which are 'neither necessary for our being well fed, well clothed, well defended against the injuries of the weather, nor for securing us against every-

[1] Adam Ferguson, *An Essay on the History of Civil Society* (1767; 4th ed., London, 1773), part vi, sect. 2, p. 375. Ferguson (1723–1816), studied Divinity at Edinburgh, served as chaplain to the Black Watch at Fontenoy; Professor of Natural Philosophy at Edinburgh (1759), then of Pneumatics and Moral Philosophy there (1764–85); after that Professor of Mathematics; Secretary to British Commissioners, Philadelphia, 1778. (*Dictionary of National Biography*.)

thing which can hurt us', is right or wrong, depends on its effect on the whole of society, and not on any arbitrary standard.[1]

On the other hand, William Temple, a Trowbridge clothier who refuted the ascetic William Bell's attacks on commerce and the arts as depopulators, in 1758, was at pains to distinguish moral principles in defining luxuries: '. . . there is a vicious luxury, and an innocent luxury . . . a Porter may be viciously luxurious on fat bacon, tobacco, red herrings, gin, malt-spirits, and with a nasty bunter, or a stinking dirty fish drab . . .'—but a nobleman living up to his income would be innocent, whatever he might consume.[2]

There are clear indications that on the Continent, too, the relative and changing nature of luxury was clearly recognized. The famous general of the French army, Herman Maurice, Marshal de Saxe, published a book in 1756 under the title *Les Rêveries, ou Mémoires sur l'art de la Guerre*. This was in fact a compilation by a French officer in the Prussian service, M. de Bonneville. Saxe had a chapter on population, to which his editor supplied a footnote which is relevant here. The Marshal had spoken of the ravages of epidemics and venereal disease. But these, the editor claims:

> have never made such desolation in the world, or have been such enemies to propagation, as that contagious malady . . . by which I mean luxury. Formerly it was confined to the palaces of the great, but now it prevails even in cottages; and it is that which multiplies our wants, and renders children a burden to their parents. . . .[3]

[1] Sir J. Steuart, *An Inquiry into the Principles of Political Economy: Being an Essay on the Science of Domestic Policy in Free Nations, in Which are Particularly Considered Population, Agriculture, Trade, Industry, Money, Corn, Interest, Circulation, Banks, Exchange, Public Credit and Taxes* (London, 1767, 2 vols.), i, bk. i, ch. vi, p. 31. See also i, bk. ii, ch. xx, pp. 306 ff. for further evidence of Steuart's ability to see 'luxury' as a relative term: what is excess to one man is moderation to another. '. . . no man can become luxurious, in our acceptation of the word . . . without encouraging emulation, industry, and agriculture', &c. He distinguished luxury, the provision of certain objects, sensuality, the act of enjoying these, and excess, an abuse of enjoyment. Obviously it was only the latter that was indefensible.

[2] I . . . B . . . (M.D.) [i.e. William Temple], *A Vindication of Commerce and the Arts, proving that they are the Source of the Greatness, Power, Riches and Populousness of a State, being an Examination of Mr. Bell's Dissertation upon Populousness, read in the Schools and honoured with the Lord Viscount Townshend's Prize, by the University of Cambridge, wherein Mr. Bell's calumnies on trade are answered, his arguments refuted, his system exploded, and the principal causes of populosity assigned* (London, 1768), reprinted in *A Select Collection of Scarce and Valuable Tracts on Commerce* (J. McCulloch, ed., London, 1859), p. 515.

[3] Translations from the English edition, published in Edinburgh in 1776 under the title *Reveries, or, Memoirs concerning the Art of War . . .*, p. 262. The work was evidently widely read, for there are two earlier editions in England—the original translation by Major-General Sir E. Fawcett (London, 1757), then an anonymous one, which seems, however,

Both the wording of the original, *le luxe et la mollesse*, which the translator simply renders as 'luxury' and the reference to cottages clearly show that what the author means is a certain amount of comfort and civilized living.

The point was well put by the German population theorist L. A. G. Schrader writing slightly later. Defining luxury, he quoted a satirical writer: 'anything more than the simplest physical necessities, anything I have more of the comforts of life than my grandfather had, that is luxury!' In view of this definition he disagreed with the better-known Prussian, Süßmilch, who was extensively quoted by Malthus. Süßmilch thought of luxury simply as a 'stream of over-abundance'. Schrader thought that what the moralists were describing was in fact human progress itself—the desire and the ability to live better than the next man—sentiments which were the very origin of all endeavour.[1]

By the nineteenth century, at any rate in England, the spread of manufactures so completely upset the old standards of what was necessary and what was not, that a complete system of graded requirements was built up by Nassau Senior and others—we shall see later what the word luxury meant to him, and to Archibald Alison and George Rickards. Only very rarely could the word be employed in its old censorious meaning. An echo is to be found in the work of the arch-apologist for the factory system, Andrew Ure, when he spoke of operatives gratifying 'luxurious habits'—on a weekly wage of, at the most, 21*s*.[2] When modern writers returned to an attack on luxury, it

to be by the same translator (Edinburgh, 1759). At one time I thought the anonymous translator might be Ferguson (see above), who was present at Saxe's victory at Fontenoy, and was working in Edinburgh, as the footnote was clearly, from internal evidence, by the editor or translator. C. E. Stangeland, *Pre-Malthusian Doctrines of Population* (New York, 1904), attributes the remark to the translator.

[1] L. A. G. Schrader, *Grundgesetze der Natur in der Geburt, dem Leben und Tode der Menschen, als ein freyer Auszug, aus Süßmilchs göttlicher Ordnung . . . in Veränderter Ordnung entworfen* (Glückstadt, 1777), p. 443. Schrader was familiar with the work of English demographers of his time, such as Thomas Short, who, like Süßmilch, was inclined to take an absolute view of the nature of luxury.

[2] A. Ure, *The Philosophy of Manufactures: Or, an Exposition of the Scientific, Moral, and Commercial Economy of the Factory System of Great Britain* (3rd ed., London, 1861), p. 364. Earlier observations (p. 349) show that he meant they could own sofas, good chairs, an eight-day clock in a mahogany case, pictures in oils, and even a barometer and a cottage piano. Ure may be regarded as an arch-apologist of the factory system. Although his knowledge was no doubt extensive, especially on the technical side, he minimized all the disadvantages. His familiarity with the mechanisms of spindles and looms gave an air of authority to such assertions as that the humid air of the mills was believed to be a positive specific for certain diseases.

was not as a depopulating factor, but as an obstacle to the achievement of a better society.[1]

Luxury condemned

Both the Greeks and the Romans had cause to condemn the habits of their ruling classes during the period of national decline. Polybius, writing in the second century B.C., found the origin of the depopulation of the country in the passion, amongst all classes, for conspicuous consumption and a life of ease—psychological explanations which contrast sharply with the physical causes adduced by more recent scholars.[2] The movement was, of course, particularly noticeable in towns; there was a widespread belief that the countryside still reproduced itself.[3] The most obvious manifestation of the disease was the failure to marry, or the habit of married men to prefer the company of other women. Artificial means were used to prevent or interrupt pregnancy.

'Tantum artes hujus, tantum medicamina possunt, Quae steriles facit' continues Juvenal from the line cited above. If, as Beloch and others claim, all this preaching against the depopulating effect of luxury is unreal, contemporary legislators at least took it seriously, and acted accordingly.[4] Already in Macedonia in the third century B.C., Philip saw himself forced to encourage procreation by law, and imported the presumably more fertile Thracians into the country for the purpose.[5] In Rome, the legislation of the Emperor Augustus in the time of Christ, the *Lex Papia Poppaea*, constituted a code of measures designed to bring back the life of the Roman family. There were not only regulations on the conditions of marriage, but also sumptuary regulations designed to prevent the conspicuous luxury and the moral deterioration that went with it. These laws aimed at nothing less than the regeneration of the Roman people as a whole, and it is significant that the prevention of luxury and the promotion of fertility were at their centre.[6] Trajan and other emperors followed in Augustus'

[1] For a modern discussion, see Baron Émile de Laveleye, *Luxury* (2nd ed., London, 1891). Other evidence for the flexibility of the term in F. S. Nitti, *Population and the Social System* (London, 1894), p. 100.

[2] For discussion of this, see M. I. Rostovtzeff, *Social and Economic History of the Hellenistic World* (Oxford, 1941, 3 vols.), ii. 623.

[3] See Polybius, *Histories*, iv, bk. cxxiii, para. 6. The reference is to Elis.

[4] J. Beloch, *Die Bevölkerung der griechisch-römischen Welt* (Leipzig, 1886), p. 503.

[5] Livy, *Histories*, bk. xxxix, para. 24.

[6] Cf. Tacitus, *Annals*, iii. 25. For details of this legislation and the evils it sought to

footsteps.[1] But the advantages of remaining single or at any rate childless were too obvious—the legacy-hunters provided a life of ease and flattery for those who had riches to leave behind, if they had no heirs; as many Roman writers from Petronius to Tertullian testify.[2] We shall return to details of these classical arguments later, when we examine some of the refinements of the luxury theory.

After the collapse of the Roman Empire, we hear very little about the evil effects of luxury. True, it was fashionable for monks to preach simplicity to court and nobility, but there is no stress on the general spread of soft habits. From what we know about medieval domestic arrangements, there does not, indeed, appear to have been much occasion for censure. Significantly, the earliest complaints in modern times appear at a time of expansion, in the Elizabethan age. England was being rebuilt, and new houses were much better than the old. Even cottages occasionally showed signs of becoming habitable. So Raphael Holinshed, the chronicler, complained in 1577 of the luxury of chimneys, replacing cracks in the roof, and earthenware and pewter instead of wooden vessels.[3] But it was not until a hundred years later that renewed fears of depopulation once more brought the matter to the foreground. The writers of the time were sufficiently steeped in the classical tradition to take up the theme in the ancient fashion. It is appropriate to start with Fénelon (1651–1715), Archbishop of Cambrai, who was instructor to Louis XIV's grandson, the Duc de Bourgogne, for whom he wrote *Télémaque* (published in 1699), a didactic novel containing many indirect criticisms of the king and his policy. There he preached the simple life and warned against the effects of superabundance which had depopulated the ancient world. Manufactures are included in the list of undesirable influences; simple peasants are shown as being most fertile.[4] It is the urban population with its multifarious wants which fails to populate the kingdom. Fénelon's intimate knowledge of court life of the *Roi Soleil* lends plausibility to the charge, to which writers of the eighteenth century frequently returned.

The word 'Mercantilism' is one which we must use with caution,

attack: P. Jörs, 'Die Ehegesetze des Augustus', in *Festschrift für Theodor Mommsen* (Marburg, 1893). See also, p. 49, n. 3.

[1] Pliny, *Panegyrics*, 26.

[2] See L. Friedländer, *Roman Life and Manners under the Early Empire* (L. A. Magnus, trans., London, 1908, 4 vols.), i. 215.

[3] Quoted in Laveleye, op. cit., p. 5. He also cites Slaney, in the nineteenth century, as condemning houses built of oak instead of the customary willow.

[4] Fénelon, *Les Aventures de Télémaque* (Chassang, ed., Paris, 1806), p. 112.

since not even Eli Heckscher's monumental work finally settled what were the origins and consequences of the policies to which the term is loosely applied. But for our purpose it is clear enough what the mercantilist outlook on population was: whatever might be the effects of concentrating on bullion as a means of enriching the kingdom, manpower was held by all of them in highest esteem. That state was powerful which had a large and healthy population at its disposal, whether for war-like purposes or civil employment. We can therefore safely equate mercantilists and pro-populationists, of whom there were many in the fifty years following the death of Colbert, Louis XIV's minister, who had initiated the policy of encouraging manufactures and exports.

Most of the eighteenth-century French writers had still the elements of the mercantilist outlook on population in them, even if they were not primarily writers on economic subjects, or even if, like the Physiocrats, they were critical of the commercial and industrial policies of mercantilism. The majority of the writers we shall have to quote here are moralists or politicians, and the word 'pro-populationist' describes them accurately in our context.

Amongst these there is, for instance, Plumard de Danguel, who showed how luxury prevented marriage, and how the women in the richer sections of society thought motherhood troublesome and nursing improper.[1] Here we have a cry which is re-echoed wherever we see a society emerging into a state of refinement—and where women take a leading role in such a society. The Romans had cause to complain—Theodoric tried to stem the rot by legislation regulating wet-nursing.[2] In the middle of the eighteenth century German princelings were aping French manners, and their subjects followed suit. Everywhere ladies who had once known their business in life shunned children or had them brought up by others.[3] Ange de Goudar saw the habit as part of

[1] N. P. de Danguel (pseud.), *Remarques sur les avantages et les désavantages de la France et de la Gr. Bretagne* (Leyden, 1754), quoted in Spengler, op. cit., pp. 82 ff. Also in Moheau, cf. J. J. Spengler, 'Moheau, prophet of depopulation', *Journal of Political Economy* (1939), xlvii. 648 ff.

[2] *Codex Theodoricus*, IX. xxxi, I. Cf. O. Seeck, *Geschichte des Untergangs der antiken Welt* (Stuttgart, 1920–2, 6 vols.), i. 356.

[3] A treatise on this was written by a Professor of Mathematics at Hamburg in 1777: J. G. Büsch, *Vermischte Abhandlungen*, 2. Teil: *Von dem Schaden für die Bevölkerung durch die Menge der Säugammen*, pp. 437 ff. In France high infant mortality was blamed on the practice in the following centuries: see J. J. Spengler, *France Faces Depopulation* (Durham, North Carolina, 1938), p. 117, note 3. For other French authors, see the same work, p. 52.

a larger disease which attacked society. 'L'humeur, le génie, les préjugés, l'esprit de société, la délicatesse, l'amour des aises et des commodités de la vie, l'esprit philosophique, la sensualité, la débauche . . .'[1] —all these sap the desire to have children. The very deference to the female sex is part of this attitude: 'On trouve mal-honnête de ne pouvoir faire paroître une femme dans le monde avec un certain éclat, et à cause de celà on conclut qu'il est plus séant de ne pas se marier.'[2]

De Maupassant was to observe the same attitude more than a hundred years later—men of refinement look with horror on a beautiful woman who is condemned to perpetual child-bearing by an insensitive husband: '. . . plus nous sommes civilisés, intelligents, raffinés, plus nous devons vaincre et dompter l'instinct animal qui représente en nous la volonté de Dieu.'[3]

Richard Cantillon, the Anglo-French economist (*c.* 1680–1734), must be reckoned as one of the precursors of the Physiocrats in his recognition of the primary importance of agricultural production, and of Adam Smith in his realization that what counted in the State was the diffusion of wealth rather than mere numbers. He did not condemn industry, trade, or consumption, but he wished these to be kept within bounds. He was amongst the first in this field to have a reasonably clear idea of the connexion between the amount of subsistence available, the customary standard of living, and the size of the population, and we shall have to deal with him in greater detail at a later stage. Here we must see him as part of the almost universal French movement against excess. The reasoning of this group was not confined to the idea that an idle life and a rich diet weaken man's reproductive power, or the psychological type of argument just mentioned, but it also included theories of distribution. Under this heading come the Physiocrats, whose ideas on population are not always easy to understand.[4]

Certainly these writers had shaken themselves free from the mercantilist attitudes which saw an advantage in a larger population as such, and therefore they would not declare any influence as evil simply because it checked population. On the other hand, they were not yet afraid of over-population and therefore did not yet welcome any of the checks in operation. On the whole, they tended to regard population

[1] Ange de Goudar, *Les Intérêts de la France mal entendus* (Amsterdam, 1757, 3 vols.), i. 172.

[2] Ibid., p. 184.

[3] G. de Maupassant, *L'Inutile beauté* (Paris, *c.* 1910), p. 40.

[4] Spengler, *French Predecessors . . .*, ch. iv, pp. 110 ff. 'Cantillon and the theory of luxury'. We follow Spengler in classifying Cantillon amongst the French writers.

as a dependent variable, the outcome of a form of economic organization. The difficulty is that they started out from a preconceived idea of what this organization should be. Therefore all influences were related to this idea, and the effect on population movements was quite incidental. Spengler, who has dealt very fully with their ideas, and with Cantillon, calls their chief spokesman Quesnay 'populationist in several senses of the term'. This means that Quesnay disliked conditions which produced depopulation, foresaw the likelihood of population and national wealth growing together, and awaited with equanimity the larger population which he thought would be produced by the policies advocated by him.

The elder Mirabeau, repeating the customary interpretations of the way in which luxurious consumption checks births, was more careful than some of his contemporaries in pointing out that the effects were not confined to the richer classes alone: 'In the lowest ranks, as in the first, that which was formerly folly to-day is become usage and almost necessity.'[1] This was not to be condemned; indeed, Cantillon himself and his followers were only too well aware of the role played by these 'secondary wants' in the economy; the question was, how far was the movement to be allowed to go, and how was the extra wealth to be distributed? The observation was clear: in France it had gone too far, and the extra wealth did not benefit great numbers. 'Ces observations', wrote Du Buat-Nançay: 'puisées dans une expérience journalière, prouvent invinciblement que l'amour excessif des richesses est très-contraire au désir de la reproduction, et par conséquent à la population . . .'.[2] Satisfaction of primary wants will increase the population; the creation of secondary wants will retard it; we must sometimes satisfy these too, to keep our population from emigrating, but the main policy remains: 'il faut multiplier les moyens, non les besoins'.[3] It is easy to invert this to a Malthusian phrase: if you cannot multiply the means of subsistence, multiply people's wants.

The worst effect, all agreed, was to be found where the habits of the few acted as a double check to population: the rich did not reproduce themselves precisely because they had too much to eat, and the vast mass of the poor were kept down by the lack of means to keep alive.[4]

[1] V. R. Mirabeau, *L'Ami des Hommes, ou traité de la Population* (Avignon, 1758 ed.), i. 146, as quoted by Spengler, *French Predecessors . . .*, p. 133.

[2] L. G. du Buat-Nançay, *Éléments de la politique; ou recherche des vrais principes de l'économie sociale* (London, 1773, 6 vols.), ii, livre iv, ch. vii, p. 66.

[3] Ibid., livre ii, chs. x, xiv, xv, *passim*.

[4] Cf. Senac de Meilhan and the Abbé Pluquet, in Spengler, op. cit., pp. 162–9.

The attack on luxury, as one would expect, took a new turn amongst the writers who prepared the way for the Revolution. For Rousseau, the unnatural life of contemporary society leads to all evils. Depopulation is but one of them. The unhealthy occupations which are necessary to satisfy man's complicated wants, like the mining of lead, mercury, and cobalt (prophetic Rousseau!) will lead to the diminution of the species which has been observed by many philosophers.[1]

Le luxe, impossible à prévenir chez des hommes avides de leurs propres commodités et de la considération des autres, achève bientôt le mal que les sociétés ont commencé, et sous prétexte de faire vivre les pauvres, qu'il n'eût pas fallu faire, il appauvrit tout le reste, et dépeuple l'Etat tôt ou tard.

We have so far mentioned only authors who conceived of a luxurious standard of living as a population check, an obstacle to national prosperity, and the cause of vice and degeneration. But there were also writers who could see beyond these obvious and old-established notions. Luxury as a stimulus to economic progress figured in the writings of Montesquieu and Voltaire. But the clearest exposition of the positive view is to be found in J. F. Melon.[2] Here luxury is what Ferguson conceived it to be: a relative term, a temporary description in a changing system of values.

Le luxe est une somptuosité extraordinaire que donnent les richesses et la sécurité d'un gouvernement, c'est une suite nécessaire de toute Société bien policée. Celui qui se trouve dans l'abondance, veut en jouir; il a là-dessus des recherches que le moins riche n'est pas en état de payer, et cette recherche est toujours relative au tem(p)s et aux personnes. Ce qui étoit luxe pour nos pères, est à présent commun; et ce qui l'est pour nous, ne le sera pas pour nos neveux. Des bas de soye étoient Luxe du tem(p)s de Henri II, et la fayance l'est autant, comparée à la terre commune, que la porcelaine comparée à la fayance.[2]

Here again we have practical evidence of the notion that the change of standard is a concomitant of industrial progress.

Le pain est de nécessité absolue; et les laines sont de seconde nécessité; mais le pain blanc et les draps fins, établis par M. Colbert, seroient de plus grand luxe sans l'habitude où nous sommes de nous en servir tous les jours. Le terme de Luxe est un vain nom, qu'il faut bannir de toutes les opérations de Police et de Commerce, parce qu'il ne porte que des idées vagues, confuses, fausses, dont l'abus peut arrêter l'industrie même dans sa source.[3]

[1] J. J. Rousseau, *Political Writings* (C. E. Vaughan, ed., Cambridge, 1915, 2 vols.), i, 'Discours sur l'inégalité' (1755), Notes, p. 205.

[2] J. F. Melon, *Essai politique sur le commerce* (Paris, 1736), pp. 106–7.

[3] Ibid., pp. 112–13.

Of course one would expect a mercantilist like Melon to justify Colbert, but he must be given credit for seeing how the absorption of new commodities into the general scheme of consumption could be operated without detriment. Since Melon was also convinced, like his contemporaries, that men tend to avoid marrying if they cannot support their families according to their accustomed standard, and since he perceived this to be rising, Spengler is surely justified in thinking that: '... he virtually conceived of a rising standard of living which presumably could or would check population growth before numbers had reached the supportable maximum'.[1]

We have so far quoted mainly from French authors. Reference to luxury exists in other languages too—but the fact remains that the theory does not seem to have been worked out so elaborately elsewhere. Almost everywhere it occurs it seems cruder by comparison, and often consists of vague generalizations, such as one might expect in authors well versed in the classical authorities. The tirade is too often purely moral in its tone. In England, the attack on luxury was mounted less vehemently than that in France. Perhaps the principal reason was that the courts of George II and George III hardly lent themselves to the type of observation justified in the reigns of Louis XV and Louis XVI. The British aristocracy of the time were not perhaps all occupied in raising turnips like Lord Townshend, or digging canals like the Duke of Bridgewater, but it was certainly a far cry from the times of Charles II and the Duke of Buckingham. The attack therefore is more general and less convincing. We may take here three representative authors: the Scots divine Robert Wallace, who crossed swords with Hume over the question of the relative magnitude of populations in the ancient and modern world; William Bell, who attacked commerce in a widely circulated prize essay; and Dr. Thomas Short, one of the shrewdest commentators on contemporary population statistics. Bell,[2] though he gained fame and had his work translated into German, had less circulation than Short and Wallace, whose works were reprinted several times and almost certainly influenced Malthus. In these works we find particular references to the habits of people in London, just as the French authors talk in Parisian terms. Presumably the life of the eighteenth-century squire was not yet a riot of high living.[3]

[1] Spengler, op. cit., pp. 54–55.

[2] Quoted in R. R. Kuczynski, 'British Demographers' Opinions on Fertility, 1660–1760', L. T. Hogben, ed., *Political Arithmetic* (London, 1938), pp. 307–8.

[3] T. Short, *A Comparative History of the Increase and Decrease of Mankind in England*

Wallace sees no check in a mere high standard of living; for him, it is: '. . . in a debauched nation, addicted to sensuality and to irregular amours, and where luxury and an high taste of delicate living prevail, the number of the people must be proportionably small'.[1] Could it be that the Rev. Dr. Wallace, 'late one of the Ministers of Edinburgh', had never in fact seen what a high standard of living means, and referred to luxury as a southern form of debauch? He certainly lacks his contemporary and compatriot Ferguson's wide approach—his authorities are ancient, since the main part of the book deals with the numbers of nations in classical times.

Adam Smith, too, was given to mere generalizations about the prolific habits of the poor and the barrenness of women of fashion. 'Luxury, in the fair sex, . . . seems always to weaken, and frequently to destroy altogether, the powers of generation.'[2]

When the post-Malthusian authors spoke of luxury, as did Gray and Moreton, it was already the luxury of the industrializing phase —of the transitory kind, which really meant a rising standard of living.

Of German authors, we have already mentioned J. P. Süßmilch, one of the important precursors of Malthus in his recognition of a geometrical ratio, who devoted several chapters to the obstacles to population growth. Here, too, luxury is treated in the severe manner one might expect from the Royal Prussian Higher Consistory Counsel, Provost of Coelln—he was in fact in favour of a higher standard of living to eliminate the positive checks to population, but he expressly warned that this movement must stop short of a standard which would mean debauchment and sterility.[3]

In the United States, we may cite Benjamin Franklin as a representative of the orthodox European school, basing his arguments in part on the observations of Short and Wallace. One suspects that his views

and Several Countries Abroad (London, 1767), may be taken as a good example of the usual straightforward anti-luxury, anti-urban view. Short, a Sheffield physician, had studied the bills of mortality in some detail, and thought they lent colour to his observations.

[1] R. Wallace, *A Dissertation On the Numbers of Mankind in Ancient and Modern Times* (2nd ed., Edinburgh, 1809), p. 19. The first edition had been published in 1753.

[2] A. Smith, *An Inquiry into the Nature and Causes of the Wealth of Nations* (1776; Cannan's ed., New York, 1937, 2 vols.), i, ch. viii, p. 79.

[3] J. P. Süßmilch, *Die göttliche Ordnung in den Veränderungen des menschlichen Geschlechts aus der Geburt, dem Tode und der Fortpflanzung desselben erwiesen* (Berlin, 1775, 3 vols.), ii, esp. ch. xvii—'Of Luxury'. The first edition was published in 1741. Süßmilch was 'Königlich Preußischer Oberconsistorialrath' and a member of the Prussian Academy of Sciences.

were coloured by European conditions, and that the life of the colonists gave little cause for complaints on that score.[1]

The luxury argument, then, may be said to have been the legacy of the ancient world to the eighteenth century. It found favour, obviously, with the moralists, but the economists and politicians had their own reasons for condemning riotous living. The attack fitted well into the system of philosophy which preached the virtues of a simple life as such—however little its advocates might themselves be disposed to follow their own advice.

A few far-sighted people, however, saw that this condemnation was altogether too simple. First of all, nobody seemed able to define clearly what was luxury, as opposed to vice. Standards were seen to change, and by the end of the century every decade saw a new assessment of what was necessary and what was not. Along with this discovery came another—that 'luxuries' were in fact the product of the rising industries; that their prohibition meant the killing of these new sources of wealth; and that it was precisely in the greater diffusion of these comforts that the hope for the future lay. With the coming of Malthus, fresh point was given to this changing attitude.

2. TOWNS

The idea of infertile towns, graveyards of a nation's manhood, is probably as old as cities themselves. There were many who had good cause to dislike towns, and this particular accusation was a handy one. It has never failed to provoke great emotional excitement. Towns rose either because there developed a seat of powerful central or regional government, or because the rise of trade and industry demanded concentration. In either case there were large injured or jealous parties. Again, it is striking to note that the Roman strictures on towns were taken up in the seventeenth century. Even discounting the more exaggerated accounts of the decline of the large cities of the ancient world, there is no doubt that they played a much lesser role in the Middle Ages. Feudal castles and great abbeys held the balance. The development of overland and overseas trade once more gave rise to powerful urban interests.

In England, the dislike of towns was always particularly strong. It would be an interesting piece of literary research to trace the perpetuation of the myth of England as a nation made strong by its agriculture,

[1] See A. Aldridge, 'Franklin as Demographer', *Journal of Economic History* (1949), ix, no. 1, pp. 25–29.

and the Englishman as John Bull, precisely during the period when trade and industry came to assume a dominant role in the economy. Whatever the causes, the English certainly came to regard the country as life-giving; escape from the towns, temporarily or every week-end, or permanently at the end of one's life, became a nation-wide obsession by the end of the nineteenth century and began to be shared actively by successive classes as their standard of living improved. It did not take the physiocratic movement to set English farmers to claim that they alone were the wealth of the nation, and their influence survived parliamentary reform and the repeal of the Corn Laws. When depression brought disaster to British farming after 1873, the appeal for active aid was, in part at least, based on the assumption that the strength of the nation would suffer materially without a flourishing agricultural population. Not only quantitatively, but qualitatively, the offspring of the country families surpassed that of the urban dwellers. This was noticed by Francis Galton, the Census of 1881, and witnesses before Royal Commissions.[1]

Just as in the case of luxury, the argument that towns depopulate is to be taken not only as an indicator of urban growth, but as a weapon in a larger dispute. Once more there are philosophical, political, and economic reasons for disliking towns and their occupations, and these are rationalized into the surest means of frightening the country at large—by saying that urban conditions depopulate.

Socrates eulogized farming as a pursuit for men of liberal feelings.[2] Virgil, in the *Georgics*, typified the Roman attitude towards farming as a wholesome occupation, contrasted with the intrigues and corruption of town life.

> non ullus aratro
> dignus honos: squalent abductis arva colonis,
> et curvae rigidum falces conflantur in ensem.

—that is the sign of the troubled times in which they live. And what has happened to the cultivators?

> vicinae ruptis inter se legibus urbes
> arma ferunt: saevit toto Mars impius orbe.[3]

[1] See J. Saville, *Rural Depopulation in England and Wales, 1851–1951* (London, 1957), pp. 125 ff. Galton's article: 'The Relative Supplies from Town and Country Families to the Population of Future Generations', *Journal of the Royal Statistical Society* (1873), xxxvi. 19.

[2] See H. Michell, *The Economics of Ancient Greece* (Cambridge, 1940), pp. 38 ff.

[3] Virgil, *Georgics*, i, lines 506–11.

Polybius was of the opinion that country districts were free of corruption and immorality, and that the country people were more prolific.[1] Tacitus, in the *Germania*, constantly contrasted the simple, healthy, fruitful life of the tribes in their villages with the decadent customs of Rome.[2] Horace waxed eloquent on the subject of the Scythians on their steppes, and the hardy Getae—innocent corn-growers, chaste, virtuous, where a 'wife on the strength of her dower' could not overrule her husband: in fact they had no dowries except their chastity. Everywhere rural life was praised as healthier in every sense than urban customs.[3]

The classical attitude survived in an unbroken tradition to modern times. As an intermediate link between Virgil and Graunt we may cite the Italian Giovanni Botero (1533–1617), whose most important work, *The Reason of State*, has recently received increased attention. In his treatise, *Of the Causes of the Magnificence and Greatness of Cities*, translated into English in 1606, he had this to say:

> . . . great cities are more subject unto dearths than the little, for they need more sustenance and victuals. The plague also afflicteth them more surely and more often, with greater loss of people. . . .
>
> So, that, although men were as apt to generation in the height and pride of the Romans' greatness as in the first beginning thereof, yet for all that the people increased not proportionably. For the virtue nutritive of that city had no power to go further, so that in success of time the inhabitants, finding much want and less means to supply their lack of victual, either forbare to marry or, if they did marry, their children oppressed with penury, their parents affording them no relief, fled their own country and sought abroad for better fortune.[4]

Several comments on this passage are necessary. The impression of the infertility of cities stands out quite clearly. But there is also the element of higher mortality to be considered, and this persists as an undertone in later writers. Not until the twentieth century could cities show a better health record than rural areas.

[1] Polybius, *Histories*, iv, bk. cxxiii, para. 6. But the ancients may have described the depopulation of 'Megalopolis' because it is more evident there than in the sparsely settled countryside. See A. Landry, 'Quelques aperçus concernant la dépopulation dans l'antiquité gréco-romaine', *Revue historique* (1936), clxxvii. 2 ff.

[2] Tacitus, *Germania*, chs. xvii and xix, 287–8 and 291–2.

[3] Horace, *Odes*, bk. iii, ode 24, 104–106, 'Moral Reformation'.

[4] G. Botero, *The Reason of State* (with a subsection *A Treatise Concerning Causes of the Magnificency and Greatness of Cities*, Robert Peterson, trans., 1606) (P. J. and D. P. Waley, trans. and eds., London, 1956). This is quoted from the subsection, bk. iii, ch. ix, pp. 277–8.

As far as the working out of the infertility of urban dwellers is concerned, Botero obviously traces it to a proper Malthusian process. Subsistence is short, so the prudent refrain from marriage, or else emigrate. The motive presumably is the fear of losing that high standard which, as he shows elsewhere, they can attain in urban occupations. The idea of an absolute limit to subsistence at the time of the Renaissance, when European densities were still very low, strikes us as incongruous, but we must not forget that the city states of Italy did, in fact, dispose of only limited territories. At the same time, London already had a highly organized food market which drew on distant areas of production. Nevertheless, the idea of such a limit persisted, even if it did not figure largely in the pre-Malthusian discussion of towns.

The idea of differential fertility, which now plays such an important role in demography, may be said to originate in the contrast of town and country. The earliest of the English demographers were well aware of it.[1] Thus John Graunt thought that marriages were less fruitful in London because of:

> the intemperance in feeding, and especially the Adulteries and Fornications, supposed more frequent in London than elsewhere . . .

and

> . . . that the minds of men in London are more thoughtful and full of business than in the Country.[2]

Similar reasons were adduced by Gregory King and Charles D'Avenant, one of the earliest 'Tory Free Traders', who added luxury and intemperance, the evil effects of coal smoke, and the greater inequality of age between husbands and wives.[3] Corbyn Morris and Wallace, half a century later, agreed; the former adds the habit of gin-drinking to the deleterious influences of urban life; both stress the large numbers of healthy children born to country people. Wallace conjures up his usual vision:

> . . . huge and overgrown cities, which are nurseries of corruption and debauchery, and prejudicial in many other respects, are in a particular manner destructive to the populousness of the world, as they cherish luxury, entice great numbers of all ranks to resort to them, and drain the rest of a country of useful labouring hands, who otherwise would be employed in agriculture and the most necessary arts.[4]

[1] For full treatment, see Kuczynski, op. cit., pp. 312 ff., from which this information is taken.

[2] J. Graunt, *Natural and Political Observations* (London, 1662), p. 46, quoted in Kuczynski, op. cit., p. 296.

[3] Kuczynski, op. cit., pp. 314–15.

[4] Wallace, op. cit., pp. 22–23.

Wallace, in his mind, connected towns with industry, as is shown by the passage immediately following the one just quoted, where he refers to the 'operose manufacture' of textiles, wooden, metal, and earthenware goods; none of which he thinks contribute much to the increase of the people. After all, they create a taste for delicacies, and make them necessary, in some degree, to the bulk of the people.[1] In turn, of course, Wallace eulogized the country occupations, basing his opinion on the Roman writers who, in the fashion of their day, praised rural simplicity, notable among them being Columella (*fl.* A.D. 20).[2]

This passion in eighteenth-century England does not, of course, spring simply from a love of classical authors. Even allowing for a fair amount of distortion and exaggeration, it has to be admitted that London, at this time, was not a good place to live in. Thomas Short, who did not go so far as his contemporaries in condemning London, and in fact thought that the expectation of life there was probably not much less than elsewhere, had a remarkable list of reasons why London should be accounted an unhealthy and infertile place. Quoting figures of baptisms and burials of 296,831 and 486,171 respectively, for the period 1738–58, he attributed this decline to the 'Shocking effects' of the excessive consumption of spirituous liquors; namely barrenness and increased adult mortality.[3] Whether we believe his figures in detail or not, there can be little doubt that the city failed to show any appreciable natural increase. It acted as a magnet, drawing people in from outside—their deaths added to the excess of burials over baptisms, since they had been born elsewhere. What Short only guessed, and most of his contemporaries do not seem to have known, is that in the first half of the eighteenth century, few areas in the country showed any appreciable surplus of births—the smallpox raged as effectively in the country as the gin-shop in London. Nevertheless, the stench and open depravity of London, its inefficient burial arrangements—all these created a general prejudice in the minds of the writers on population.

To some extent, the writers quoted realized that the growth of towns and their baneful influence was in itself a consequence of new economic

[1] Ibid., p. 25. Similar ideas at the time in the works of Dr. Price and J. Howlett. See Stangeland, op. cit., pp. 346, 348.

[2] Wallace, op. cit., pp. 98 ff.

[3] Short, op. cit., p. 21. Amongst his less-inspired proposals to end immorality was that of cashiering officers who 'needlessly or unnecessarily' frequented women, 'especially at unreasonable Hours, or in private Places' (ibid., p. 29). (See also his *New Observations, Natural, Moral, Civil, Political, and Medical, on City, Town and Country Bills of Mortality* (London, 1750), esp. p. 121: 'In general Country Breeders are more fruitful in proportion to their Numbers, than in large Towns' (quoted in Kuczynski, op. cit., p. 315).)

developments. It is curious to note, however, that Thomas Short saw these developments as resulting in the comparative decline of London: he cited the rise of other ports which had attracted some of the trade which London formerly possessed, and 'The late great Improvement in, and Increase of, our Manufactories, which now supply both home and foreign Marts' is quoted as having an adverse influence on London's population. In this he was certainly wrong; London continued to grow and to be the principal port of the kingdom. More accurate was his observation that London itself was losing in relative importance through suburbanization: 'A great Number of new Villas or Country-Seats within a moderate Day's Journey of London.' For these and other reasons he thought he could subscribe to Sir William Petty's vision of London 'at its full Zenith at or before the Year 1800'.[1] If one takes the City of London alone, they were right. Otherwise, it has to be taken as wishful thinking.

We find similar ideas in eighteenth-century France. The times were much addicted to pastoral poetry; the rich loved to appear in the guise of simple shepherd folk, and however urban their tastes, a country retreat and landed estates were the order of the day. Fénelon already pointed out the stability of a society based on agriculture:

> La nature seule tirerait de son sein fécond tout ce qu'il faudrait pour un nombre infini d'hommes modérés et laborieux; mais c'est l'orgueil et la mollesse de certains hommes, qui en mettent tant d'autres dans une affreuse pauvreté.[2]

The first statement would acquire a different significance in the post-Malthusian controversy—for the eighteenth century, it is simply an opinion that all mankind could be well fed, numerous, and happy, if only towns did not drain away men and wealth.

The idea is further elaborated in the writings of many authors of the mid-century. Amongst them we may mention C. J. Herbert, who saw one of the chief contrasts between town and countryside in the absence of *ambition* amongst simple folk:

> It is not in the Cities, nor in the highest ranks, that a resource for posterity must be sought. The manner of living, the passions, concern, delicacy, are obstacles to population. Human nature unfolds all her fecundity only in the flourishing country districts, and amongst those who, without any ambition, work only just to live. . . .[3]

[1] Short, *A Comparative History* . . ., pp. 19–20. [2] Fénelon, op. cit., p. 170.

[3] Quoted by Spengler, *French Predecessors* . . ., p. 70, from C. J. Herbert, *Essai sur la police générale des grains, sur leurs prix, et sur les effets d'agriculture* (1753; Berlin, 1755 ed.). For the significance of ambition, see Ch. IV below.

We now have cities characterized, not only as seats of the courts and their dissipations, but as the natural habitat of those who want to get on—to whom children are obstacles. With the Physiocrats, the argument becomes a little less direct and simple. Agriculture is the source of wealth; population can only increase if wealth increases, therefore a flourishing agriculture will lead to an increase in population. The growth of towns thus acts as an 'intermediate' check, i.e. one which, though not in itself to be condemned as evil, may be traced back to policies which are to be condemned in any case as being unfavourable to agriculture.[1]

Mirabeau, on the other hand, saw an advantage in agriculture not only on the grounds we have just mentioned, but also because he was aware of some differential in fertility. He called the countryside 'the sole source of Population'. Country people, he thought, were healthier and simpler in their habits. He advocated, therefore, that the government should take measures to support agriculture, so as to encourage more hands to this pursuit.[2]

The general attitude to the problem was one of the time. It is shared alike by non-physiocrats and anti-physiocrats—Herrenschwand, Linguet, Moheau, and many others cited by Spengler. One of them is worth quoting in a little more detail because he observed urban effects more closely: Du Buat-Nançay distinguished between rural and urban artisans, i.e. between people of the same social standing and occupation. This is helpful to us in isolating what were thought to be the purely urban factors in the situation (in contrast with a writer like Herbert, who constantly mixes location, occupation, and social class). Thus, Du Buat-Nançay thought that a rural artisan was inclined to marry because a wife was a help in his work. He was property-less, and had no great prospects, and so would not be able to afford a servant. (He did admit that sometimes these people did pass into the ranks of the proprietors, but it is not clear whether he thought that was an incentive to marry or not.) At any rate the town artisan was altogether disinclined to marry:

> . . . le superflu peut être aussi aisément contraire que favorable à la résolution de se marier, parce qu'il ne peut que diminuer par la société, que du moins il y a peu d'espérance qu'il s'accroisse, et parce qu'aussi ce superflu, qui n'est le plus souvent que pécuniaire, met un artisan en état de se passer de femme.[3]

[1] See Spengler, op. cit., pp. 180–2.

[2] Mirabeau, op. cit. i. 17; iii. 117. Quoted in Spengler, op. cit., p. 355.

[3] Du Buat-Nançay, op. cit. ii. 355.

He also mentioned the effect of the general instability of urban occupations, owing to intense competition—but the important observation relates to the notion of an urban standard of living which marriage threatens. Under such conditions, a servant is a more economical form of help. Once again, we must see in *le superflu*, not riotous living and waste, but the excess of comfort over absolute necessity which the town affords. We shall return to Du Buat-Nançay when we discuss the growing concern for the prospects of children.[1]

Let us take the story forward into the nineteenth century—England in the stage of industrialization. Malthus's opponents were anxious to show the causes which were at work in checking the headlong progress of population. These checks are all preventive—not only that, they are in themselves mostly evidences of desirable changes in society.[2] By the second decade of the century, inquiring minds had the figures of two census returns to compare. They had an opportunity of observing, in the mass, the habits of those engaged in commerce and industry, in all social classes. Towns are part of the general transformation: the urban mentality is the spirit of commerce. Hence all the psychological factors which keep down population are presented as urban phenomena. One example of this is Sir Archibald Alison's emulation—'the desire to keep up with the Joneses'—this operates more easily in towns, where people live in close contact with each other:

> The extension of artificial wants among the inhabitants of towns is of course more immediate than what takes place in the country, in consequence of the close proximity of the higher and the lower orders, and the rapid progress of improvements, where luxury, invention, talent, and opulence are brought together.[3]

[1] For additional similar views on the effects of towns, in Italy, see Reynaud, *La Théorie de la population en Italie du XVIe au XVIIIe siècle* (Lyon, 1904), p. 54 (Giambattista d'Arco) and p. 38 (Beccaria): luxury, expensive weddings, heavy dowries, and the growth of cities. Moheau suggested differential fertility of town and countryside in a less imprecise manner than some others. He distinguished also between these differences and those attributable to social class. See Spengler, op. cit., p. 103, and *Journal of Political Economy* (1936), xlvii. 657. Jaubert particularly stressed that towns caused illness (Spengler, *France Faces Depopulation*, p. 94). Rousseau commented on the comparative infertility of urban women (Spengler, *French Predecessors* . . ., pp. 345–50). This is also quoted by Michael Sadler in support of his own *Law of Population* (London, 1830), ii. 360. In Germany, J. P. Süßmilch, op. cit. (1748 ed.), p. 50, noted that peasants were in theory subject to the same heavy expenses as others, yet hardly any of them remained unmarried.

[2] Not all of them. Thus John Weyland, jnr., F.R.S., in *The Principles of Population and Production, as They Are Affected by the Progress of Society; with a View to Moral and Political Consequences* (London, 1816), knew that the atmosphere of towns weakened health, necessary for healthy progeny, and therefore diminished births, and also increased deaths (pp. 63, 157).

[3] Sir A. Alison, *The Principles of Population and Their Connection with Human Happiness*

Alison went on to prescribe the same cure for rural districts: if only landed proprietors could be persuaded to live on their estates, and if the properties were smaller, so that more gentry could live closer to the people, the agricultural labourer would then be subjected to the same salutary influences as the townsman.

Thomas Rowe Edmonds was probably one of the most competent statisticians of the middle of the nineteenth century, with an extensive practical knowledge of conditions in London, where he worked for many years as an actuary. His *Enquiry into the Principles of Population* was published anonymously in 1832, and has perhaps the best description of the urban situation at the time. Population was increasing there at a slower rate than in the country. He ascribed this not only to the sickliness of town life—because in fact there was better medical attendance to be had there, '... and there are more comforts and foreign commodities, considered now as necessaries rather than as luxuries, procured with facility'. It is rather the 'greater efficacy of the preventive check' which distinguishes town life, at least where it has a chance to operate. Not in the very poor and crowded quarters, where privations are as great as ever, but in the new salubrious outer districts where wealth and respectability grow, there will prudence lead to a slower rate of increase. So far from any tendency of the population to diminish where it is densest, it grows fastest where most congregate:

> In St. Giles's, Shoreditch, the most crowded parts of the Borough, indeed in all the most populous parts of large towns, a greater number of persons are born than in other parts less densely inhabited. Where the people enjoy greater room in their dwellings observation is more sedulously fixed upon their actions, and, attending more to the comforts and decencies of life, they postpone marriage.[1]

(Edinburgh, 1840, 2 vols.), i. 107. (We shall return to the desire for emulation below, Ch. IV, sect. 2, when discussing the general topic of ambition in a mobile society.) Alison was a Tory, author of a vast *History of Europe*. He was Sheriff of Lanarkshire, presiding daily over his court at Glasgow. *The Principles* ... were written as early as 1828. Despite his acute remarks here on the population question, he was a defender of the Corn Laws and of slavery. The work has a bad reputation, probably thanks to Sir Leslie Stephen, who wrote the notice in the *D.N.B.* and comments on him in *The English Utilitarians* (London, 1900, 3 vols.), iii. 180.

[1] *An Enquiry into the Principles of Population, Exhibiting a System of Regulations for the Poor; Designed Immediately to Lessen, and Finally To Remove, the Evils Which Have Hitherto Pressed upon the Labouring Classes of Society* (London, 1832), pp. 86–87. (The attribution to Edmonds is made by J. A. Field and others.) T. R. Edmonds was born in Cornwall in 1803. He was Actuary to the Legal and General Life Assurance Society from 1832 to 1866. He had already written a *Practical Moral and Political Economy* (London 1828), and later compiled life-tables.

These ideas are interesting because they are in exact opposition to Sadler's law, published two years earlier, that fertility varies inversely with density. Nevertheless, the outcome of Sadler's theory may be said to describe the same urban phenomena as Edmonds's. On the whole, urban density was greater than rural density—so towns would have less fertility than the countryside. Sadler (1780–1835), a much less careful author than Edmonds, did not inquire into differential fertility within towns. He was above all a controversialist, an effective social reformer, and a propagandist for good causes. As an economist he was less effective. When attempting to make some point in an argument, he would often adduce a curious collection of authorities for his views, ranging from the Bible and Hippocrates to Francis Bacon and Dr. Perceval, the Manchester statistician of the late eighteenth century.[1] Often these quotations cannot be traced, or the passage to which he refers conveys a different meaning from that which he claimed. He had a taste for mathematics in the abstract, but apparently little gift for the application of statistics. His massive two-volume 'refutation' of Malthus was not taken very seriously, although he himself was quite convinced, as were so many other authors, that the work would provide a final answer.

There is an echo of the difference between Edmonds and Sadler in later writings. Already in 1839 a Frenchman, H. Passy, investigating the effects of the law relating to the division of inheritances, noticed that the cities of the *bourgeoisie* (like Le Mans and Tours) were relatively infertile, with about 2½ children to each marriage, whereas the cities of the proletariat could show as many as 4·6 children (as at Saint-Étienne).[2] At the beginning of the twentieth century David Heron, a statistician associated with Galton and Pearson at University College, London, investigated inter-urban fertility and mortality differentials, and in his work on London there are striking similarities to T. R. Edmonds's investigation.[3] The three Southwark parishes and St. Giles's, in 1851,

[1] Sadler, op. cit. i. 577–8. Macaulay attacked this work in the *Edinburgh Review* and elsewhere. It is interesting to note that he described the town argument as a matter of common knowledge, accepted by Malthus among the positive checks, and therefore hardly worth a chapter. See L. Stephen, op. cit. iii. 181.

[2] H. Passy, 'De la division des héritages et de l'influence qu'elle exerce sur la distribution des richesses', *L'Académie des sciences morales et politiques* (2e série, 1839), tome ii, 291 ff. Quoted in J. Goldstein, *Bevölkerungsprobleme und Berufsgliederung in Frankreich* (Berlin, 1900), p. 133.

[3] D. Heron, *On the Relation of Fertility in Man to Social Status, and on the Changes in this Relation that have taken place during the last fifty years* (Drapers' Company Memoirs, Studies in National Deterioration, I, London, 1906).

had the highest infant mortality rates, though not particularly high birth-rates. Shoreditch had a very much higher birth-rate than, for instance, Hampstead, although the infant mortality rates were not so dissimilar. In 1901, Shoreditch had the third highest rate of overcrowding on the basis of people per room.[1]

Still more recently, Raymond Pearl, in his *Biology of Population Growth*, maintained that density reduced rates of growth, yet gave figures to show that in towns the wealthy (with their ample gardens) had fewer children than the overcrowded poor. One of his opponents, F. Hankins, thought that the true explanation lay in the fact that towns in general reduced fertility through the excessive nerve strain they impose, a strain which would operate more heavily on those with cares of business and property.[2]

This last idea was not new. As we saw, John Graunt and Du Buat-Nançay had already referred to it. One who used this theory in the post-Malthusian debate was John Weyland. He distinguished sharply between the townsman and the countryman, with essentially different tendencies to contribute to the increase in population.[3] Generally speaking, he thought, civilization as such diminished the power of increase—but greater mental exertion would lead in any case to fewer marriages through incapacity or indisposition to rear families. Towns, too, would always abound in the type of people who, in any case, would not reproduce themselves—soldiers, sailors, men of good families but small fortunes, and the domestic servants and dependants of the wealthy.[4] Life in the towns was becoming too soft, some argued; there was a lack of healthy exercise, and too much food. Simon Gray, who had written an anti-Malthusian book, *The Happiness of States*, in 1804, published a further volume, *The Principles of Population and Production investigated*, under the pseudonym George Purves. One of the principal ideas in these works was the notion that 'Superabundance reduces fecundity and population'. Urbanization was a special case of this.[5] He compared the rates of increase of population of Middlesex and

[1] Ibid., pp. 6–8.

[2] F. H. Hankins, 'Does Advancing Civilisation Involve a Decline in Natural Fertility?', *Publications of the American Sociology Society* (May, 1930), xxiv. 119, for analysis and criticism of Pearl. For his own views: 'Has the reproductive power of western peoples declined?', *Problems of Population* (Pitt-Rivers, ed., London, 1932), pp. 187–8.

[3] Weyland, op. cit., p. 62.

[4] Ibid., p. 84.

[5] G. Purves (Simon Gray), *Gray versus Malthus. The Principles of Population and Production Investigated, and the Question: Does Population Regulate Subsistence, or Subsistence Population? . . . etc., Discussed* (London and Edinburgh, 1818), bk. ii, ch. vii.

Kentucky to prove his point. Thomas Jarrold, at the same time, claimed that the Americans increased faster because they were farmers, not philosophers, and did not shine in literature or science![1]

Some Americans of this period, at any rate, were aware of the differential—George Tucker, for instance, saw the same kind of checks in civilization and urbanization as contemporary Englishmen.[2] Benjamin Franklin expressed the view that cities were apt to show a high standard of living, and thus provided a dis-incentive to marriage: '... cities do not, by natural generation, supply themselves with inhabitants; the deaths are more than the births'.[3] Jefferson appears to have held like views.[4]

Later in the nineteenth century, very few writers elevated the influence of urbanization to the position of a population check in its own right. But nearly all of them listed the habits of city dwellers, their fears and opportunities, amongst the causes of diminishing fertility. Some stressed this factor more than others, and the condemnation of the evil influence of large cities has had the same sort of attraction for writers on the fringe of science as the earlier moral onslaught on luxury. An interesting example of this type of theory is provided in the work of Georg Hanssen (1809–94), a Göttingen Professor of Economics who studied the history and structure of German agriculture and appears to have held views which in some ways provide a nineteenth-century equivalent to those of the Physiocrats. He thought there were three *Stufen* or degrees of population development.[5] The landowners and farmers formed the first, and only permanent degree. From amongst the surpluses of this class were recruited the second and third degrees, middle classes and citizen traders on one hand, and property-less workers on the other. These two latter groups, left without the infusion of fresh blood from the rich countryside, would die out in two or three generations.[6] The process described here, although obviously not a tenable

[1] T. Jarrold, *Dissertations on Man, Philosophical, Physiological and Political; in Answer to Mr. Malthus' 'Essay on the Principle of Population'* (London, 1806), p. 281.

[2] J. J. Spengler, 'Population Doctrines in the United States', *Journal of Political Economy* (Aug.–Oct. 1933), xli, no. 4, pp. 433–67, 639–72.

[3] B. Franklin, *The Complete Works, in Philosophy, Politics, and Morals, . . . with Memoirs of His Early Life, Written by Himself* (London, 1806, 3 vols.), ii. 384. See also Aldridge, op. cit., pp. 25–27.

[4] See J. J. Spengler, 'The Political Economy of Jefferson, Adams, and Madison', *American Studies in Honor of W. K. Boyd* (Durham, North Carolina, 1940).

[5] G. Hanssen, *Die drei Bevölkerungsstufen. Ein Versuch, die Ursachen für das Blühen und Altern der Völker nachzuweisen* (Munich, 1889).

[6] Ibid., p. 173. Much of his material relating to cities was taken from an earlier work: A. v. Öttingen, *Die Moralstatistik in ihrer Bedeutung für eine Sozialethik* (3rd ed., Erlangen, 1882).

explanation of the long-term movements, bears a striking resemblance to some of the known facts about the recruitment of the entrepreneurs and workers of the British industrial revolution. The yeoman farmers who became cotton-spinners, and the displaced small copyholders who became urban labourers figure largely in the histories of the textile industries in particular.

Hanssen's thesis is also interesting because it demonstrates a movement opposite to the more usual idea of upward social mobility, the one that Arsène Dumont was to term 'social capillarity'. The effect was held to be the same; a decline of population. Hanssen's theories were kept alive in a number of writers who may be described as 'culture pessimists'—as indeed at all times authors have described urban growth in terms of general decadence. We shall have to come back to these general cultural explanations later, and will see in Spengler's *Decline of the West* some echoes of the urban theories.[1]

As in the case of luxury, we see that towards the end of the eighteenth century it becomes more and more difficult to find views which blame a decline in fertility on the single cause of the level of consumption or the physical environment. As luxury came to mean diffusion of comforts through increasing numbers of people in all ranks of society, so urbanization became synonymous with civilization, industrialization, and physical and social mobility of population. The temptation is therefore to plunge at once into the history of the more complex economic, political, and social theories. But one argument deserves a short scrutiny, which was also once used in isolation, and later merges into the general stream of theory. This concerns the habits of aristocracies.

3. ARISTOCRACIES

Most societies have some form of aristocracy, whether in the shape of an hereditary nobility, or a class of large proprietors, or of officials who may pass on their high position to their sons. The essential characteristic in each case is the possession of considerable power in society, whether wielded by wealth, prestige, or privilege, and the ability to

[1] For further discussion of urban theories, see: G. Mackenroth, *Bevölkerungslehre; Theorie, Soziologie und Statistik der Bevölkerung* (Enzyklopädie der Rechts- und Staatswissenschaft. Abteilung Staatswissenschaft, Berlin, 1953), pp. 262 ff., and S. Budge, *Das Malthus'sche Bevölkerungsgesetz und die theoretische Nationalökonomie der letzten Jahrzehnte* (Karlsruhe, 1912). This work examines Cauderlier, Bertillon, Oldenburg, and others.

transmit that power to their bodily or spiritual, but self-chosen, heirs. The view has for long been held that such aristocracies die out rapidly, or at least that they are constantly faced with the problem of the absence of a male heir. Such a view seems to imply that ordinary families always perpetuate themselves, which is manifestly untrue. It is well known that even rural populations in medieval England showed no permanent family structure: out of each generation, only perhaps half the names are transmitted to the next, and so on, until, in a hundred years, barely any of the original names survive.[1] But we are not here concerned, primarily, with the correctness of this view, but only with the fact that it was widely held. The explanations offered are of two kinds: they either blame the system of primogeniture and laws of inheritance, or they link aristocracies to the ideas on soft living and urbanization with which we have already dealt. On the first problem, a good deal of imprecise reasoning exists. The prevailing view was that since only the eldest could inherit the estate, additional children would be a burden, a permanent charge on the revenues falling on the eldest. But the opposite view was also possible: that since the law of inheritance kept the estate intact in any case, there was no need to worry about how many other children there were. This was to become of crucial importance when the Napoleonic code decreed the equal division of property amongst all heirs, a system already in partial operation in France before his time. In either case the main question is whether the undivided estate, or the parts into which it is split on the father's decease, are capable of supporting other children in the accustomed manner, enabling them to marry and have children in their turn.[2]

Moheau and others in eighteenth-century France who considered primogeniture unfavourable to population did so on the grounds that it prevented the spread of small proprietorship, which was favourable to population.[3] The idea that such proprietorship had exactly the opposite effect did not emerge till later.

Michael Sadler thought that the earliest mention of the idea of an infertile aristocracy occurred in the Bible, and in support cited the 49th Psalm:

[1] See E. J. Buckatzsch, 'The Constancy of Local Populations and Migration in England before 1800', *Population Studies* (1952), v. 62–69.

[2] This is a point which J. A. Field seemed to misunderstand. J. A. Field, *Essays on Population and Other Papers* (H. F. Hohman, ed. and comp., Chicago, 1931), p. 62.

[3] See Spengler, 'Moheau, prophet of depopulation', *Journal of Political Economy* (1939), xlvii. 664.

They that trust in their wealth, and boast themselves in the multitude of their riches. . . .

Their inward thought is, that their houses shall continue for ever, and their dwelling places to all generations: they call their lands after their own names.

But man abideth not in honour: he is like the beasts that perish.

Whether or not this passage is capable of such an interpretation, Sadler certainly believed that aristocracies were doomed to a short and infertile life, and cited in support also the works of Tacitus, Vestergan, Chastellux, and Addison. His interpretation of the psalm rests on the earlier verse—taken by itself, the last verse simply means that the great and the rich die and are forgotten as quickly as brutes and fools.[1]

The Bible apart, Aristotle provides us with an early and detailed account of a dying aristocracy or oligarchy. The Spartiates, the ruling class of the Lacedaemonian polity, once numerous, had died out very quickly. Aristotle ascribed this to the inequality of property, habits of giving large dowries which left little land for male heirs, and the failure to admit non-citizens to civic rights. Aristotle would have preferred the problem to be solved by an equalization of property, which would have led to a numerous and strong citizenry in the state. But if this could not be done, then, distasteful as this expedient was to a man of Aristotle's susceptibilities, he would have kept up the strength of the country by the admission of inferior classes to the rights and duties of the ruling class. Out of this discussion there emerges clearly the concept of an upper stratum of society which would have to be artificially encouraged to keep it alive.[2] The dowries question will arise again later. The idea of recruitment from below is, of course, central to the whole problem. Even if Aristotle disliked it, it certainly pervaded the ancient world: slaves were enfranchised, and lower orders admitted to higher categories.

The lamentation of the classical authors, as well as the struggles over disputed successions in their own century, would make the writers of the eighteenth century perfectly familiar with the phenomenon.[3] One of the most quoted passages was one from Tacitus:

The freedmen were a numerous body. From them the number of the

[1] M. T. Sadler, *The Law of Population: a Treatise, in Six Books; in Disproof of the Super-fecundity of Human Beings, and Developing the Real Principle of Their Increase* (London, 1830, 2 vols.), ii, ch. xxiii, pp. 596 ff.

[2] Aristotle, *Politics*, bk. ii, ch. ix. Malthus quoted this passage, *An Essay on the Principle of Population* (Everyman ed., 1914, 2 vols.), i. 144.

[3] See W. W. Tarn, *Hellenistic Civilisation* (London, 1927), pp. 86 ff.; R. F. Willetts, 'The Neodamodeis', *Classical Philology* (Jan. 1954), xlix, i. 28; M. I. Rostovtzeff, *The Social and Economic History of the Roman Empire* (Oxford, 1926), pp. 175, 177. The *Lex Papia Poppaea* of Augustus sought to arrest the extinction of the *ingenii* by allowing them

tribes was completed, the magistrates were supplied with inferior officers, the sacerdotal orders with assistants, and the praetorian cohort with recruits. Many of the Roman knights, and even the Senators, had no other origin. Deduct the men whose fathers were enfranchised, and the number of free-born citizens will dwindle into nothing. When the ranks of society were established at Rome, it was the wisdom of the old republic to make liberty the common right of all, not the prerogative of the few.[1]

Although Tacitus does not say so, the implication clearly is that the upper classes of the republic failed to produce sons who could carry on the offices traditionally reserved for them. The only remedy was to admit more from below. As we shall see, there are further assumptions in such a system regarding the origin and effect of social mobility.

In the eighteenth century Wallace, harking back to the glories of an ancient world more populous than his own, spoke of the evils of the laws of succession, and especially the right of primogeniture, as being unknown in the ancient world and common in his period. At Venice, he thought, only the eldest son (in a patrician family presumably) married—the others could not live at the accustomed level if they raised a family.[2] Wallace indeed favoured a 'splendid nobility or gentry' to counterbalance the powers of a monarch. He did not mind if there were just a few such families, who might well keep their numbers down —what he feared was the spread of these aristocratic habits to lower orders of society.

Cantillon provides a link between the traditional view of the aristocracy and the later standard-of-living argument:

In Europe the Children of the Nobility are brought up in affluence; and as the largest share of the Property is usually given to the Eldest sons, the younger Sons are in no hurry to marry. They usually live as Bachelors, either in the Army or in the Cloisters, but will seldom be found unwilling to marry if they are offered Heiresses and Fortunes, or the means of supporting a

to marry the *liberatae*. Cf. Jörs, 'Die Ehegesetze des Augustus', in *Festschrift für Theodor Mommsen* (Marburg, 1893), p. 20. Also in D. Hume, 'Population of Ancient Nations', *Essays and Treatises on Several Subjects* (1742; new ed., Edinburgh, 1825, 2 vols.), i. 383. The Augustan legislation had a respectable ancestry, both in Greece and Rome. See Stangeland, op. cit., pp. 21, 32. For the extinction of noble Roman families see also B. G. Niebuhr, *Römische Geschichte* (Berlin, 1828–32), i. 417 ff. Michael Sadler was one of the many participants in the main Malthusian controversy who used evidence from classical sources (op. cit. i. 280–1, quoting from Cicero and Tacitus; only the admission of freedmen could keep up the numbers of the Republic).

[1] Tacitus, *Annals*, xiii. 27.

[2] Wallace, op. cit., pp. 93–94.

Family on the footing which they have in view and without which they would consider themselves to make their Children wretched.[1]

Like Wallace, he saw the habit gradually spreading downwards.

Malthus, collecting evidence of the operation of the preventive check in history, did not miss the effect. The *bourgeoisie* of Berne, which he described as being constantly in danger of extinction, was a comparatively small and certainly wealthy oligarchy. But Malthus failed to interpret the movement correctly, even though he knew of the way in which new families were recruited. To him, it was just another example of the preventive check operating in a group with a *given* standard of living.

George Ensor (1769–1843), a political writer of advanced views and well-known expert on Ireland, writing at the same time as Malthus, seized on these same facts and interpreted them differently, making them in effect part of a larger theory, where fruitfulness is related to wealth and social position. Like Wallace, he was aware of the extinction ot noble families in Venice, and he used the story to better effect.[2] But perhaps the best exposition is that of Thomas Doubleday (1790–1870), the Newcastle radical and poet, in his *True Law of Population*, devoted to the idea that a rich diet causes sterility. The over-fed peerage, he observed, never lasted long. But the same applied to any other oligarchy which did not take care to replenish its ranks from below. He cited particularly the Newcastle burgesses[3] who were several times threatened with extinction until they relaxed the rules of admission. At Bristol, where the franchise was easily obtained, the class of freemen not only maintained their numbers, but actually increased.[4]

Sismondi, one of the first to recognize the fact that, as he put it: 'La multiplication de l'espèce dépend de la volonté, c'est dans cette volonté qu'elle a les bornes',[5] was quick to see that these limits would be the

[1] R. Cantillon, *Essai sur la nature du commerce en général* (H. Higgs, trans. and ed., London, 1931), pp. 77–79. Moheau also thought that the 'nobility do not people' (Spengler on Moheau, op. cit., p. 658).

[2] G. Ensor, *An Inquiry Concerning the Population of Nations: Containing a Refutation of Mr. Malthus' 'Essay on Population'* (London, 1818), pp. 145, 147.

[3] T. Doubleday, *The True Law of Population Shewn To Be Connected with the Food of the People* (London, 1841; 3rd ed., 1853), pp. 44 ff.

[4] Ibid., p. 63. T. S. Ashton has noted that at Preston, while marriage was restricted for sons and daughters of Gild members, their numbers declined. When these restrictions fell into disuse, many of those who could not otherwise have found partners, began to do so, and population increased; *Economic History of England: the Eighteenth Century* (London, 1955), p. 5.

[5] J. C. L. S. de Sismondi, *Les Nouveaux Principes d'économie politique ou de la richesse dans ses rapports avec la population* (2nd ed., Paris, 1827), ii. 252.

narrower, the greater the intelligence, or the higher the social position of the family. Recruitment from below is the natural corollary: '. . . la population de toutes les classes supérieures de la société tendrait . . . constamment à s'éteindre si elle n'était recrutée par les classes inférieures'.[1] The clearest evidence of this was provided by the fate of ancient families. Sismondi quoted the Montmorencys: if they had multiplied in the Malthusian way, there would have been over sixteen million of them by 1600, and over 2,000 million by 1800—instead, they were practically extinct. Yet a rich, powerful family like this could not be subject to positive checks! Sismondi's reasoning is, of course, fallacious in every way, but his point was clear enough.[2]

Richard Jones (1790–1855), the London economist who gained fame as an expert on the tithe question, seeking to prove that the desire for secondary wants grew greater as he surveyed ever higher ranks of society, pointed to the record of the oligarchies:

> So far from their numbers increasing with undesirable rapidity, the annals of all the corporate towns in Europe show that the families of the citizens admitted to their freedom, offices and honours, are constantly fading away and disappearing. We may remark it, as a merciful dispensation, that it is the wealthier who disappear and the poorer who rise in their places.[3]

We note that Jones, like others, demonstrates clearly the link between these old-established beliefs and the newer idea of a constant upward movement between the classes.

Archibald Alison also drew his illustrations of the thesis that prudence increases in proportion to rank from the highest classes of society:

> The common observation, that the nobility of every country are on the decline, and would speedily become extinct, if not recruited by new creations from the sovereign, shows how universally the truth of this observation has been experienced. . . . Whatever may be the rapidity with which population is advancing in some parts of the British empire, in the class which composes the House of Peers and Commons, it is stationary, if not declining.[4]

As we would expect, the prejudices of the earlier social scientists were subjected to more stringent statistical tests in the mid-nineteenth century. Among the earliest investigations of differential mortality was that

[1] J. C. L. S. de Sismondi, op. cit., p. 265. [2] Ibid., p. 274.

[3] R. Jones, *Literary Remains, Consisting of Lectures and Tracts on Political Economy* (W. Whewell and Cazenove, eds., London, 1859), p. 103.

[4] Alison, op. cit. i. 111. See also J. Lowe, *The Present State of England in Regard to Agriculture, Trade and Finance* (2nd ed., London, 1823), p. 202, quoted by J. A. Field, *Essays on Population and Other Papers* (H. F. Hohman, ed. and comp., Chicago, 1931), p. 61. (The reference is to continental nobility.)

of Bailey and Day in 1863[1] and of fertility that of Benoiston de Chateauneuf in France.[2]

It is worth noting that already Joshua Milne, the author of *A Treatise on the Valuation of Annuities*, published in 1815, had precise views on this subject. Milne was not addicted to guess-work. His work for insurance companies was the first to be based entirely on reputable life-tables which he derived from those compiled by John Heysham of Carlisle. He said (quoted by Bailey and Day) that there could be 'no doubt but that mortality is greater amongst the higher than the middle classes of society'—but figures were not then available for a comparative study. But it was the Chateauneuf study which focused attention again on what was the core of the problem—not their higher mortality, but their failure to produce heirs in the male line (or any heirs at all, where descent, as so often in European countries, could be through the female line).

Amongst German authors, we have already mentioned Georg Hanssen. He also refers to Berne, and in addition quotes Augsburg, Nuremberg, and Lübeck as cities where the ruling classes died out. More scientific studies belong to the present century, such as those by Fahlbeck and Savorgnan.[3] The demographic decline of ruling castes is part of the general tradition of Western social thinking. But it was not until the end of the nineteenth century that its true significance was realized—and then it became part of a wider theory of differential fertility.

This concludes our survey of theories held widely at different times and in different countries. As we have shown, they had a certain validity in preindustrial societies. If they survived into the modern framework of theory, it is mostly because we now see luxury, urbanization, and the infertility of a ruling class as part of more intricate changes. The important feature they all have in common is that they were not merely philosophical speculations, but the basis for demands for action. Fear of depopulation dictated the social and economic policy advocated by these writers, from Aristotle's wish for an equalization of property to the demand for the reform of the court voiced by the *philosophes* of the era before the French Revolution.

[1] A. H. Bailey and A. Day, 'On the Rate of Mortality Prevailing amongst the Families of the Peerage during the Nineteenth Century', *Journal of the Royal Statistical Society* (1863), xxvi. 49–71.

[2] B. de Chateauneuf, 'De la durée des familles nobles en France', *Académie des Sciences Morales et Politiques* (Paris, 1845), p. 224. He had made earlier more general investigations beginning in 1824. See Spengler, *France Faces Depopulation*, pp. 117, 157, 173.

[3] P. E. Fahlbeck, *Der Adel Schwedens (und Finlands): Eine demographische Studie* (Jena, 1903), and F. Savorgnan, *La Fecondità dell' aristocrazia* (Pisa, 1942).

III

THE ECONOMIC BASIS OF MORAL RESTRAINT IN A STATIC SOCIETY

I. POVERTY BREEDS MEN

'Foecunda virorum/Paupertas fugitur.' (LUCANUS)[1]

ONCE again we start with an observation which is probably as old as inequality in society. It is never, by implication, a completely isolated statement. If we say that the poor have many children, we imply that the rich have few. Yet it seems worth while singling out those authors who have stressed the first part of the argument more than its corollary. There is an assumption, in many of the early writers, that there is some sort of standard fertility, from which there are deviations. It makes some difference then where the deviation lies: one may assume that the rich have the normal number of children (because they are reasonable) and the poor have too many, because they do not care. That is implied in Malthus's first *Essay*, when he speaks of the preventive check operating in England amongst the prudent classes. They have obviously arrived at some happy medium which enables them to reproduce themselves without having to sink into penury. The poor, encouraged by a bad poor law, have too many.

The other attitude is the one which assumes that the poor, having no artificial restraints like a taste for luxury, give full vent to their powers of reproduction, and only the rich, selfishly fearing consequences, artificially reduce the size of their families. These two attitudes are to some extent bound up with the period in which they originate. If over-population is feared, the poor are blamed. If depopulation is the spectre, the moralist censures the rich. In between are those authors who are less interested in preaching one fear or another, but who try to work out the laws of population. Finally, the two attitudes are merged in more recent writers until they are merely two manifestations of the same general phenomenon—the restraining influence of the standard of living.

Perhaps Sadler was right when he claimed that the best evidence for the ancient belief in the fertility of the poor is etymological—the word

[1] M. Annaeus Lucanus, *De bello civili*, i. 165–6.

proletarius and its widespread use in many languages. The proletarian was one who served the state, not by his non-existent wealth, but by his numerous offspring (*proles*). Thus poverty and fertility are indissolubly linked: '... qui aut non plus mille quingentos aeris aut omnino nihil in suum censum praeter caput attulissent, proletarios nominavit, ut ex iis quasi proles, id est quasi progenies civitatis, exspectari videretur'.[1] A number of authors have clearly formed the view that the poor continued to be fertile whilst the rich failed to reproduce themselves. This, for instance, is one interpretation of the laws of Augustus: that they were a sort of eugenic measure, an attempt to promote births amongst the more refined sections of the population, perhaps to prevent their being drowned in the general flood of children of the poor.[2] Similarly, a passage written by Dionysius of Halicarnassus, implying a scarcity of marriage amongst labourers, is interpreted by some as referring only to rural, not urban, labourers.[3] Again, a number of classical authors and scholars refer to the prolific habits of slaves and freedmen, who had to provide a compensating increase for the decline of the ranks of citizens. Others believed that slave populations were sterile, and that owners discouraged breeding from them.[4] Amongst those who thought that slaves were barren was David Hume, in his essay *Of the Populousness of Ancient Nations*, published in 1752. This

[1] Cicero, *De re publica*, ii. 22. 40. The sum named (perhaps £4) compared with the senatorial or equestrian assessment of several thousand pounds, clearly defines the completely property-less section of the population.

[2] See L. Friedländer, *Roman Life and Manners under the Early Empire* (L. A. Magnus *et al.*, trans., London, 1908–13, 4 vols.), iv, (note) 20. The simple view that the poor did not need encouraging, but the rich did, was expressed by R. v. Pöhlmann, *Die Übervölkerung der antiken Großstädte im Zusammenhange mit der Gesammtentwicklung städtischer Civilisation dargestellt* (Leipzig, 1884), p. 48, a work I have not consulted.

[3] Dionysius of Halicarnassus, *Roman Antiquities*, bk. ix, 51. The interpretation is Pöhlmann's and it is quoted in Friedländer, ibid. For the quarrels between different learned authorities (mostly German) on the significance of these assertions, see *Jahrbücher für Nationalökonomik und Statistik* (1897), iii. Folge, xiii. Band, 161 ff.: O. Seeck, 'Die Statistik in der alten Geschichte', and Julius Beloch's rejoinder, 'Zur Bevölkerungsgeschichte des Altertums', ibid. 321 ff. They accuse each other of fanciful interpretations, and then proceed to do likewise. But Beloch was more cautious, and competent as an economist, than many of the others, and one may sympathize with his strictures, e.g. on the famous U. v. Wilamowitz-Möllendorff, of whom he said 'Wenn selbst ein Mann wie Wilamowitz "es für illusorisch hält, mit statistischen Wahrscheinlichkeitsrechnungen zu operieren" (Arist. v. Athen, ii. 707), und daraufhin über die Bevölkerung von Athen ins Blaue hinein einen Exkurs schreibt, was ist dann von anderen zu erwarten?' (ibid., p. 321).

[4] Cf. M. I. Rostovtzeff, *The Social and Economic History of the Hellenistic World* (Oxford, 1941, 3 vols.), ii. 1464, and Sir W. W. Tarn, *Hellenistic Civilisation* (London, 1927), pp. 92 ff.

work moved Wallace to publish an 'Appendix, containing additional observations', to his *Dissertation*, and Part 1 of this Appendix is particularly devoted to the proof that slave populations were very fertile. Wallace's reasoning is cumbrous, and the evidence is thinnest just where we would most like to have it—i.e. on whether slaves did in fact multiply mostly by propagation rather than fresh imports, as Hume had claimed.[1]

The discussions about the relative fertility of slaves, proletarians, and rich Roman citizens strike us, in many ways, as being rather remote from the problem as it emerged again in the eighteenth century. Where, in the ancient world, arguments had been chiefly socio-political—concerning the structure of society in relation to the distribution of power—the tendency of the later period was to stress the moral aspects and the economic implications. Was the poverty of the masses their own fault? Were their large numbers the result of moral turpitude? Were the decently restrained families of the well-to-do signs of virtue? Did the economic system need the poverty-stricken masses? Were they truly an asset to the kingdom? Against the background of these questions we read the colourful answers of the English writers of the Georgian age. Thus Thomas Short:

> The most laborious Part of Mankind are also the most fruitful in proportion to their Numbers, and the most voluptuous, idle, effeminate and luxurious are the barrenest . . . hard Labour makes the Poor most fruitful . . . they are less Slaves to the sensual Passion, are more fruitful, their Progeny more vigorous and healthy, have fewer hereditary Diseases. . . .[2]

William Temple, the Trowbridge clothier, stressed both the moral degradation of the poverty-stricken, and the advantages of a Spartan existence:

> The consideration of the cares of a family does not prevent one in a thousand from marrying. When does the fear of hunger extinguish the incitements and allurements of lust? . . . we find that the Hebrews lived under a

[1] R. Wallace, *A Dissertation on the Numbers of Mankind, in Ancient and Modern Times* (Edinburgh, 1809), pp. 171 ff., esp. pp. 205–9. For more recent views on the slavery problem, see O. Seeck, *Geschichte des Untergangs der antiken Welt* (Stuttgart, 1920–2, 6 vols.), i. 351, which refers to evidence of continuous replacement of native population by slaves; and J. E. Wappäus, *Allgemeine Bevölkerungsstatistik* (1859, 2 vols.), i. 157, where it is claimed that the birth-rates of slaves were generally low. For French discussion, see J. J. Spengler, *French Predecessors of Malthus* (Durham, North Carolina, 1942), esp. on Herrenschwand, pp. 291 ff. Malthus agreed with Hume, *An Essay on Population* (Everyman ed., 1914, 2 vols.), i. 150.

[2] T. Short, *New Observations, Natural, Moral, Civil, Political, and Medical on City, Town and Country Bills of Mortality* (London, 1750), pp. 143–5, quoted in R. R. Kuczynski, 'British Demographers' Opinions on Fertility, 1660–1760', *Political Arithmetic* (L. T. Hogben, ed., London, 1938), p. 317.

hard slavery in Egypt, and were rewarded for all their toil with only onions and garlick. And yet those hardships did not destroy their fecundity or prevent marriages, for they grew and multiplied exceedingly. . . .[1]

Both these authors foreshadow the later theories connecting rich food with barrenness.

The improvidence of the poor becomes a fruitful theme with moralizing authors. This may have been partly due to fears of countries being swamped with idle paupers—fears which explain the enthusiastic reception Malthus experienced at the end of the century. Adam Smith would have observed the fertility of the poor Highlanders and the Glasgow tenement-dwellers: 'Poverty, though it no doubt discourages, does not always prevent marriage. It seems even to be favourable to generation.'[2] Dr. Johnson, discussing the rumoured rapid growth of the population of poverty-stricken Russia, thought the explanation was simple: 'A man is poor—he thinks—I cannot be worse, so I'll e'en take Peggy.'[3] We find echoes of this theory in Cantillon. He knew that the Chinese multiplied fast, and that they lived almost naked, on a diet of rice and rice-water. Since they had such low standards, they could well raise a large number of children. Since little subsistence was required, in fact, positive checks through lack of food would be few. Only in years of crop failure would they resort to infanticide. This could mean, perhaps, that we have a prudent nation—but since their prudence is related to infinitesimal wants, they can multiply fast. Here 'poor' has a slightly different connotation. The differential is not between classes of the same nation, but between one nation and another. Nevertheless, the meaning is the same: if your wants are fixed, and easily satisfied, there is no sense in restriction.[4]

Montesquieu granted the application of the general idea only in the case of those without hope:

Les gens qui n'ont absolument rien, comme les mendiants, ont beaucoup

[1] I . . . B . . . (M.D.) [W. Temple], *A Vindication of Commerce and the Arts* . . . (1768; reprinted in *A Select Collection of Scarce and Valuable Tracts on Commerce* (J. McCulloch, ed., London, 1859)), pp. 498–9.

[2] A. Smith, *An Inquiry into the Nature and Causes of the Wealth of Nations* (11th ed., London, 1805; E. Cannan, ed., New York, 1937, 2 vols.), i, bk. i, ch. viii. See also J. Townsend, *Dissertation on the Poor Laws* (1787, reprint London, 1817), quoted in C. E. Stangeland, *Pre-Malthusian Doctrines of Population; a Study in the History of Economic Theory* (New York, 1904), p. 344. 'The procreative powers of the lower orders are astounding.'

[3] J. Boswell, *Life of Johnson* (G. B. Hill, ed., revised ed. by L. F. Powell, Oxford, 1934–50, 6 vols.), ii. 101.

[4] R. Cantillon, *Essai sur la nature du commerce en général* (H. Higgs, trans. and ed., London, 1931), pp. 39, 67.

d'enfants. C'est qu'ils sont dans le cas des peuples naissants: il n'en coûte rien au père pour donner son art à ses enfants, qui même sont, en naissant, des instruments de cet art.[1]

He contrasted this with the position of peasants under a bad government, who have few children. He explicitly rejected the theory that poverty in general leads to large families. This is a myth, he said, like the one which supposes that men work the harder the more you tax them. One must interpret these peasants then as beings who have something to lose, a standard of living to maintain, or an inheritance to preserve, in contrast with those who have nothing to lose at all. Once again, 'poverty' is qualified by reference to customs and prospects rather than absolute income.

The post-Malthusian age subjected the habits of the poor to much more searching light than the previous one. If Marie Antoinette's injunction to the poor to eat cake if they had no bread is an extreme and legendary example of ignorance of conditions amongst the lower orders, we cannot help feeling that the later approach went far nearer the root of the matter. One early distinction was that between fertility of families and size of surviving families. Where, especially in urban areas, infant mortality rates were high (and in some districts, notably western Germany, it climbed to 50 per cent. of all new-born babies), it might not be apparent, without precise investigation, that the poor were liable to have more children than the rich. Moreover, it became necessary to distinguish more clearly between those who had many children simply because they were improvident, and those who were in any case condemned to a standard of living where a child more or less could not affect their comfort.

The early nineteenth century saw not only more precise investigations of working-class habits (starting with Sir Frederic Eden's great work, *The State of the Poor*), but it also saw the beginning of the formation of different political schools of social analysis. In the previous century we do not notice much shading of opinion in the observations of the lower orders. Most writers seemed undecided in their minds whether the poor were in that state by their own fault, or by divine ordering, or both. In neither case did any responsibility descend on their betters to alter their state. With the emergence of practical socialist thought from the utopian writings of the revolutionary period, it was natural that such bad habits as the working classes

[1] Montesquieu, C.-L. de Secondat, Baron de la Brède et de, *De l'Esprit des Lois* (*Œuvres complètes de Montesquieu*, E. Laboulaye, ed., tome 5, Paris, 1877), p. 72.

were observed to have, should be blamed on the system under which they lived. Improvidence came to be regarded as the result of an order of society in which all hope was taken from the workers. Some even went so far as to deny that it existed at all, and to claim that family size varied directly, not inversely, with comfort. This was to be a mainstay of socialist thinking.

In fact, when the liberal sociologists evolved a comforting *Wohlstandstheorie*, or prosperity theory of population increase, their socialist colleagues countered with an *Armutstheorie*, or poverty theory. Of these the most important was Ferdinand Lassalles's Iron Law of Wages. The prosperity theory established once again that the normal fertility was that experienced by the poor, and that the deviation occurred as the level of welfare increased. The poverty theory, by contrast, seems to assume that the normal patterns of fertility occur amongst the better-off, the bourgeois and the capitalists. It is only amongst the poor that any small changes in subsistence are, following Malthus, taken out in family increases. Hence the Law of Wages: the poor can never improve their lot in the long run. Every time a relative shortage of labour leads to slightly higher money wages, an increase in labour supply follows, with consequent renewed reductions of wages to the old subsistence level. This is, of course, a variant on an important Marxian theme, which will once again occupy us in the last chapter.

In England the natural starting-point for the theory that poverty was a cause of fertility, under the new economic conditions, was provided by the Speenhamland system, whereby relief was given to paupers on a scale commensurate with their family responsibility. The supposed degrading results form the theme of every Malthusian writer, and the belief that the system was responsible for a rise in the birth-rate survived to modern times. What can hardly be disputed is the fact that the subsistence provided would have saved the life of many a new-born child. It may be argued that this method ensured in fact a form of wealth, not poverty—but essentially any increase in (voluntary) fertility, caused, principally, by earlier marriages, would be due to the same sort of improvidence as that of Montesquieu's beggars, or the Irish potato-eating peasant.

Much more important was the new realization that the way to combat the evil of population was to raise the standard of living of the poor to check the headlong rush. The poor have nothing to lose—that was the operative phrase: give them something, and they will be careful. This was the thought which ran through the pages of the main anti-Malthusian school of socialists. While it is true that most of the Marxists subscribed to the other theory (that the amount of available subsistence regulates the numbers directly—i.e. a Malthusian proposition), others were in favour of the inverse relationship between social and economic advancement and the fertility of the working classes. This latter view was represented by such writers as August Bebel, who concentrated his attention on the low status of the women under the existing system.[1]

The general sentiment in England is perhaps best expressed in an anonymous essay, *On the Means of Retaining the Population*, published in 1820:

> Is it not evident... that misery, far from preventing, is the principal cause by which the pressure of the population against the means of subsistence is produced?... I am most fully persuaded, that it is by promoting the comfort, the happiness and the virtue of the community at large, instead of having a large portion of our fellow-creatures in a state of misery and vice, that we can ever hope to obviate the evil said to arise from the principle of population.[2]

The hopelessness of the poor is stressed—the very fact that they have no chance of rising. Godwin's first answer to Malthus claimed that the poor were too desperately oppressed under the existing order ever to cultivate prudence,[3] Malthus, in the 1803 edition of the *Essay*, accepted this at least theoretically by oblique references to the existence of such classes of people even in civilized countries[4]—but in general, of course, he persisted in the notion that efforts from outside would never succeed; the poor would have to cultivate the habit of moral restraint themselves, or perish.

John Stuart Mill, however, was as certain as Godwin that prudence cannot operate without hope:

> But the preventive remedy seldom, I believe, consists in the unaided operation of prudential motives on a class wholly or mainly composed of labourers for hire, and looking forward to no other lot. In England, for example, I much doubt if the generality of agricultural labourers practise any prudential restraint whatever.[5]

By the middle of the century, Ireland provided the best evidence that

[1] A. Bebel, *Die Frau und der Sozialismus* (Stuttgart, 1911), p. 503.

[2] *The Pamphleteer* (London, 1813–28, 29 vols.) (1820), xvi. 414–15. Author unknown.

[3] W. Godwin, *Thoughts Occasioned by the Perusal of Dr. Parr's Spital Sermon Preached ... 1800* (6th ed., London, 1801), p. 73.

[4] Malthus, *Essay* (1803 ed.), p. 475.

[5] J. S. Mill, *Principles of Political Economy* (6th ed., London, 1902), bk. ii, ch. xi, sect. 3, p. 213.

where there was no hope, there was no fear.[1] Thomas Doubleday of Newcastle, the radical economist, who thought that fertility stood in inverse relation to the quantity and quality of food consumed, attributed this phenomenon to the poor Irish diet, but the end result was the same: the poorer the people are, the more children they will have.[2]

Irish observers themselves were not slow to point out the same connexion between poverty and fertility. James Doyle, the Catholic bishop of Kildare and Leitrim, echoed Dr. Johnson:

> The poverty of the people contributes to this result [their fast increase] also; for the poor people are less solicitous about an establishment in the world than those who already have a competency. They say of marriage, as of other changes in their life, that it 'cannot make them worse', but that it may give them a helpmate in distress, or at least a companion in suffering.[3]

Only action to remove poverty would end the reckless marriages, facilitated by enforced familiarity in overcrowded conditions. Similar evidence was given in the Reports of the Commissioners who inquired into the conditions of the Irish poor. A Leitrim priest testified that those who were a little above poverty level were slower to marry. 'The poor man cannot be a chooser.'[4] In fact we know that prudence did not come to Ireland until the worst was over, but even after 1850 the differential fertility of labourers was still worthy of remark.[5]

All the evidence of the time pointed to the conclusion that Malthus's positive checks were not very effective amongst the poor (quite apart from the absence of restraint), and they were actually increasing their numbers more rapidly than the wealthy. A differential increase was added to differential restraint (to use Field's distinction).

Edwin Chadwick, the most famous of the nineteenth-century sanitary reformers, who probably knew more about the life of the poor in detail than any other man of his age, was quite sure about the matter:

> If, in the most crowded districts, the inference is found to be erroneous,

[1] Sir G. Rickards, *Population and Capital: Being a Course of Lectures Delivered before the University of Oxford in 1853–54* (London, 1854), p. 249.

[2] T. Doubleday, *The True Law of Population Shewn To Be Connected with the Food of the People* (London, 1841; 3rd ed., 1853), pp. 25–26.

[3] J. K. L. (i.e. James Doyle, Bishop of Kildare and Leitrim), *Letters on the State of Ireland, Addressed by J. K. L. to a Friend in England* (Dublin, 1825), p. 110. I owe this and most of the other Irish references to Dr. Kenneth Connell of Belfast.

[4] *Reports of Commissioners for Inquiring into the Condition of the Poorer Classes in Ireland* (1836, xxx–xxxiv, Appendix F (xxxiii)), p. 40, see also p. 49.

[5] R. Lynd, *Home Life in Ireland* (3rd ed., London, 1910), p. 4, and M. MacDonagh, *Irish Life and Character* (London, 1905), p. 207.

that the extent of sickness and mortality is indicative of the pressure of population on the means of subsistence, so is the inference that the ravages act to the extent supposed, as a positive check to the increase of the numbers of the population. In such districts the fact is observable, that where the mortality is the highest, the number of births are more than sufficient to replace the deaths, however numerous they may be.[1]

The natural conclusion is that not only did the wretches survive, but they even lived to push their way upwards into the higher ranks of society. This provides something of a contrast to the assumption with which we started—that it was principally the hopelessly poor who were so fertile. We may reconcile the views of the authors who share basically the same conviction about the effect of poverty on population by saying that it would be agreed that for the vast majority of the labouring classes in England there were no prospects of a rise. But a lucky few would indeed supply the gaps left in the ranks of the better-off who failed to reproduce themselves, and these social climbers in turn would then become less fertile. 'The reproductive part of the people are principally the lower orders who . . . must, therefore, do the same now in order to make up for the deficiencies left by the non-reproductive part of the people.'[2]

This was the observation of John Weyland (1774–1854), a lawyer and member of the last unreformed parliament, whose *Principles of Production and Population* was one of the few treatises to draw a reply in one of Malthus's later editions. While he accepted the existence of many of the Malthusian checks, he had a much more elaborate model of the progress of society in which both disasters and moral evolution had their place. Like Marx after him, he held that there was not one law of population, but different rules applicable according to methods of production and government.

There were others who saw that conditions might change. William Ferguson Lloyd (1794–1852), a Fellow of the Royal Society, who

[1] *Report from the Poor Law Commissioners on an Inquiry into the Sanitary Condition of the Labouring Population of Great Britain* (E. Chadwick, secretary), London, 1842, p. 177.

[2] J. Weyland, jnr., *The Principles of Population and Production* . . . (London, 1816), p. 410. Similar views were expressed by S. Gray, *The Happiness of States: or an Inquiry Concerning Population* . . . (2nd ed., London, 1819), p. 451; W. Thompson, *An Inquiry into the Principles of the Distribution of Wealth Most Conducive to Human Happiness: Applied to the Newly Proposed System of Voluntary Equality of Wealth* (London, 1824), pp. 537, 544; A. Alison, *The Principles of Population* . . . (Edinburgh, 1840, 2 vols.), i. 112. It is noteworthy that socialists like Thompson stressed the possibility of the poorer classes rising, even under a capitalist system. This was left out in later socialist population theories.

successively lectured on Greek, mathematics, and political economy at Oxford (occupying the Drummond chair in the latter subject from 1832 to 1837), wrote a number of treatises on the Poor Laws and on the checks to population. He particularly observed the position of the English labourer in the early thirties, and perceived clearly what removed the incentive to prudence: the outlook for employment and prices was too uncertain. He had some notions of the trade cycle, and he saw that the employment of women and children weakened the responsibility of the male wage-earner. His position was often without hopes or prospects. Yet children might be an asset. Sometimes there was a demand for child labour, or juvenile labour, when adults were unemployed. This was the position when prices were low or falling. At times of rising prices and at the height of the boom the demand for hands might be so great that the children might be employed in addition to their parents. Prudence was still a virtue, but a man had to consider the matter on balance.[1] Obviously here again we have poverty acting as a stimulus to fertility under certain circumstances. Lloyd's view of the operation of the demand for labour on population movements is similar to that of many of the classical and neo-classical economists, and rather in contrast to the sociological view. The English-speaking world of Malthus's time referred to the working classes almost invariably as 'the poor', and in this period we may well interpret theories incorporating the word 'poor', not in a class sense, but as describing the working of an economic system.

We may end our account of English authors with a fine counterblast to Malthus by the younger Samuel Laing, one of those enthusiastically radical tories who wished to redistribute property and incomes as a means of checking the growth of imprudence and population:

> . . . it is distinctly true, that duty and expediency, the means of raising the conditions of the labouring classes, and the means of rightly proportioning their numbers to the supply of food, go hand in hand, and that in applying ourselves zealously to the task imposed upon us by religion and humanity, of relieving immediate distress, and promoting the welfare and improvement of the poorer classes, we are at the same time adopting the only effectual means of limiting the morbid and unhealthy increase of a destitute population.[2]

Turning to writers in French, we find the differential fertility

[1] W. F. Lloyd, *Two Lectures on the Checks to Population, Delivered before the University of Oxford in Michaelmas Term, 1832* (Oxford, 1833), pp. 47, 68.

[2] S. Laing (the younger), *National Distress: Its Causes and Remedies* (London, 1844), p. 70.

problem most clearly recognized by the socialists, who relate their explanation to their general philosophy. Already Sismondi saw the demoralization of the working man as one of the crimes of society:

> The more the poor man is robbed of his property, the more he is in danger of being mistaken as to his income, and contributing to the growth of the population in a measure which bears no relation to his position in life . . . the unfortunate factory worker who earns no more than eight sous a day, and often suffers from hunger, will not voluntarily withhold from marriage: we have accustomed him to look no further than Saturday, when the week's pay is given out; we have so blunted his feelings of sympathy and morality and let him suffer present pain, that the future pain which may be felt by his wife and family causes him little worry . . . his family will become more numerous, the more they are a burden on society, and the nation will groan under the weight of a population which stands in no relationship to the necessities of life.[1]

For Sismondi, the remedy lay in a new system of peasant proprietorship, to restore those checks to over-population which the capitalist system had destroyed.[2] There are allusions to similar ideas in the writings of Louis Blanc, who believed that free competition had created the misery which made the worker reckless; Fourier and Proudhon, all of whom envisage some form of higher existence for the lowest classes in a socialist society, which will produce a measure of restraint.[3]

More accurate than the work of these political philosophers is the statistician Adolphe Quételet's *Treatise on Man*, which we shall have to discuss again later in another context. Basing his assertions on a number of contemporary observations, he is sure that lack of hope and foresight amongst poor populations are a sure way of increasing populations.[4]

In Germany the fertility of the hopelessly poor was described by the Suabian administrator Robert v. Mohl, but since he quoted Thornton

[1] J. C. L. S. de Sismondi, *Les Nouveaux Principes d'économie politique ou de la richesse dans ses rapports avec la population* (2nd ed., Paris, 1827), ii, pp. 263–7 (C. M. Lovatt, trans.).

[2] Note that W. T. Thornton, the chief English advocate of peasant proprietorship as a remedy to over-population, is also one of those who particularly stress the impotence of the prudential check amongst the very poor. W. T. Thornton, *Over-population and Its Remedy; Or, an Inquiry into the Extent and Causes of Distress Prevailing Among the Labouring Classes of the British Islands, and into the Means of Remedying It* (London, 1846), p. 121.

[3] For accounts of these writers, see J. J. Spengler, 'French Population Theory Since 1800', *Journal of Political Economy* (1936), xliv. 749 ff., and L. Elster, in 'Bevölkerungswesen', *Handwörterbuch der Staatswissenschaften* (4th ed., Jena, 1924), ii. 775.

[4] L. A. J. Quételet, *Sur l'homme et le développement de ses facultés, ou Essai de physique sociale* (Brussels, 1836), pp. 114 ff.

as his authority, just as he quoted Alison for the effect of social mobility, we may well conclude that preindustrial Germany did not easily lend itself to such observations.[1]

With the spread of statistical methods in England, and the growth of an urban proletariat in other countries, more scientific studies became available, which stressed the general fertility differential of income groups, but none of these were guilty of the extreme simplifications of the earlier writers. They generally pointed out that other factors than absolute income (or degree of social mobility) determined the number of births.[2]

We must reserve the considerations of these complex theories for a later stage, when we have examined some more of their component parts. Hitherto we have drawn attention mainly to the state of the very poor. The idea that the best remedy for their fertility is the possession of wealth or income above the absolute minimum, provides the transition to the general argument that the chief check to fertility lies in the desire to preserve one's standard of living.

2. WHAT WE HAVE, WE HOLD

In a simple society consisting of feudal overlords and serfs, rich and poor, exploiters and exploited, there is no room for observations on the habits of families on the margin of social classes. The upper strata's status is not dependent on their conduct: the lower strata remain where they are, irrespective of their habits. But such a society we meet but rarely. In those nations we have here considered, there have always been families on the brink of poverty, or of affluence. The number of such families naturally increases when particularly violent economic changes occur, as they did in England in the eighteenth century. The emergence of an urban middle class, in fact, is the phenomenon which gave rise to the most acute observations on this score.

Once again, we may trace an integral part of the general theory which we are examining to an observation so commonplace that we

[1] R. v. Mohl, *Die Polizeiwissenschaft nach den Grundsätzen des Rechtsstaates* (Tübingen, 1866, 3 vols.), i. 114.

[2] A number of these are cited in United Nations, *The Determinants and Consequences of Population Trends* (New York, 1953), pp. 86–87. See also J. Goldstein, *Bevölkerungsprobleme und Berufsgliederung in Frankreich* (Berlin, 1900), where more than 300 titles are cited. He analysed France by the wealth of the *départements*. For a late nineteenth-century view of the connexion between misery and a high birth-rate, see M. Schippel, *Das moderne Elend und die moderne Übervölkerung* (Leipzig, 1883), quoted in Goldstein, ibid., p. 48.

may almost regard it as folk-lore. A few general conditions for the existence of this line of reasoning must be stated first. Inequalities of wealth and income rather than status are prerequisites. Property must be private, inheritable, and alienable. Class barriers must not be rigid in a downward direction—the fear of falling cannot exist where national sinecures or pensions are the prerogative of any particular section of the population.

Unless the raising of a child or children is a positive charge on income, the fear will not operate. This we have already noted in connexion with the imprudence of the very poor. It now assumes a new significance. To take the extreme ends of the scale: to a couple living in two furnished rooms, both of them working, the appearance of a child may mean a reduction of income by one-half, a loss of all savings or capital in acquiring new accommodation, and a violent fall in their standard of living. To a family in a primitive society, living in a one-roomed hut, on the proceeds of hunting and fishing expeditions, an extra child may mean more squalor in the hut, and perhaps fewer days of idleness for the father, but no positive charge on income results. The more elastic the type of accommodation usual in the class and society under review, the less important this factor becomes. (Equally so, whether the house is a baronial mansion or a cave.) The greater the care usually bestowed upon the upbringing of the children, the more important it will be. Cheap indoor servants or slaves, absence of organized schooling outside the house, and absence of positive costs of launching children into marriage or career—all these mean that the check will not operate. But given the institution of a boarding-school, the habit of giving dowries, or the purchase of commissions for younger sons, the operation of the check will be very forceful indeed.

In tracing the emergence of awareness of this factor, we shall at first omit the consideration of the children's welfare itself, and begin with the purely selfish point of view, that the expense involved, however caused, will lead to a diminution of one's own standard of living, and hence a desire to limit or prevent births.

The first period in which we meet the charge that men restrict their fertility because of their fear of falling into a lower social class is that epoch of Greek history which drew the complaints of the historians and philosophers about the decaying manners of the times. Polybius, a writer suspect in the role of unbiased observer, described abortion and exposure as the usual means of limiting one's family, though this is challenged by modern authors. Rostovtzeff, discussing the whole problem, showed that the practice had been alleged in earlier periods by such authors as Poseidippus and Menander. But it had not, then, been the prerogative of the wealthy. Even the proletariat had resorted to this means of reducing their burdens.[1]

Nevertheless, Polybius is specific on the fact that in his day the middle and upper classes were afraid of losing their status. Admittedly, he alleged that the reason was that they were more frightened for their children's future than their own, and his explanation may therefore justly be cited amongst those authors who thought this concern one of the chief checks to fertility, but the whole tenor of his attack suggests that he is concerned with selfishness, with the *amour propre* of an impious generation. In any case, one can hardly say that to expose one's children in a mountain fastness is a way of demonstrating one's solicitude for them.[2]

Documentary evidence of the survival of this theory of infertility arising from the fear of falling is, as in other cases, hard to procure until the eighteenth century. But it is unlikely to have been absent from people's minds. G. G. Coulton, in his work on *The Medieval Village*, quoted a fourteenth-century Franciscan friar as indicting the peasantry because, amongst other things, '. . . they often abstain from knowing their own wives lest children should be born, fearing that they could not bring up so many, under pretext of poverty'.[3] But on the whole, though medieval moralists have much to say on the sins of the flesh, the pride and extravagance of the fashionable society of courts and castles, the effect of this system on the fertility of the knights and ladies does not seem to come into the picture at all. One may surmise that the arrival or lack of children made little difference to the pleasures of that society. One reads of the results of indiscreet amours, the lack of chastity amongst the women. It does not seem to have been suggested that anyone refrained from marriage for fear of the consequences. Much of the worst extravagance was found in episcopal courts and monastic establishments. There, by definition, the problem as such did not arise.

The post-medieval period is hardly more rewarding. True, the censure on loose and rich living is no less pronounced in Puritan America or England; but only when the numbers of the King's subjects

[1] Rostovtzeff, op. cit. ii. 63.

[2] Ibid. ii. 626. He does not accept Polybius's charge of selfishness—he prefers to call it an instinct of self-preservation under very difficult economic circumstances.

[3] G. G. Coulton, *The Medieval Village* (Cambridge, 1925), p. 244, quoted in S. H. Coontz, *Population Theories and the Economic Interpretation* (London, 1957), p. 149.

form an object of deliberate national policy do we begin to hear of the disastrous consequences of a high standard of living on fertility. Some of these views have already been discussed with reference to urban conditions, and luxury. The change in emphasis in the writers of the eighteenth century is pronounced. One must ascribe this to the fact that the society described by Wallace or Archdeacon Paley was much more clearly stratified.

At the same time, the way down, the slide into the next lower social class, was much more easily accomplished. Where a comparatively small accretion of wealth and a few modish mannerisms could soon gain an *entrée* into polite society, the temporary loss of the means of competitive existence would soon ensure the loss of the coveted position. The Puritan squire could lose most of his wealth, and keep his position in his society so long as he kept his character. But in the world of Molière already, and much more strongly in that of Sheridan and Voltaire, in that whirl of impostors, and half-acknowledged bastards of noble stock, when a measure of vulgarity might even procure admission into the royal circles of more than one country, the fear of falling from one's perch becomes an overwhelming preoccupation.

The writers of the age were themselves deeply steeped in classical literature, and were able to draw on the classical example to make their point. Amongst these was Robert Wallace, Hume's adversary and pessimistic critic of his age, who regretted the lack of laws, such as those in force in Rome, which favoured marriage and punished bachelors.

> In modern times . . . the laugh is often against matrimony; married persons have no privileges; and a prevailing luxury often makes it be thought imprudent to marry at the most proper season of life: men must first purchase such an estate, and be able to live in such a manner, as they cannot often afford to do till they are grown old.[1]

We have already stated that the 'luxuries' of eighteenth-century writers may not amount to much. Wallace himself spoke of manufactures producing:

> . . . trifles [which] will become more necessary for the bulk of the people. . . . Hence living even in the most simple manner will become more expensive; consequently, mankind be less able to support families, and be less encouraged to marry.[2]

The first statement was general, the second applied particularly to the lower orders. His observation on the rich was:

> Many, . . . particularly the younger sons of the richer families, either

[1] Wallace, op. cit., p. 96.

[2] Ibid., p. 24.

imagine themselves not to be, or in reality are not, able to maintain families suitably to their birth; or, though able during their own life, yet cannot leave a sufficient provision for their families after their death; and thus are discouraged from marrying.[1]

In France, Cantillon observed the same point. He extended the principle of the Chinese peasants which we quoted earlier, to the small proprietors of his own country. Men would marry, he thought, once they were in a position to keep their families in the same style as they kept themselves. That decision would be based on a given available quantity of land. But let him set his sights higher, and he will not marry until he can assure the new standard not only for himself, but for his children also.[2]

The same held true in towns:

> When Labourers and Mechanicks do not marry it is because they wait till they save something to enable them to set up a household or to find some young woman who brings a little capital for the purpose, since they see every day others like them who for lack of such precaution start housekeeping and fall into the most frightful poverty, being obliged to deprive themselves of their own food in order to nourish their Children.... Therefore they do not all marry or marry so late that of six Women, or at least four, who should produce a child every year there is actually only one in six who becomes a Mother.[3]

Many other French authors of the time are full of instances of wealthy people dispensing with marriage, or avoiding children, whether on account of their own expenditure in extravagant living, or because of the cost of bringing up children. The effect is the same: marriages are barren because in this way the greatest possible sum is available for spending on oneself.[4]

[1] Ibid., p. 151.

[2] Cantillon, op. cit., p. 77. A number of modern authors, e.g. A. Landry, 'Trois Théories de la population', *La Révolution démographique* (Paris, 1934), have elevated the Cantillon theory to the dignity of a separate category. Landry speaks of the original pre-Malthusian pure subsistence theory, as represented by Townsend and Wallace, which was followed by the more advanced theory, that population is governed by the widespread notion of a proper standard of living.

[3] Cantillon, ibid., pp. 79–81.

[4] See Spengler, *French Predecessors...*, esp. pp. 82–94, on Plumard de Danguel, Goyon de la Plombaine, and the Abbé Jaubert. Plombaine is interesting because he proposed to stop the rot in noble and some bourgeois families by a system of life pensions to be paid to male children of those who had been in the king's service—300 livres a year in some cases. An interesting anticipation of family allowances. See the remarks at the head of this section: the fear of falling cannot operate where sinecures or pensions automatically keep classes intact.

At the end of the century Archdeacon Paley, both a precursor and later a follower of Malthus, stated quite clearly what had become the rules of conduct in his day. Had he only thought more deeply about what was implied in the rules he might have hesitated to embrace the Malthus doctrine. If he did so, it was probably because he agreed with the *Essay on Population* on one central point—that the more subsistence is available, the more people will marry and consequently produce offspring. But he himself had considerably modified this picture as the full statement of his proposition on population shows:

> Wherever the commerce between the sexes is regulated by marriage, and a provision for that mode of subsistence, to which each class of the community is accustomed, can be procured with ease and certainty, there the number of people will increase; and the rapidity, as well as the extent of the increase, will be proportioned to the degree in which these causes exist.[1]

He amplified this notion of a customary standard by saying it was not enough that man's *natural* wants should be supplied—he must have those things which 'in the present relaxed state of morals and discipline' make sure that they stay where they are, do not

> degrade their condition, reduce their mode of living, deprive them of the accommodations to which they have been accustomed, or even of those ornaments or appendages of rank and station, which they have been taught to regard as belonging to their birth, or class, or profession, or place in society. The same consideration, namely, a view to their accustomed mode of life, which is so apparent in the superior orders of the people, has no less influence upon those ranks which compose the mass of the community. The kind and quality of food and liquor, the species of habitation, furniture and clothing, to which the common people of each country are habituated, must be attainable with ease and certainty before marriages will be sufficiently early and general, to carry the progress of population to its just extent. It is in vain to allege, that a more simple diet, ruder habitations, or coarser apparel, would be sufficient for the purpose of life and health, or even of physical ease and pleasure. Men will not marry with this encouragement. For instance, when the common people of a country are accustomed to eat a large proportion of animal food, to drink wine, spirits, or beer, to wear shoes and stockings, to dwell in stone houses, they will not marry to live in clay cottages, upon roots and milk, with no other clothing than skins, or what is necessary to defend the trunk of the body from the effects of cold. . . .[2]

He then goes on to say how these standards are created, and how the needs are satisfied. Some of his ideas on these subjects will occupy us

[1] W. Paley, *The Principles of Moral and Political Philosophy* (9th ed., London, 1793, 2 vols.), ii. 350.

[2] Ibid., pp. 352–3.

later. But we note the essential message of the passage just quoted: that in fact everyone has a measure of prudence, except the people who wear skins! From that it would have been only one step to the assertion that, provided everyone has something which they would be afraid to lose, there is no fear even of the population developing 'to its just extent'. He did not think it necessary to make this point in 1785, since in fact few people were worried about over-expansion—but he should have made it again after 1798!

Malthus himself cannot in fact have been totally unaware of what went on in his country, as even the first edition shows. Like Paley, he seems to have lacked the courage to follow through the implications of his own observations. For, after all, if he believed what he wrote to be true, he should have heartily agreed with those who wanted to banish the spectre he had raised by improving everyone's income, not cutting off relief:

> . . . a foresight of the difficulties attending the rearing of a family acts as a preventive check; . . . England, as one of the most flourishing states of Europe, may be fairly taken for an example, and the observations made, will apply with but little variation to any other country where the population increases slowly.
>
> The preventive check appears to operate in some degree through all the ranks of society in England. There are some men, even in the highest rank, who are prevented from marrying by the idea of the expences that they must retrench, and the fancied pleasures that they must deprive themselves of, on the supposition of having a family. These considerations are certainly trivial; but a preventive foresight of this kind has objects of much greater weight for its contemplation as we go lower.[1]

That is to say, the fear of going without decencies or even necessities, to use Senior's phrase, is much stronger than that of going without luxuries. Malthus enlarged the point in the following paragraphs. A gentleman with only just sufficient means would have to mix with moderate farmers and tradespeople if he married. How awkward for a wife brought up with similar pretensions!

> Two or three steps of descent in society, particularly at this round of the ladder, where education ends, and ignorance begins, will not be considered by the generality of people, as a fancied and chimerical, but a real and essential evil.[2]

It may, of course, be objected that Malthus did not attach much total

[1] Malthus, op. cit. (1st ed., 1798), ch. iv, pp. 62–64.
[2] Ibid., p. 65.

significance to the operation of this check, since there would always be large sections of the community (if not the great majority), who were not subject to such influences, and that to redistribute incomes so as to give these people some standard worth preserving, would have been an impossible task. For in the short run, it is claimed, all extra subsistence provided at once defeats its aims as it is swallowed up by a larger family. But there is evidence that Malthus himself saw this fear of degradation operating at very low income levels, and if what he wrote was based on observation, one would say that in his day a very slight raising of the wages (as opposed to the relief) given to the poorest workers would have put them on an equal footing with his decent labourer.

After showing how the fear of descent affected tradesmen and farmers, who might find it difficult to get a holding, he went on to apply the sentiment to this labourer, not a poor man in Malthus's estimation, since he earns eighteenpence a day and has some degree of comfort. Malthus pointed out that should this man have a large family, and any ill luck whatever, he would see his children starve, or 'being obliged to the parish for their support'.[1] Now the year 1798, when the first *Essay* was written, was one of very rapidly rising food prices. In fact, according to Silberling's index, the rise in the annual index of prices was greatest between 1798 and 1799—from 121 in the former year to 143 in the latter, taking 1790 as 100.[2] The Speenhamland system was just coming into fairly general operation, but it had by no means become so universal and demoralizing as it was when Malthus castigated it in his later editions. Malthus's recognition of a prudential check, therefore, was based on the grim fact that a man with nine shillings a week, even in regular work, needed no worse luck than a continuation in the disastrous price rises of the last decade to make him starve. Had the labourers of England in fact acted universally on Malthus's advice, without the general application of the Speenhamland system, the next generation would not have been born until after 1813.

Malthus never changed the paragraphs just quoted, except to amend his 'eighteenpence' by adding the alternative 'two shillings'.[3] But even twelve shillings a week was really too little to marry on, whether at the

[1] Malthus, op. cit., p. 67.

[2] N. J. Silberling, 'British Prices and Business Cycles, 1779–1850', *Review of Economic Statistics* (1923), quoted in Sir J. H. Clapham, *An Economic History of Modern Britain* (Cambridge, 1926–38, 3 vols.), i. 602.

[3] This was added in the second edition and survived in the final text (Everyman ed., 1914), ii. 38.

time of the second edition in 1803 or the fifth in 1817.[1] The conclusion therefore is obvious. The higher ranks of society would be prevented from marrying prematurely by the fear of becoming petty bourgeois. The lower middle classes would equally fear to sink to the status of labourers, and the labourers themselves would try to avoid the stigma of pauperism. It was a neat system—rigid, and static, incapable of progressing economically or of abolishing injustices. Yet this system was the pattern for thought on the subject of prudence for a century ahead. Malthus's opponents are distinguished by the fact that they at least add the hope of rising to the fear of falling—the hope that Malthus contemptuously dismissed as being 'perfectly feeble, compared with the tendency of the population to increase'.[2] Godwin's hope rested on that rise:

> . . . one of the great operative checks upon an increasing population arises from virtue, prudence or pride. . . . The more men are raised above poverty and a life of expedients, the more decency will prevail in their conduct, and sobriety in their sentiments.[3]

The hope of rising itself as a check will form the subject of another section. Meanwhile we may note a few others who were also concerned with the fear of falling in the world. J. R. McCulloch (1789–1864) was one of the most versatile of classical economists, Richard Jones's immediate predecessor in the London chair, and prolific author and editor in the field of statistics, applied economics, and history of doctrine. In his earlier works he manifested an excessive regard for the Malthusian power of population to outrun subsistence, but later, no doubt influenced by Senior and other critics, he inserted a paragraph in the third edition of his *Principles of Political Economy*, stressing the importance of the 'circumstances' in which the population was placed, that is to say, he assumed a scale of standards which dictated the attitude to children.[4] This acknowledgement, published in 1843, eighteen years after the first edition, is perhaps symptomatic of a general change of

[1] He was sufficiently frightened by the spectre he himself had raised, that he would have been quite happy not to have labourers marry at all, until the scarcity of the human commodity had raised wages sufficiently, and caused prices to fall, so that the custom of marriage might be resumed. At a later stage in his work he formulated his wage-fund theories —but these were mostly devoted to the uselessness of trying to raise money wage-rates (and he again refers there to 'eighteenpence or two shillings a day').

[2] Letters from Malthus to Senior, 23 Mar. 1829, printed as appendix to N. W. Senior, *Two Lectures on Population* (London, 1831), p. 63.

[3] Godwin, op. cit., pp. 73–74.

[4] J. R. McCulloch, *The Principles of Political Economy* (new ed., Edinburgh, 1843), part i, ch. xiii, p. 229.

attitude in that generation of economists. In a sense, all the liberals were Malthusians, but they had all come to qualify the bare thesis by reference to the modifying influence of the standard of living. This is perhaps not surprising if one recalls that in the forty-five years since the first *Essay*, the population of England and Wales had doubled itself and not only showed few signs of pressing against the means of subsistence but was in point of fact improving its standard of living, as McCulloch himself showed in successive editions of his *Dictionary of Commerce*. A severe set-back occurred shortly after he had made his concession to Malthus's critics, but on the whole he and his contemporaries had more occasion to observe the operation of moral restraint than to lament the unchecked expansion of population.

Some writers were anxious to point out the essentially economic character of this check, divorcing it in the process from the epithet 'moral' which Malthus had bestowed upon it.[1] Thus, for instance, T. R. Edmonds, author of *An Enquiry into the Principles of Population*, published in 1832, talks about restraints which work with powerful efficacy 'not associated with the word moral'. These relate in part to the amusements of a bachelor, such as his club, and partly to habits of society, such as display of dress, 'which it becomes discreditable to leave ungratified'. None of these, the book continues, operate in the labouring orders—they have neither diversions nor appointments. The particular classes cited as being susceptible to this non-moral preventive check are notably clerks, and to a lesser extent warehousemen and printers—their low incomes and genteel manners induce habits which, if universally applied, should make us fear depopulation at a rapid rate. Common day-labourers, however, are not observed to exercise any restraint whatever. Yet, it is noted, if only we could provide for these people some necessity for display, however small, they would soon learn caution. The author considers that this would be particularly beneficial in the case of a temporary trade recession: if then people had only married when they judged they could maintain some cherished habit, a decency rather than a necessity, they could give it up when in want of immediate employment, and yet not starve. 'It is illiberal', he says, 'to confine the lower classes to an undeviating standard.' He wants each individual to be able to rise in the social scale, and thus acquire the basis of prudence. The very worst contributors to the population problem are those for whom 'sexual intercourse is the only gratification'. 'To better the condition of the labouring classes,

[1] See discussion of this question in the last chapter.

that is, to place more food and comforts before them, however paradoxical it may appear, is the wisest mode to check redundancy.'[1] Paradoxical—but only to a generation imbued with the spirit of Malthus. In this case the author had sufficient confidence in his prescription to recommend its immediate application in Ireland, where the increase of births was directly blamed on increased poverty—the clearest possible perversion of Malthus. The whole book is full of methods of making the life of the labourer more pleasant—even the provision of public parks is included, and the extension of life insurance to the working classes.[2]

Archibald Alison saw the desire to cling to a given standard as part of the larger process of an ever rising standard of life and an upward movement of individuals through society. Then

> The incessant desire of every succeeding generation becomes to preserve the advantages which their predecessors had gained, and to raise itself above the level to which it was destined by its birth; and a fall from those advantages is felt as the severest penalty of imprudence or guilt.[3]

Another of the observers of this check (they are frequent in the England of the eighteen-thirties) was Richard Jones, Malthus's successor at Haileybury and at one time Professor of Political Economy at King's College, London. We shall meet him again in connexion with many of the more important 'modern' arguments. Here we need only say that he saw farther than the crude advantages resulting from prudence at a higher standard of living. Restraint elevated and purified character, he thought—but there were evils, too, in an abstinence based on the indulgence in secondary wants.[4]

The Laings, father and son, each contributed something to this new theory of economic restraint. The father, in 1842, criticized a volume by Sir Francis d'Ivernois[5] which had sought to show the operation of

[1] [T. R. Edmonds,] *An Enquiry into the Principles of Population* . . . (London, 1832), pp. 79–86.

[2] Ibid., pp. 209–15.

[3] Alison, op. cit. i. 105.

[4] R. Jones, *Literary Remains, Consisting of Lectures and Tracts on Political Economy* (W. Whewell and Cazenove, eds., London, 1859), pp. 96, 101, 105, 154 ff.

[5] Sir F. d'Ivernois, *Enquête sur les causes patentes ou occultes de la faible proportion des naissances à Montreux* (Geneva, 1837). Sir Francis d'Ivernois was a French refugee knighted by George III, who later settled in Switzerland and wrote a number of interesting economic treatises. In addition to the *Enquête*, one may cite *Matériaux pour aider à la recherche des effets du morcellement de la propriété foncière en France* (Geneva and Paris, 1826). This was left unfinished and the statistics showing the reduction of population through subdivision remain unpublished.

In *Sur la mortalité proportionnelle de quelques populations, considérée comme mesure de leur*

moral restraint in certain parts of Switzerland. Laing, having visited the place, found there was no question of morality; simply a system of limited and fixed holdings, making marriage impossible until one fell vacant: a state of no change and no progress.[1] This state is suspiciously like Malthus's dream of a society where all are contented with their lot without a chance of moving. (Malthus in fact was very fond of quoting examples of moral restraint in Switzerland.)

The *Atlas* was a newspaper of liberal pretensions, which offered a prize for an essay to be adjudicated by Herman Merivale and Thomas Tooke amongst others. The winner was Samuel Laing, jnr., and his effort was published under the title *National Distress; Its Causes and Remedies*, in 1844. When discussing the population problem, he quoted Chadwick's reports with approbation, where the reference is to the improvident marriages of the poor and their high birth-rate in the face of disastrous mortality. The great checks on premature marriages in other classes, he declared, were due to the pressure of 'public opinion' in any particular class—the need for a certain income and establishment before marriage, under penalty of losing caste.[2] We have now moved into the world of Queen Victoria—conventions become even stronger than personal preferences.[3]

At this point we must note how much the basis of the argument has changed since the eighteenth century. In the earlier period the wants which restrained population were, on the whole, condemned by the moralists—they were artificial, many of them were termed vicious. The simple, prolific life was equated with virtue. But now the tone has changed. The minimum requirements whose possible loss is now such an obstacle to marriage with decent people, look suspiciously like

aisance et de leur civilisation (Geneva, 1832, reprinted from the *Bibliothèque Universelle*) he continued the work begun by the Pastor Muret, whom Malthus had already quoted, investigating especially the parish of Leysin: there were no illegitimate births, a high expectation of life, and a very slowly growing population. D'Ivernois called it a beautiful example of moral restraint (ibid., p. 19). At Montreux he found the same state of affairs.

Malthus cites d'Ivernois's work on French population losses in his *Essay* (Everyman ed., 1914), i. 218.

[1] S. Laing (the elder), *Notes of a Traveller on the Social and Political State of France, Prussia, Switzerland, Italy, and Other Parts of Europe, During the Present Century* (London, 1842), pp. 338 ff. His views on the significance of the acquisition of property will be discussed below. Laing was a radical of the old school, something after the manner of Cobbett, i.e. with some tory affiliations.

[2] S. Laing (the younger), op. cit., part ii, ch. iv, p. 68.

[3] See J. A. Banks, *Prosperity and Parenthood; a Study of Family Planning among the Victorian Middle Classes* (London, 1954), for the power of these conventions and their changes.

some of the extravagances of the previous century, not, perhaps, in substance, but in their relative place in the hierarchy of possessions. The question that arises again, as it does throughout the history of population theories, is this: Was there a fundamental change of attitude towards the working classes, or did the changed demographic situation persuade the ruling classes of the wisdom of allowing the labouring masses to gain a measure of comfort? There is probably no one clear answer. Godwin turned his concern for the welfare of his fellow men into an argument which he thought would appeal to the anxious men of property; Chadwick and the other utilitarians stated the effect of the economic check as an indisputable fact, of which those who had the power could, if they wished, make use. The economists, on the whole, strike us as having made an exceedingly convenient discovery—that without resort to any undue egalitarianism, one of the evil forces threatening the existing fabric of society can be staved off.

Sir George Rickards (1812–89), a barrister who for six years held the chair of Political Economy at Oxford, had wide knowledge, for his time, on labour questions and the significance of social changes which followed mechanization and the concentration of industry. In his Oxford lectures, *Population and Capital*, published in 1854 and dedicated to Gladstone, he discussed the stresses and strains of competition for places in the middle rank of society, which are constantly receiving recruits from below, and pointed to the restraints imposed by the need to maintain a situation once acquired. There, he said, it is not the actual fear of distress, but the stimulus of social emulation which animates families.[1] He, too, stressed the need to place more people in a situation where they had something to lose—production must be cheapened so that the labourer may have, at a trifling cost, conveniences and luxuries which in former times even the high-born and wealthy could not command—once superfluities, now indispensable.[2] Presumably if the rich will not marry precipitately through want of a coach and pair, the poor can be induced to react similarly to the absence of an elegant gas chandelier. In fact he agrees with Malthus that this would be a perfect world if only we were all middle class! We should then have 'regard for comfort and creditable appearances, a taste for order, neatness, and the simpler luxuries of life'.[3]

[1] Rickards, op. cit., p. 248.

[2] Ibid., p. 251. Note again how flexible is the word 'luxury'.

[3] Ibid., p. 252. An interesting early mention of the force of public opinion occurs in R. Torrens, *An Essay on the Influence of the External Corn Trade upon the Production and Distribution of National Wealth* (2nd ed., London, 1820), quoted by L. Robbins, 'On a

We have now shown that the emergence of the economic type of prudence as a powerful force belongs already to the industrialized stage. It is a hallmark of a mobile society, with a strong middle-class element, and accepted standards of proper behaviour—as a substitute, perhaps, for the blue blood or landed property which once made families acceptable in society.

In France, where the decline in fertility was already most evident by the mid-century, the type of argument we have outlined in England was not likely to be used in a similar way. In England the economic checks were largely answers to Malthus's fears, but in France they became explanations of an existing trend. In England a description of these movements was generally a panegyric on a progressive society inhabited by virtuous citizens. In France the same virtues were not held to be desirable. Malthus had a strong following in France for the first forty years of the century. Then, rather abruptly, the spectre of depopulation replaced that of over-population. It is in the short intervening period that we would look for a development of population theory similar to the one we have described in Great Britain.

Adolphe Quételet, author of one of the first statistical theories of population growth, gave due weight to the existence of foresight, especially where there prevailed: 'une certaine aisance à laquelle [la famille] était habituée'. He contrasted this with a population where there was no hope, and consequently no foresight.[1] The spirit of order and foresight was also the theme of A. Legoyt, another statistician. His contribution is notable because it stresses that this kind of foresight is characteristic of post-feudal, industrializing, and highly competitive society. This is a world where there is no charity from château or monastery; where wealth is more equally distributed, and economic change more rapid.[2] He contrasted this state of affairs with countries where population growth was rapid, but pauperism also increased quickly. Amongst these he included Prussia and Saxony—but also England![3] By 1857 Léonce de Lavergne, basically a Malthusian, found

Certain Ambiguity in the Conception of Stationary Equilibrium', *The Economic Journal* (June 1930), vol. xl, no. 158, p. 196. Torrens saw that people regarded the prospect of rearing their families according to the accustomed standard—so that labourers must obtain not only what the climate demands, but what the habits of the country, operating as a second nature, may require. *Essay on the . . . Corn Trade* (4th ed., 1827), pp. 87 ff.

[1] Quételet, op. cit., pp. 114–16. He too referred to writings on the economic check in Switzerland by d'Ivernois, published in the *Bibliothèque Universelle de Genève* (1830).

[2] A. Legoyt, in *Journal des Économistes* (1st series, 1847), xvii. 176–90, quoted in J. J. Spengler, *France Faces Depopulation* (Durham, North Carolina, 1938), pp. 110–11.

[3] Ibid.

it necessary to quibble about the difference between the 'voluntary continence' of Malthus and the 'shameful calculations of egoism' which were vicious.[1] From 1860 onwards numerous French writers described these calculations. In most cases the phenomenon was related to the general social picture. We shall return to this again later.

In Germany we find the emergence of a clear theory of economic restraint only at the end of the nineteenth century. This is not surprising: for neither did Germany suffer from the kind of demographic decline which the French feared, nor, until after 1870, did a process of industrialization and an increase in foreign trade create a new middle class with habits of excessive prudence. The repressive Malthusianist population policies of German states[2] are a good indication of the fact that the prudential checks were not yet sufficiently visible to obtrude themselves into the field of vision of governments or economists. For one thing, Germany was so obviously under-developed industrially that the writers were too full of the potential needs of the industries they desired, to look for people whose opportunities were limited.[3]

But after 1870 many German writers described and classified the checks which were so obvious in England fifty years earlier—indeed, Germany became the home of some of the most elaborate *Wohlstandstheorien* such as those of Brentano, Johannes Conrad, and C. J. Fuchs. The latter, like Sismondi, believed that the poor, deprived of property, were the cause of over-population. Social reform would at once remove the excess of births, and the frightful infant mortality which was particularly noticeable in some German areas, e.g. the Bavarian Palatinate, at the time.[4]

Similar theories and studies are to be found in most countries after about 1890, and are fully classified in the standard reference works quoted in the Introduction. One may add that these studies became increasingly statistical, e.g. Tallquist, *Recherches statistiques sur la tendance à une moindre fécondité des mariages* (Helsingfors, 1886), and therefore less given to simple unitary explanations of the phenomenon.[5]

[1] Ibid., p. 112.

[2] Elster, op. cit., pp. 770 ff.

[3] Cf. F. List, *The National System of Political Economy* (S. S. Lloyd, trans., new ed., London, 1904), pp. 341–9.

[4] On Conrad and Fuchs, see Elster, op. cit., pp. 792 and 799.

[5] For an assessment of Tallquist and related works, see R. v. Ungern-Sternberg, *The Causes of the Decline of the Birth-rate within the European Sphere of Civilization* (Cold Spring Harbor, 1931). Also G. Mackenroth, *Bevölkerungslehre; Theorie, Soziologie und*

3. THE CONCERN FOR CHILDREN

Philippe Ariès, in his *Histoire des populations françaises*, stressed that in the eighteenth century Western society discovered the Child, and that the nineteenth made it into a tyrant.[1] The inference is that if the child has the status of an individual in the family, the instinct will be to limit the number of children so as to give each one of them the best possible food, entertainment, and so on. It also follows that if the child is treated in this way, its chances of survival into adult age will be much better. Once infant mortality is reduced, as other authors have argued, there is no need to go on having children if one's desire is simply to have an heir; or, as the Norman proverb went: 'Désir de roi: garçon et fille.'[2] Still less could caution be thrown to the winds on the assumption that the end-result would, through losses, still be manageable. It would be possible to disregard Ariès's assumption, therefore, that the discovery of the child was a moral or philosophical event; for if medical science improved in any case, then children would have a greater chance of survival, and hence cease to be regarded as of little account. There is literary evidence that once mothers trained themselves not to become too attached to their children, since these were not likely to live long in any case. One should point out that the English mother even of a century ago still took the early death of a child to be a usual, rather than an exceptional, occurrence. The very habit of calling a number of boys in succession by the same name, as happened in the family of Edward Gibbon, each of whom died after a short time and was at once replaced by another Edward, shows an absence of individual recognition based clearly on failure to survive.[3] Nevertheless, Ariès's main point undoubtedly stands, as one may perceive by a comparison of the position of children, say, in Regency England, and in contemporary America.[4]

Statistik der Bevölkerung (Enzyklopädie der Rechts- und Staatswissenschaft. Abteilung Staatswissenschaft, Berlin, 1953), pp. 317 ff., &c.; United Nations, *Determinants and Consequences* . . ., esp. ch. v, pp. 71 ff., and others.

[1] P. Ariès, *Histoire des populations françaises et de leurs attitudes devant la vie depuis le XVIIIe siècle* (Paris, 1948), pp. 473 ff.

[2] J. Bertillon, *La Dépopulation de la France* (Paris, 1911), p. 108.

[3] The effect on births of greater survival rates will be taken up again below.

[4] Examples of attitudes are bound to be many and contradictory. Certainly English society in the eighteenth century provides views of spoilt children. See, for instance, Ambrose Philips (died 1749): To Charlotte Poultenay:

Timely blossom, Infant fair,
Fondling of a happy pair,
Every morn and every night,
Their solicitous delight . . .

It is, of course, exceedingly difficult to differentiate between a genuine regard for the person of the child and a large number of selfish motives which may, incidentally, furnish the occasion for bettering the position of the child. The nineteenth century saw the complete revolution for which the eighteenth had laid the sentimental foundations.

The expansion of the educational system, a complete code of factory legislation, the advances in pediatrics and psychology—all these represent an inextricable mixture of economic necessity, political expediency, and genuine humanitarian feeling. One need only look at the battles for the ten-hour day in the 1840's to realize that selfish motives often brought greater advances than pure philanthropy. From Robert Raikes to Robert Lowe, men and women strove to bring salutary influences to bear on the child. Yet what a range of horrors lay behind the provision made, from Dotheboys Hall down to the unsung and insanitary board school; from Dr. Blimber's Academy up to the finishing schools for young ladies at Montreux. To say that the concern for children acted as a strong delaying factor to marriage and, later on, as one of the principal reasons for trying to restrict the number of children after marriage, is merely to follow the prevailing fashion in pushing forward the universal sentimental appeal to cloak a rag-bag of motives, from the highest to the lowest.

Thus apart from the regard for children as individuals, we have it as a natural extension of the feeling outlined in the last section, that the status and income of any possible children become one's main anxiety. Here we have the desire to avoid the disgrace of seeing sons having to take employment in trade, or as hired servants; or daughters marrying 'beneath themselves' for want of a dowry that will attract a high-born suitor. We distinguish it from the simple fear of losing one's own status, because the extension to children is conditional upon a certain set of new social requirements, such as education, in all its aspects of learning and accomplishments, dowries, or even the débutante's 'coming out'.

We begin by citing in full the celebrated passage of Polybius, to which we have already alluded. The historian devoted a chapter to the question of how far everything that happens in human affairs is the result of divine providence. Droughts and frosts, he conceded, may be acts of the gods. But depopulation is not in that category, and it is no

The family died out soon after. Both Charles and Mary Lamb wrote poems mourning the death of children—Charles's 'On an Infant Dying as Soon as Born', calls it 'a nameless piece of Babyhood'. Mary's 'In Memoriam' is full of genuine feeling—it is not the sentimental gushing of a mad spinster. Wordsworth's relations with children have been discussed too much to require comment here.

use trying to alter the tendency by supplication and sacrifices. The cause of this scourge is all too human:

For this evil grew upon us rapidly, and without attracting attention, by our men becoming perverted to a passion for show and money and the pleasures of an idle life, and accordingly either not marrying at all, or, if they did marry, refusing to rear the children that were born, or at most one or two out of a great number, for the sake of leaving them well off or bringing them up in extravagant luxury. For when there are only one or two sons, it is evident that, if war or pestilence carries off one, the houses must be left heirless: and, like swarms of bees, little by little the cities become sparsely inhabited and weak. On this subject there is no need to ask the gods how we are to be relieved from such a curse: for any one in the world will tell you that it is by the men themselves if possible changing their objects of ambitions; or if that cannot be done, by passing laws for the preservation of infants.[1]

A modern writer has doubted whether this description, assuming it to be correct at all, would have applied to anyone except wealthy citizens, and have been significant for the country as a whole.[2] That is, of course, difficult to determine with the sparseness of the material. But we have Plutarch's testimony at a later date. At the end of an essay devoted to the natural love of one's children, he said:

. . . poor people do not rear their children, fearing that, if they should not be well educated, they would prove slavish, clownish and destitute of all things commendable: since they cannot endure to entail poverty, which they look upon as the worst of all evils or distresses, upon their posterity.[3]

Dowries

The habit of giving large dowries was stated by Aristotle to have been detrimental to population growth. Describing the polity of Lacedaemon, he criticized the inequality of property in that state. To some extent that was the result of giving large dowries, so that two-fifths of the land came to be owned by women. Daughters of wealthy men then have large estates, whether at marriage or when the father dies, and only those lucky enough to marry one of these girls are likely to be able to rear the children which the law encourages. (If there were four, this carried exemption from all public burdens.) The rest cannot get land, and perish as paupers. Thus the state was reduced from its former greatness to a mere thousand warriors.[4]

[1] Polybius, *Histories*, bk. xxxvii. 9.

[2] A. B. Wolfe, 'The Economics of Population in Ancient Greece', *Facts and Factors in Economic History* (Cambridge, Mass., 1932).

[3] Plutarch, *De amore prolis*, iv. 197.

[4] Aristotle, *Politics*, bk. ii, ch. ix.

Dowries have been common in many civilizations. But the eighteenth century was possibly the period of their greatest significance, at least in Europe. Men judged it impossible to launch out into life and society without the help of an heiress; and a daughter without portion was a disgrace as well as a spinster for life. In eighteenth-century England the fashionable journals of the day, such as the *Gentleman's Magazine*, usually printed the brides' fortunes as part of the minimum information required: it was not necessary to know who their fathers were, but vital to state the size of the dowry. This seems to have been mentioned particularly by the Italian writers listed by Reynaud.[1]

Other references to dowries are frequent—they are usually linked to general censures of luxurious habits. Alison, in 1840, observed that the higher ranks of society voiced the universal complaint of the excessive difficulty of getting young women established in life.[2] The reader may gain further information by inspecting marriage settlements of the eighteenth century, which show the appalling price fathers even of the 'middling ranks of society' had to pay to get their daughters off their hands. We are justified in treating the habit of giving dowries as one of the 'accepted' checks to population increase.

One of the earliest and shrewdest observations on the effect of a higher standard of living, in whatever form it is encountered, on the size of the family, is that of Sir William Temple, who in the seventeenth century observed the extinction of families of fashionable habits:

> The weakness of children, both in their bodies and minds, proceeds not only from such constitutions or qualities in the parents, but also from the ill consequences upon generation, by marriages contracted without affection, choice or inclination . . . these contracts would never be made, but by men's avarice, and greediness of portions with the women they marry, which is grown among us to that degree, as to surmount and extinguish all other regards or desires: so that our marriages are made, just like other common bargains and sales, by the meer consideration of interest or gain, without any love or esteem, of birth or of beauty itself . . . this public grievance, which has since ruined so many estates by the necessity of giving great portions to daughters; impaired many families by the weak or mean productions of

[1] P. Reynaud, *La Théorie de la population en Italie du XVIe au XVIIIe siècle* (Lyon, 1904), p. 34. He quotes the Abbé Genovesi de Castiglione, *Delle lezione di commercio ossia d'economia civile* (Naples, 1765, 2 vols.), condemning heavy dowries and elaborate marriage ceremonies. F. Villano, *L'ozio autunnale, ovvero discorsi economici politici* (Naples, 1768), also correlates marriage frequency with absence of dowries. Similarly in Beccaria, *Della Popolazione*; Reynaud, ibid., p. 138.

[2] Alison, op. cit. i. 111.

marriage . . . and extinguished many great ones by the aversion of the persons who should have continued them. . . .[1]

This line of reasoning has received much attention from sociologists and anthropologists. There is a sharp distinction between countries where women work before and possibly during marriage, and others where women bring in a dowry and then stay at home. The former marriage may be based on mutual attraction; under the latter system, economic considerations may prevail. Max Scheler considered the rational marriage of social classes (*Standesehe*) or of economic interests (*Mitgiftehe*) as biologically harmful. He quoted sociologists who attributed the high value of the Anglo-Saxon peoples to the absence amongst them of such marriages. (He was speaking of the post-1800 period.)[2]

Other authors, again, consider that the economic or social marriage is inherently more stable than the romantic Anglo-Saxon marriage, or that a marriage not based on the physical attraction of the wife is likely to be more fertile since a large number of children do not destroy the *raison d'être* of the union. This view was already held in the eighteenth century by one of the shrewdest of the German cameralists, J. H. G. von Justi, who wrote under the *nom de plume* 'Anaxagoras von Occident'. His *Physicalische und Politische Betrachtungen* on demographic subjects included detailed studies of human fertility.[3] Although he complains against dowries, and claims that they are prejudicial to marital happiness, he also felt that a love-marriage was not conducive to generation, and that cool, and even calculated ones, were much more fertile.[4] The inherent contradiction was perhaps typical of the period of transition in which Justi wrote. Brought up in the cameralist tradition of the old Prussia, his inclinations brought him nearer to the French encyclopaedists, and the physiocrats, and so finally to a position where he could whole-heartedly approve of the love-match.

[1] Sir W. Temple, *The Works of Sir William Temple, Of Popular Discontents* (new ed., London, 1757, 4 vols.), iii. 61 ff.

[2] M. Scheler, *Schriften zur Soziologie und Weltanschauungslehre* (Leipzig, 1924, 3 vols.), iii, part ii, 152. See also Mackenroth, op. cit., pp. 364, 374, on marriage patterns. See also the article 'Dowry' in the *Encyclopaedia of Social Sciences*, v. 230 ff., and F. Müller-Lyer, *The Evolution of Modern Marriage* (Isabella Wigglesworth, trans., London, 1930), p. 128. These last two are quoted in Coontz, op. cit., p. 148; see also there for a discussion of the economic factor in altering the purposes of the family and marriage, and consequent effects on fertility.

[3] Anaxagoras von Occident [i.e. J. H. G. v. Justi], *Physicalische und politische Betrachtungen über die Erzeugung des Menschen und Bevölkerung der Länder* (Smirna, i.e. Karlsruhe, 1769), pp. 123 ff.

[4] Ibid., pp. 21 ff. He also thought that 'soft' women did not conceive as readily as 'hard' ones—cold baths were a sure specific.

Education

Next to dowries, the education of children has always been put forward as a great expense in civilized society. Short saw in this a bar to marriage:

As when Parents breed up their Daughters, and give them an Education much superior to their Circumstance, or Fortune they intend to give them, or a Match suitable to their Patrimony . . . (instead of being given instruction in Christian virtues). They are . . . too often brought up the very reverse; being taught to mind and affect Gaiety, Dress and Modes, . . . As soon as they are grown up a little, Misses are packed off to Boarding-Schools to learn Dancing, Musick, *French*, Gaming, and withal get well tinctured with Pride, etc. . . . When married the way is paved, for Dress, Idleness, Luxury, Voluptuousness and Pleasures. . . . [The result is that even Rakes won't look at them, for fear of saddling themselves with expense, and a virtuous youth has to resort to a country girl.][1]

We have a double check here: parents will shun children since the fashionable expense of bringing them up is excessive, and the notions they acquire in the process will deter potential husbands.

Cantillon observed the situation in all ranks of society: 'All the lower orders wish to live and bring up Children who can live like themselves.' If they cannot do it on their own capital, they postpone marriage until they find 'some young woman who brings a little capital for that purpose'. In the upper classes, younger sons are in no hurry to marry unless 'they are offered Heiresses and Fortunes'.[2]

The irony of Ange de Goudar makes us feel that the 'education' under discussion was as extravagant in France as in Short's England. 'Comment donner une éducation honnête à six enfans, dit-on, si on n'a un gros revenu? Et parce qu'on n'a pas ce gros revenu, on prive l'Etat de six enfans.'[3] But as we have seen in the case of the word 'luxury', the extravagance of one generation may be a reasonable expense in the next. We have already quoted a footnote in the Marshal de Saxe's *Rêveries*—it also says that the multiplication of wants renders children a burden to their parents, because to educate them becomes attended with extraordinary expenses: 'The son of a peasant is now brought up with more pride and delicacy than a prince.'[4] So, too,

[1] Short, op. cit., pp. 164–6, quoted in Kuczynski, op. cit., pp. 308–9.

[2] Cantillon, op. cit., p. 79.

[3] A. de Goudar, *Les Intérêts de la France mal entendus* (Amsterdam, 1757, 3 vols.), i. 185.

[4] Herman Maurice, Marshal de Saxe, *Reveries, or, Memoirs concerning the Art of War* . . . (Edinburgh, 1776), p. 262. On the authorship of the footnote, see section on Luxury.

Forbonnais noticed that poor parents would avoid children if it were difficult to apprentice them.[1] We are familiar with the excessive premiums required by some English masters in the eighteenth century. It seems clear that there is little fundamental difference between the necessity of buying a younger son a sinecure, or of apprenticing him to a woolcomber.

Many writers ceased to distinguish between income groups when describing this sort of feeling. It applied to anyone who wanted to be 'somebody in the world' as Süßmilch said—whatever little world he inhabited.[2] The very desire to have children becomes subordinated to one's notion of well-being—one does not deliberately create obstacles to that condition.[3]

> ... however humble his desires [wrote Nassau Senior], he cannot contemplate without anxiety a probability that the income which supported his social rank, while single, may be insufficient to maintain it when he is married; that he may be unable to give his children the advantages of education which he enjoyed himself; in short, that he may lose his caste.[4]

Presumably that would be true whether the education consisted in attendance at a dame school at 2*d.* a week, or the factory school of some enlightened employer, where elementary instruction was thrown in with some paltry employment at two shillings a week, or complete education on a charitable foundation which meant failure to earn until late adolescence.

The dilemma of the man who wants children had already been clearly stated by Moheau in the eighteenth century:

> ... on a des enfants par une impulsion de la nature, on les éléve par attachement; mais un calcul des charges auxquelles ils assujetissent, demontreroit que, dans la classe des gens de peine, un enfant, avant qu'il puisse rendre

[1] F. V. de Forbonnais, *Élémens du commerce* (Leyden, 1754), i. 276. Quoted in Spengler, *French Predecessors* . . ., p. 271.

[2] J. P. Süßmilch, *Die göttliche Ordnung in den Veränderungen des menschlichen Geschlechts aus der Geburt, dem Tode und der Fortpflanzung desselben erwiesen* (Berlin, 1775, 3 vols.), i. 50. 'Die so sich aus Furcht, um nicht arme Kinder zu haben, nicht verheyratheten, wären solche, die gerne in der Welt was vorstellen wollten.'

[3] L. G. Du Buat-Nançay, *Éléments de la politique ou recherche des vrais principes de l'économie sociale* (London, 1773, 6 vols.), ii. 67: '. . . l'amour de la postérité naît du sentiment du bien-être'.

[4] N. W. Senior, *An Outline of the Science of Political Economy* (London, 1938 ed.), p. 38. Cf. also T. R. Malthus, *Principles of Political Economy* . . . (London, 1820), p. 250: where higher wages tend to a higher standard of comfort, without a 'proportionate acceleration in the rate of increase', we find 'all the circumstances which tend to elevate the character of the lower classes of society, which makes them approach the nearest to beings who "look before and after" '.

quelque service, a beaucoup plus coûté que les gages d'un homme fait et instruit; dans les autres classes, les enfants sont onéreux à leurs parens par leur institution & leur établissement; devenus adultes, ils se détachent d'eux, & quelquefois sont leur malheur par leurs désordres et leurs vices. Ainsi la réflexion et l'esprit de calcul ne conduiroient point à la propagation de l'éspece . . .[1]

It needs an altogether higher conception of family life than these sordid calculations to make sure of posterity. Yet what Moheau described soon became a common opinion.

So, almost imperceptibly, another change takes place: the nineteenth century goes beyond the rationalization of self-love which found expression in supposed love for one's children: the feeling is sublimated into an active desire to surround the children with affection and comfort. When Proudhon described the more perfect society which he envisaged, he could see the love of one's children contributing to the general decline in fertility: it 'purges conjugal affection of eroticism; the respect that they inspire is the sign that passion is about to die in the heart of the fathers'.[2]

We find Lujo Brentano in the direct line of succession of those who caricatured contemporary foppishness. In primitive society, he said, the love of children is no obstacle to their creation. But with increased well-being and at higher levels of culture, man begins a sort of marginal utility calculation, and he sets the satisfaction of his sexual urges (or the maternal instinct) against other enjoyments and satisfactions—amongst which the desire for healthy children, and their thorough preparation for the struggle for existence, ranks high.[3]

The boundary between what is permissible affection for one's children, and gratification of vanity, is so nebulous as to defy definition in any objective sense. Just as the motives of education can be mixed, so the provision of any physical comforts for members of one's family may spring from pure affection or pure egotism—but much more likely the two are mixed. But just because such an array of calculations and

[1] M. Moheau, *Recherches et considérations sur la population de la France* (Paris, 1778), part ii, p. 98.

[2] P. J. Proudhon, *De la Justice dans la révolution et dans l'église* (Paris, 1858), quoted in Spengler, 'French Population Theory since 1800', *Journal of Political Economy* (1936), xliv. 752.

[3] L. Brentano, 'Die Malthus'sche Lehre und die Bevölkerungsbewegung der letzten Dezennien', *Abhandlungen der historischen Klasse der Königlich Bayerischen Akademie der Wissenschaften* (Munich, 1909), xxiv. 605 ff. For further modern treatments of the same phenomenon, see references in United Nations, *Determinants and Consequences . . .*, pp. 80–81. We shall link up with these ideas again later when discussing general theories.

emotions propels parents in this same direction, sociologists of all ages have found the concern for children one of the most powerful causes of abstinence from marriage, and limitation of children after it. Undoubtedly such considerations apply most strongly in a rapidly developing society, where it is possible for individuals, and *a fortiori* their children, to rise in the world, and where calculations of advantages become a common feature of family life. In France it appears that a disastrous trend of a century was only reversed when the state provided an economic incentive to produce children which was greater than the advantage of remaining unmarried, childless, or with but a single child for which to make provision.

To understand the significance of these old ideas against the background of a nineteenth-century society, we must re-examine our terms as they apply to a changing society.

IV

THE ECONOMIC BASIS OF VOLUNTARY RESTRAINT IN A CHANGING SOCIETY

I. NECESSITIES, DECENCIES, LUXURIES

WE have so far discussed the economic checks to population growth only in terms of the preservation of a *status quo*. It is true that the fear of falling expressed in early nineteenth-century England presupposes some social mobility—it is precisely the *nouveaux-arrivés* who fear most the possibility of sliding back into their former status. We have also urged strongly that the word 'luxury' has no fixed meaning, and varies according to the standard of the observer. The notion of a constantly dying aristocracy involves the corollary of the recruitment of rising classes. Yet, on the whole, most of the checks so far described could quite easily operate in a society which has an unchanging standard of living or civilization. We need not assume a process of industrialization or changes in foreign trade—the urban-rural differential remains an argument in static theory unless it is advanced as one of the automatic checks on population at a time of increasing urbanization of the country, due to industrial or commercial developments.

We must now investigate the characteristic movement of an expanding society in particular: the results of a widespread prospect of economic advancement. We do so in three sections—first we add to our vocabulary by defining the different possible levels at which man can exist, then we trace views on the influence of a prospect of rising on the industrial world, and lastly we discuss the whole system of social capillarity and vertical mobility.

We have already seen the distinctions made by Ferguson, the Marshal de Saxe, Sir Archibald Alison, and Sir George Rickards between the standards of one age and those of another, and between different civilizations.

Cantillon had elevated these differences to the dignity of a whole system controlling the size of the population. The clearest statement of the eighteenth century, again, comes from Archdeacon Paley. We saw in the last chapter how accurately he had observed the fact that even the masses of the people have wants beyond the absolute subsistence minimum, and how these proved a bar to marriage. But these wants, he thought, were not fixed: they were likely to increase. Paley considered this point under the heading of 'luxury'—by which he meant, of course, introducing 'superfluities into general reception'. He said that this process would make people forgo marriage rather than 'forego those indulgences, which their own habits, or what they observe amongst their equals, have rendered necessary to their satisfaction'.[1] This effect applies to every form of expenditure and every class of society.

. . . hitherto . . . the effects are beneficial; and were these the only effects, such elegancies, or, if you please to call them so, such luxuries, could not be too universal. But here follows the mischief: when once fashion hath annexed the use of these articles of dress to any certain class, the middling ranks, for example, of the community, each individual of that rank finds them to be *necessaries* of life. . . .[2]

So that, of course, the barrier to marriage grows. Luxury then, it turns out, has two opposite effects, and it is difficult to determine the point at which it begins (as Wallace had said). It is not a straightforward arithmetical problem, but one depending upon 'circumstances too numerous, intricate, and undefined, to admit of a precise solution'. Paley then goes on to examine the general rules by which a judgement may be made, and it is the second of these which strikes us most forcibly:

2ndly. That it is the *diffusion*, rather than the *degree of luxury*, which is to be dreaded as a national evil. The mischief of luxury consists, as we have seen, in the obstruction that it forms to marriage . . . (so long as it affects only the rich no great harm is done to population). But when the imitation of the same manners descends, as it always will do, into the mass of the people, when it advances the requisites of living beyond what it adds to men's abilities to purchase them, then it is that luxury checks the formation of families, in a degree that ought to alarm the public fears.[3]

'When the imitation of the same manners descends, as it always will do'—that is the crux of the matter. Introduce, at the top, what refinements you will, and they must percolate to the masses. How then could Paley come to share Malthus's fears? His were still the opposite ones, normal to the century in which he wrote. His short answer to Malthus

[1] W. Paley, *The Principles of Moral and Political Philosophy* (9th ed., London, 1793, 2 vols.), ii. 356.
[2] Ibid., p. 357.
[3] Ibid., p. 359.

ought to have been: Given the technical progress now prevailing, you need only let matters take their natural course, and you will soon see the springs of population drying up. The reason for his failure to see this point probably lies in his own preoccupation (later in his book) with soil productivity and employment.

It might be said that the more rigid distinctions adopted by other writers of the eighteenth century were to some extent a retrograde step from Paley, and in fact they were abandoned again under the impact of the ever more rapid distribution of refinements throughout all ranks of society. This phenomenon was to be explained by the emergence of large-scale, cost-reducing industry.

J. F. Melon had already observed this. It is worth quoting again his threefold division: 'Le pain est de nécessité absolue, et les laines sont de seconde nécessité; mais le pain blanc et les draps fins . . . seroient de plus grands luxes sans l'habitude où nous sommes de nous en servir tous les jours.'[1] His conclusion had been that luxuries were necessary for economic progress—but even some of those who did not agree with this view could not help admitting that progress was being made. 'In the lowest ranks as in the first, that which was formerly folly today is become usage and almost necessity'[2]—complained the austere Mirabeau. It was a moral as well as an economic question. As Ferguson pointed out, the 'faculty of physic as well as of morality' ought to be consulted. For Wallace, the whole question became something of a dilemma:

> In general, it must be confessed, that a taste of beauty, and a desire of grandeur in objects of this kind, must have been highly advantageous at first. . . . But it is difficult to ascertain the proper boundary within which it ought to be confined in theory; it is much more difficult not to transgress it in practice. Happy should we be! happy should be society! could we find out and preserve that golden mediocrity which in a great measure constitutes the peace and tranquillity of human life.[3]

Some sort of refinement must be expected—we cannot conceive of any age where man has not somehow supplemented absolute necessities. Anything which is less than the full measure of 'elegance', indeed,

[1] J. F. Melon, *Essai politique sur le commerce* (Paris, 1736), pp. 112–13.

[2] V. R. Mirabeau, *L'Ami des hommes, ou traité de la population* (Avignon, 1756, 3 parts), i. 146. Quoted in J. J. Spengler, *French Predecessors of Malthus* (Durham, North Carolina, 1942), p. 133.

[3] This and the following quotations and summaries: R. Wallace, *A Dissertation on the Numbers of Mankind, in Ancient and Modern Times* (Edinburgh, 1809), pp. 336–8. (Conclusion of the Appendix.)

means something akin to 'fierceness and superstition'. If the standard just attains the right measure, paradise will be found on earth: it contributes to the perfection of human society. 'But so soon as it o'erleaps the proper limit, it introduces effeminacy and softness among mankind . . . it enervates both the mind and the body. . . .'

And so there follow the well-known characteristics of luxury, complete with debauch and corruption. And lastly:

> It introduces numberless superfluities and wants, the satisfaction of which is preferred to the discharge of the most important duties. It must of course prevent marriage, give check to the increase of mankind, and hinder millions from ever seeing the light.

Having stated his optimum theory, Wallace wrote 'finis' and did not inquire how we might know when we had reached this happy mean.

Nassau Senior

Wallace's fears were not voiced again in the nineteenth century. For that at least the credit must go to Malthus and his followers on the one hand, and to the industrial revolution on the other. Since it was not possible to write on population, or civilization, after 1800, without frequent reference to Malthus, and in fact most treatises on the subject were framed as apologies or counterblasts, none of the authors saw the need to warn against possible excess of 'elegant amenities' as checks to population. Moreover, though Wallace had seen some new inventions in his own time, it was only the age of Senior which daily saw new devices spreading into the homes of the poor—piped water, gas-lighting, and Andrew Ure's barometer and cottage piano. Meanwhile, the middle classes acquired water-closets, fresh milk brought by train from Wiltshire, and other luxuries, which would no doubt filter downwards in due course, only to be replaced by still more cunning devices at the top. We are familiar with the Victorian idea of Progress, and the spirit of the Great Exhibition of 1851. We must therefore regard the population theories of the time as a special manifestation of a universal view.

Senior's contribution was first made in two lectures delivered before the University of Oxford in 1828, and printed, together with some correspondence with Malthus, in 1829 (2nd ed. in 1831). His views were restated in his *Political Economy*, first published in the *Encyclopaedia Metropolitana* in 1836, and frequently reprinted since. The idea that the goods which man consumes are not all equally necessary to him, and that the grades established accordingly are subject to changes in the long run, was not a new one. But Senior elevated these considerations to the role of a principal check on the growth of population:

> It appears . . . that habits of considerable superfluous expenditure afford the only permanent protection against a population pressing so closely on the means of subsistence, as to be continually incurring the misery of positive checks.[1]

The surplus of which he spoke fell into two categories—decencies and luxuries. What substances were included in each was a matter of time and place and individual preference. But logically they were precise categories. Supposing necessities to be things '. . . the use of which is requisite to keep a given individual in the health and strength essential to his going through his habitual occupations', decencies would then be those 'which a given individual must use in order to preserve his existing rank in society'. All else beyond that was luxury.[2]

It will be seen that the definition of necessaries is very close to that required in Adam Smith's 'subsistence theory', or Lassalle's Iron Law of Wages, whereas Senior clearly meant that 'decencies' were also the rule amongst English workers. This is clear from the fact that Senior did not think that the fear of losing necessaries acted as a prudential check in England—there was always the Poor Law to fall back on. But the loss of decencies (or the fear of losing them)—that was the great preventive check operating in England. To marry before one had an income which would ensure the continuation of the existence of decencies for oneself and one's children, was also to thwart for ever the secret desire of all men: '. . . to acquire . . . the means of purchasing the decencies which give a higher social rank'.[3]

The word decency is here evidently used to describe something like a badge or symbol—the parlour is the decency of the petty bourgeois, but to marry with a parlour is to forgo the chance of ever marrying with a first-floor drawing-room. Since the word is so flexible, one begins to wonder what becomes of the third category of luxuries—the things which are not essential either for health or the maintenance of rank. In the highly competitive society in which Senior made his observations, everything was done because it was the proper thing to do. Only secret

[1] N. W. Senior, *Two Lectures on Population, Delivered Before the University of Oxford in Easter Term, 1828* (London, 1831), p. 34.

[2] N. W. Senior, *An Outline of the Science of Political Economy* (London, 1938 ed.), p. 36.

[3] Ibid.

vices of gluttony and indulgence could then be classed as luxuries—surely not what Senior had in mind.

In any case, he firmly concluded that in civilized societies (and the more so, the more civilized and opulent they became) men postponed marriage not only because they feared to sink, but because they hoped to rise in an 'unincumbered state'.[1] In fact it might go too far, because: 'as they mount the horizon of their ambition keeps receding'—until sometimes it is too late. We see clearly that the tripartite system was connected with a developing society. The whole principle depended not only on the condition that this society should have reached a certain state, but that it should be continually advancing. In this state

> as wealth increases, what were the luxuries of one generation become the decencies of their successors. Not only a taste for additional comfort and convenience, but a feeling of degradation in their absence becomes more and more widely diffused.

As productivity rises, so these advantages may be enjoyed by ever-increasing numbers. This is a sort of insurance against a recurrence of the positive checks (whose existence Senior did not doubt); for the more superfluities man acquired in his daily life, the less was he likely to starve because of some temporary misfortune like a bad harvest or a trade recession.

Malthus was not convinced. Senior wrote to him in March 1824, inviting him to say that they were actually in substantial agreement, but for the little matter of emphasis on *tendencies*. For Senior, the desire to preserve one's standards, or the hope of rising, were instincts as strong as those leading to marriage and procreation; to Malthus, they were not. In actual fact, Senior said, population and subsistence are so balanced, at least in old countries, that both may increase, the latter slightly faster than the former, so that standards of living increase, and consequently further checks are placed on population increase.[2]

Malthus replied with the phrase already quoted, that he believed the desire for bettering our condition to be perfectly feeble, compared with the tendency of the population to increase.[3] In any case, he believed, the labouring classes did not share this desire at all. Yet they were just the people who held the great power of increase. One rather

[1] N. W. Senior, op. cit., p. 38.

[2] N. W. Senior, *Two Lectures on Population*. . . . Correspondence with Malthus printed as an Appendix. Senior had sent copies of his lectures to Malthus with this first letter.

[3] Ibid., p. 63.

feels that Malthus is here being unnecessarily obstinate, since he is here denying a principle he had previously stated in the third book of the second *Essay*:

> The scanty relief granted to persons in distress . . . and the natural and becoming pride, not yet quite extinct among the peasantry of England, have deterred the more thinking and virtuous part of them from venturing on marriage without some better prospect of maintaining their families than mere parish assistance. The desire of bettering our condition, and the fear of making it worse . . . is the *vis medicatrix reipublicae* . . . it operates as a preventive check to increase; and happy for the country it is that it does so.[1]

But then Malthus felt it always his duty not to give any ground in arguments of this sort, and would oppose to some theoretical concession his practical doubt of its importance. He admitted that in some 'civilised and populous' countries restraint and self-denial might operate, and more so at certain times than at others, but on the whole he denied the practical importance of this feeling. Even if it were true, he concluded, it would be no service to their common object of increasing mankind's happiness, to draw attention to the existence of such inefficient means of checking population as improving the standard of living of the labouring classes, when we ought all to concentrate on preaching moral restraint. (Senior denied having implied that all would be well automatically.)

Senior's further remonstrances finally persuaded Malthus to yield a little ground in his second letter—at times of comparative abundance he had observed that then the labouring classes might be given 'a taste for such a mode of living as will tend to increase their prudential habits'.[2] But he did not believe that one ought to rely on such a fortuitous circumstance. Moral and religious habits must be improved first. So in the end the two economists stood almost where they had begun. But it was Senior's argument which was further developed by later writers, not Malthus's. Even the Malthusians came more and more to lay stress on the fact that the education of which their master had spoken would very largely have to take the form of instilling a taste for the 'comforts and decencies' of life into the people. This was often linked with an appeal, not only to self-respect, but to self-preservation, through a naïve belief in the wage-fund theories of the time: if they will only keep down their numbers, they will have higher wages, to indulge

[1] T. R. Malthus, *An Essay on the Principle of Population* (Everyman ed., 1914, 2 vols.), ii. 53.
[2] N. W. Senior, *Two Lectures on Population* . . ., pp. 85–86.

then in the consumption of commodities which in turn will make them want to restrict the numbers of their children.[1]

Richard Jones

Richard Jones, Malthus's successor at Haileybury, was also one of his most determined opponents. Early in his first lecture on population he postulated the existence of neutral checks (i.e. those which were neither vice, nor misery, nor moral restraint) and these he believed to be sufficiently powerful to lead him to declare categorically that: 'Population does not outstrip the supplies of food.'[2]

The main reason for this happy state of affairs was this: mankind does indeed increase until its numbers are limited by the means available, not only to feed the people, but 'to satisfy the cravings . . . for commodities necessary to supply all the wants and gratifications which are essential to maintain them in comfort and contentment'. In fact, even agricultural labourers, the worst-paid class in England, only spent two-thirds of their wages on food—and as we go higher up the social scale, so the proportion becomes ever smaller. Therefore a series of steps of deprivation will have to be passed through before anyone can claim that actual want of food limits numbers.

> What it is that prevents the power of increase from pushing all nations to these extremes, what causes are at work to check the full exercise of the mere physical power of the human race to multiply indefinitely, is the chief object of our enquiry.[3]

In answering his own question, Jones at once used the Malthusian classification, substituting only 'voluntary' for 'moral' restraint, and adding the *neutral* causes, which defied classification though their effect was evident. The operation of the voluntary restraint rested on two facts: first, that man is endowed with foresight, and second, that he has secondary wants. This distinguishes man from animals, for in no society

[1] See, for instance, T. Chalmers, *On Political Economy in Connexion with the Moral State and Moral Prospects of Society* (2nd ed., Glasgow, 1832), p. 552. I have not dealt with the wage-fund theory as a whole in this work, since it was, after all, something of a red herring. It formed simply a special case of the general arguments of economic restraint. Rickards in England, and Cantillon in France, had population theories linked to a recognition of the wage fund. There are echoes of it in J. S. Mill, *Principles of Political Economy* (6th ed., London, 1902), bk. ii, ch. xx, para. 3.

[2] R. Jones, *Literary Remains, Consisting of Lectures and Tracts on Political Economy* (W. Whewell and Cazenove, eds., London, 1859). The lectures were probably given in the early thirties.

[3] Ibid., p. 100.

does puberty coincide with marriage. Jones then went on to specify goods which fell into the classes of primary or secondary wants—the former limited, the latter unlimited. Moreover, whereas any check due to the fear of not being able to satisfy primary wants is fixed in relation to any one nation, the check relating to secondary wants is movable, depending on the degree of comfort already attained in the class under discussion.[1]

Jones thought that despite the fact that the highest classes would also often have the means of satisfying the appropriate standards, they would also show relatively many cases where income was not commensurate with what was expected of them, and failure a public event. Therefore prudence, or fear, would be greatest in those classes, and consequently they would be the ones most liable to early extinction. This in turn would mean replacement from below. The structure of society which is based on this idea will be discussed in the next section. But Jones's main contribution to the notion under review here is his constant awareness of the fact that the meaning, and the influence, of the terms used in population theory is never fixed, but must be related to the state of development of the individual or the society. Thus, in discussing misery, he points out that Alexander was miserable because he had no more worlds to conquer. The same applies, *a fortiori*, to lesser demands. The only real misery is that which shows in physical suffering—all else is the imagined suffering of a man deprived of the satisfaction of some secondary want.[2] But physical suffering apart, there is no absolute criterion for this feeling of being deprived of some essential—we just know that as societies develop, so the number of essentials becomes greater. In his own time, Jones noticed the contrast between the unvarying minimum standards of the Irish peasantry and the ever-rising requirements of the English labourer. Jones was emphatic that those who, like Malthus, regarded the operation of the check afforded by these desires as being confined to the upper ranks of society were mistaken, and were being proved more wrong every day.[3] This view naturally assumes rising real wages, and Jones was at pains to point out that it was possible for this to happen—there was no question of accepting the classical view that such a rise would lead

[1] Ibid., pp. 102–3. The parlour is here mentioned as being the hallmark of the shopkeeper and tradesman.

[2] He was careful to state (ibid., p. 159) that even people who were not miserable might easily be living in a state less healthy than that which would prevail if they knew how to feed themselves properly—in fact he considered that to be the case in most countries.

[3] Ibid., p. 107.

automatically to an increase in population. On the contrary, the effect he would expect would be the opposite: the greater the rise, the less the likelihood of its being frittered away by greater numbers.[1] To Malthus's laws of geometrical and arithmetical increase, he opposed a law relating to checks: 'As secondary wants multiply among the different classes of society, motives to prudence in regard to marriage multiply with them. The weights are increased in one scale while those in the other continue stationary.'[2] A similar state of affairs existed, he thought, with regard to the effects of postponing marriages. With every year that marriage was put off in the first place, the chances of further voluntary restraint being exercised increased.[3]

We thus see that Richard Jones made an even greater contribution than Senior in taking the subject of population checks out of the crude controversy about facts which had characterized the Malthusian era. The unnecessary distinction between 'decencies' and 'luxuries' was abolished. Senior's 'decencies' and Jones's 'secondary wants' henceforth became established categories in the discussion. The first step had been taken towards systems of explanation which would be independent of the bias of contemporary observation. It might be argued that Malthus, too, aimed at such a system, and that in fact he was too little bound by the things which he himself might observe in his own age. But when modern demographers construct models of population movements, it is more along Jones's or Senior's lines, not Malthus's.

One further point needs stressing. One may look at the relationship between population, subsistence, and the standard of living in two ways. Either one emphasizes the supply side, as Malthus invariably did, and assumes a constant pattern of demand, or one lays stress on the importance of the level and composition of demand, consciously or unconsciously taking the level of supplies as fixed, at least in the short run. In the first case it is necessary to think primarily of checks which bring population and subsistence into long-term balance. In the second, one finds the adjustment or rates in population growth treated as the natural consequence of changing 'secondary wants'. In practice, the two approaches are often found together. Nevertheless, the distinction remains important, because in the first case the analysis requires principally an economic investigation into systems of production and distribution, and in the second a more sociological approach to the

[1] R. Jones, op. cit., p. 148. He did not say this would never happen.

[2] Ibid., p. 164.

[3] Ibid., pp. 176–7.

influences which shape demand. Moreover, the two approaches often colour the whole outlook of the writer. Malthus was sceptical, not to say pessimistic, since there was, apparently, no easy road out of his predicament. Richard Jones, on the other hand, described a system which not only offered a solution to the Malthusian problem, but also described this solution in the most glowing terms. This optimism was the keynote of the sociological approach at least until the end of the nineteenth century, when the fear of decadence became paramount in some quarters.

Alison, Rickards, and Bagehot

Sir Archibald Alison clearly stressed that the extension of wants from generation to generation produced a progressively operating check. The father communicates to his children the habits, not of his own struggling youth, but of his own most successful period in life.

> The gratifications which were considered as the highest objects of ambition, or the last step of luxury during the best years of his life, are regarded as mere necessaries by his posterity. . . . They in their turn fix their affections upon still higher gratifications, which are seen and envied from the elevated ground from which they commence their career; . . .[1]

and so on *ad infinitum*. We recognize that no boundary could be fixed to the extension of human comfort. Moreover, it is no rigid system; the gradations on the scale are infinite, unlike the sharp distinctions, he thought, of feudal society, where the lowest could never hope to emulate the highest. Here, of course, we once again come to the question of social mobility, which will occupy us later.

We have already seen that Sir George Rickards quoted Ireland as a place without hope, and therefore without fear. His contrast was with England, where people were afraid of losing the 'necessary provision' —but this led him at once to consider that this was not a fixed term.[2]

[1] Sir A. Alison, *The Principles of Population and Their Connection with Human Happiness* (Edinburgh, 1840, 2 vols.), i. 104.

[2] Sir G. Rickards, *Population and Capital: Being a Course of Lectures delivered before the University of Oxford in 1853–54* (London, 1854), p. 250. As his authority, he quotes F. Bastiat, *Harmonies économiques* (2ᵉ éd., Paris, 1851) (proving God's wisdom in ordering the world as it is, so that all forces, left to themselves, harmonize for the universal good). The point of the third chapter (Paris, 1850 éd., pp. 73 ff.) was to show that the concept of 'needs' varied not only from person to person, but that even the common idea of what was necessary was constantly changing, and that this was indeed fortunate, for were it not so, much of the incentive to work, effort, and progress would be lacking. Progress, of course, is self-begetting: a new goal is set, and the effort to reach it in itself will generate new ideas and aims.

For the upper and middle classes, the effect was obvious enough. But the lower orders could only be reached in a steadily advancing society. As productive powers improved, *pari passu* with the application of science and the arts to industry, so commodities are cheapened and real wages automatically raised. This 'places within the labourer's reach, at a trifling cost, conveniences and luxuries, which in former times even the high-born and wealthy could not command', and so superfluities become indispensable, and population is checked. But in addition to this simple effect, he observed a more complicated process. As more and more machines are introduced, the hardest physical work is gradually taken off the human worker—his intelligence and skill must be developed rather than his muscles. 'Not only in manufactures but in agriculture, steam power is the BRIARAEUS that is tending to supersede the employment of human muscles and sinews.'[1] The whole process leads to refinement, better pay, and hence to changing standards of values in a labour force which is undergoing organic changes in its composition. In fact the middle class is being enlarged by an influx of technicians.

Walter Bagehot was equally certain that so far as modern society is concerned, the fear that additional subsistence would create additional population is quite groundless. This can only happen if people are at the subsistence minimum (as they were in India), or in a country where people were at what he calls a 'moral minimum'. This rather curious concept describes a people who have a fixed, though not minimal standard, below which they will not fall. But as incomes increase, they will use the additional subsistence for children they would not otherwise have had. 'But there is no sort of necessity in this; as has been explained, the "moral minimum" is very movable; the people may change their standard.'[2] And they are very likely to do so.

The changing standards, then, and their implications were clearly seen by most economists. What did the socialists think of it all? Surely those who thought like Marx must have been rather blind if they ignored this progress? Some of them did comment, and provided their own interpretations of the trend. Already Rodbertus, writing in 1850, had called poverty a social, i.e. a relative term, and this meant to him that the proper claims of labour to an existence minimum constantly

[1] Sir G. Rickards, op. cit., p. 251. Briaraeus (or Aegaeon) was a hundred-armed giant of classical mythology.

[2] W. Bagehot, *Economic Studies* (R. H. Hutton, ed., London, 1888), pp. 146–7, quoted in H. A. Boner, *Hungry Generations; the Nineteenth-Century Case Against Malthusianism* (New York, 1955), p. 187.

had to change. But if they changed, it meant that despite great material progress larger numbers than previously could be said to be 'worse off': 'es würde unrichtig sein . . . heute, wo sie diese höhere Stellung eingenommen haben, selbst bei gleichgebliebenem Lohne nicht von einer Verschlimmerung ihrer materiellen Lage zu sprechen'.[1]

So, too, Ferdinand Lassalle and Karl Kautsky realized that wants, deprivation, suffering, misery, all were relative terms. Kautsky distinguished between physical misery, measured in physiological terms, and social misery, measured by surveying contemporary ideas.[2] Only in such terms could Kautsky hope to save Marx's *Verelendungstheorie* against the onslaughts of non-Marxist socialists and liberals. But the distinction was by then becoming unreal. Everyone could see that there was comparative misery in Millionaires' Row. It was repugnant to common sense to speak of increasing misery when the standard of comfort even of the lowest ranks was constantly rising, even if the gap between them and the top layers was becoming larger—for that is the only mathematical explanation of Rodbertus's situation, where increasing numbers fall below the prevailing opinion of a minimum, whilst actually increasing their standards.

The whole problem of what is meant by a given standard of living and the interaction of population size, economic activity, and customary standards will occupy us again at the end of this book, largely as it is seen through the eyes of more recent writers. At this stage we may well leave the matter at the point where the nature of the problem began to be understood, and absolute terms were abandoned.

2. THE PROSPECT OF RISING

'A cheerful ascent is the movement which characterizes the progress of civilized society. The dolorous descent is the exceptional movement.' (RICHARD JONES)[3]

A completely closed class system would be difficult to imagine in any society. Even where the existence of castes introduces severe social differentiation, economic changes may well make members of 'lower' castes wealthier and thus enable them to some extent to be independent of the disadvantages which arise from their birth. But Western societies were never classified in this way even in theory. In practice, as we have

[1] K. Rodbertus, letter to J. v. Kirchmann, quoted by R. Michels, *Zur Beleuchtung der sozialen Frage* (1850), part i, p. 50, quoted in P. Mombert, *Bevölkerungslehre* (Grundrisse zum Studium der Nationalökonomie, Bd. 15, Jena, 1929), p. 446.

[2] Ibid., p. 447.

[3] Jones, op. cit., pp. 103–4.

seen, aristocracies died out and were replaced from below. Emperors had favourites, ghetto Jews became court physicians and financed bankrupt princes. Scriveners became bankers, and peasants' sons cardinals. Nevertheless, mobility was either insignificant, or at any rate not noticed by contemporaries, in most European societies until the end of the eighteenth century, so that the prospect of rising could not, in general, be listed as an important reason why men did not marry.[1]

But some acute observers could see the effects of ambition even then. Thus L. A. G. Schrader, in his *Grundgesetze der Natur*, published in 1777, a more profound work than the title, typical of its time, would indicate, describes quite accurately the process of 'keeping up with the Joneses'. As the lower ranks try to catch up with the standard of living of the higher ranks, so these in turn have to invent some new distinctions beyond the reach of their inferiors. But the upward press continues owing to the general desire to distinguish oneself. Is that not, he asked, the short history of all human endeavours, even in the field of scholarship?[2] This general desire to improve one's lot, which Malthus also noticed, is possibly universal, and it is certainly a powerful motive force in a society. But without some definite hope that such ambitions may be fulfilled, the effects are likely to be confined to a few exceptional people.

It is not possible to say with any precision what degree of mobility would be required to induce a given degree of reluctance to marry. At one end of the scale, the eighteenth-century Oxford scholar would know that marriage meant he would lose the chance of a fellowship, and at the other end an Austrian serf would not refrain from marriage because it might spoil his prospect of acquiring the domain. The higher the prize in the lottery, the greater may be the odds against winning without deterring a large number of gamblers. Where the degree of possible advancement is but slight, the vacancies would have to be many to instill prudence into any substantial number of men. But if the possibilities are infinite, such as they might well be in a revolutionary situation, even the fact that only very few of these glittering prizes

[1] The view that no human society was ever completely closed is advanced by many sociologists. See P. Sorokin, *Social Mobility* (New York, 1927), p. 139. This does not alter the fact that it is the degree of mobility, and the number of opportunities in relation to the total population, which determine any possible effects on marriage- and birth-rates.

[2] L. A. G. Schrader, *Grundgesetze der Natur in der Geburt, dem Leben und Tode der Menschen, als ein freyer Auszug, aus Süßmilchs göttlicher Ordnung in den Veränderungen des menschlichen Geschlechtes u. s. w. in veränderter Ordnung entworfen* (Glückstadt, 1777), p. 443.

might be available, would hardly fail to create ambitions in large numbers of men. We do not really know very much, as yet, about the exact degree of mobility attained in different societies in the last 200 years. One assumes that revolutionary France offered more chances of rapid promotion even than revolutionary America. But did the better prospects, say, of a non-commissioned officer in Napoleon's army mean that more of them remained unmarried, compared with their predecessors under Louis XVI or their contemporaries in the armies of Wellington or Blücher?

Looking at the history of the idea here examined, one can hazard a few guesses about the nature of this lottery. The 'exceptional gains', which have become so famous in the literature of economic history, almost invariably consisted of speculations, ranging from the comparatively innocent pastime of fitting out ships to trade in spices, to the devices of the feverish gambling period in the early eighteenth century. State and private lotteries, the Million Bank, the Tontines, the private gambling hells—these paths to advancement contained no marriage bar. To be successful one needed a certain amount of initial capital, but an abstemious mode of living was neither necessary nor, in the nature of things, desirable. We may pass over those who rose by personal favouritism in a corrupt society. How then did advancement come to be associated with honesty, thrift, independence, and all the virtues of the calendar, of which abstinence from marriage was only one? The answer lies in the economic development of the eighteenth century, which opened a way to wealth despised by those who waited for fortune by other routes, and therefore open to those who had little capital or vice. Not surprisingly, we look to Scotland to provide some of the earliest examples of the new attitude. But England, too, provided opportunities; and so in turn did each country where development took place. The necessary precondition for this general opportunity, of course, was a measure of reform. In the days of Elizabeth and the early years of James I, the successful exploitation of a patent was a matter of obtaining a crown monopoly, usually by corrupt means. Even when the worst abuses of the patent system were remedied, capital was readily obtainable only with the aid of wealthy patrons. The banking mechanism was not adapted to give credit to struggling inventors. Above all, opportunities were lacking for the small man, in the absence of a large home market. Large fortunes could be made by those with much initial capital out of the East India trade, or at home in the production of basic raw materials such as coal or iron. The real opportunity to rise by one's own efforts came when a growing population and improved transport facilities created a home market, an outlet for mass-produced consumer goods, and for services. It was a characteristic of this period of economic development that many of the new processes demanded very little capital at the start—in cotton, or hardware, or pottery, a man might start with the savings from a labourer's wage. Savings, that is, provided he did not marry. There is not space here to discuss the process in detail. But it is fairly clear that it was precisely when these opportunities arose to gain considerable economic advancement with very little capital, that observers began to note the new incentive for restraint.

The policy of the Scottish banks of advancing capital to young men chiefly on the security of a good character and a sound proposition helped to make the upward path easier.[1] By contrast, the English banks of the eighteenth century were criticized for not accepting small deposits from those who wished to save, and for refusing to lend except on elaborate guarantees. Adam Smith correctly saw the connexion between saving and the hope of rising:

> The principle which prompts to save is the desire of bettering our condition, a desire which . . . comes with us from the womb and never leaves us till we go into the grave. . . . An augmentation of fortune is the means by which the greater part of men propose and wish to better their condition.[2]

Smith did not go on to say that he thought this sort of ambition restrained population, but Adam Ferguson, his colleague at Edinburgh, included it amongst his checks:

> While arts improve, and riches increase; while the possessions of individuals, or their prospects of gain, come up to their opinion of what is required to settle a family, they enter on its cares with alacrity. But if this is not so, population is checked, or begins to decline.[3]

The Sheriff of Lanark was more explicit: after explaining that the

[1] See Sir J. H. Clapham, *An Economic History of Modern Britain* (Cambridge, 1926–38, 3 vols.), i. 269, quoting from *Select Committee on Promissory Notes in Scotland and Ireland, Report* (1826), p. 272, Evidence of a Scottish banker: '[Men could start with] a mere trifle, which trifle they have been known to make by their own industry.' This led to 'young men . . . from low situations . . . servants . . . farm-servants even . . . that . . . have raised themselves by becoming farmers of considerable extent, or manufacturers in a way highly creditable to themselves and beneficial to their country'.

[2] A. Smith, *An Inquiry into the Nature and Causes of the Wealth of Nations* (11th ed., London, 1805; E. Cannan, ed., New York, 1937, 2 vols.), ii, bk. ii, ch. iii, 20.

[3] A. Ferguson, *An Essay on the History of Civil Society* (1767; 4th ed., London 1773), p. 218.

descent to a lower rank in life is the greatest calamity that can befall an individual, he described it as 'the great object in life, in all ranks, to avoid this calamity: to rise to the enjoyments of a higher sphere . . .'.[1] An imprudent marriage is the surest way to defeat that hope. In the middle classes, the desire of rising further is the chief cause of moral restraint. (Alison does not trouble to distinguish, as Jones did, between moral and economic restraint.) So strongly, indeed, does it operate, that these classes are only kept in being by the continuous influx from below. The resulting society is mobile indeed, and the very hopes which led to restraint in the first place are dashed by the excessive competition of those crowding in from below.[2]

In France, as we have already seen, the prospects of a rise in social class were dim before the revolution. Only a few of the authors quoted by Spengler make more than a slight allusion to this phenomenon as a population check. Luxury, of course, is universally condemned, and one often finds the idea that men forbear to marry because they hope to drive their luxurious consumption to yet greater heights. But this does not involve any change in the composition of society. Thus Mirabeau seems to have grouped 'the desire for more goods and for higher social status for themselves and their children' in a general attack on concentrated wealth as a depopulating agent.[3] Only C. F. J. Auxiron may be said to have seen the problem clearly enough. It is significant that he, too, is the only one of the eighteenth-century authors to have discussed social mobility as such. He approved of such movement, and sanctioned postponement of marriage if its object was the desire to improve one's condition, but condemned it if the motive was fear of the future (i.e. presumably the fear of falling).[4] On the other hand he seems to have regarded this 'ascensional' movement as so strong already, that he condemned further artificial encouragement by excessive provision for the education of the lower classes and their consequent transfer to the higher classes—to the detriment of the latter, for they behaved in the way which Alison described, and suffered in consequence. The whole picture is in complete contrast to the rigid class structure assumed by most other writers of the time: Cantillon, Garnier, Helvetius, and Necker, to name only a few. It is true that some

[1] Alison, op. cit. i. 110.

[2] Ibid. i. 112.

[3] Spengler, *French Predecessors . . .*, p. 133.

[4] C. F. J. Auxiron, *Principes de tout gouvernment, ou Examen des causes de la splendeur ou de la foiblesse de tout état consideré en lui-même, et indépendamment des mœurs* (Paris, 1766, 2 vols.), ii. 306–14.

of the *philosophes* in particular thought of a society with more equal property distribution leading to prudential checks, and we shall discuss this in the appropriate section. Nevertheless, Auxiron remains somewhat isolated in his view.[1]

Turning to nineteenth-century England, we must begin with Malthus. We have already quoted his deprecating references to the hope of rising in the world—but we have also stated that he knew it to exist and to operate in the England of his own day. The Poor Laws, he thought, were bad—but they would be much worse if it were not for the fact that many people hope to do better than maintain their family on parish assistance. This was the famous *vis medicatrix rei publicae*. That it was not a mere afterthought is shown by the fact that it has its place again as the heading for the last chapter of the later editions: 'Of our rational expectations respecting the future improvement of society.' He stated blandly that marriages are not as frequent as they were in the days of constant wars and plagues. In England, especially, things had become much better since towns ceased to be the filthy places they had been.[2] (He seems to have known little about the new towns of the North, or the unimproved portions of those in the South.) The reason, he said, was that 'Universally, the practice of mankind on the subject of marriage has been much superior to their theories ...'. However much moralists preached the necessity of marriage, individuals acted differently. Once again he refers to the desire of bettering our condition in the sonorous Latin phrase. In his final peroration, all his hopes for the future were based on this wish:

> To the laws of property and marriage, and to the apparently narrow principle of self-interest which prompts each individual to exert himself in bettering his condition, we are indebted for all the noblest exertions of human genius, for everything that distinguishes the civilised from the savage state. A strict inquiry into the principle of population obliges us to conclude that we shall never be able to throw down the ladder by which we have risen to this eminence; but it by no means proves that we may not rise higher by the same means. The structure of society, in its great features, will probably always remain unchanged. We have every reason to believe that it will always consist of a class of proprietors and a class of labourers; but the condition of

[1] L. G. Du Buat-Nançay, *Éléments de la politique ou recherche des vrais principes de l'économie sociale* (London, 1773, 6 vols.), ii. 353 ff., had some reference to movements between the classes of day-labourers and very small proprietors and consequent prudence from fear or hope. But it is clear that he regards this as of limited importance. He also alludes to the desire of the wealthy to advance still further—but once again the whole picture is hardly that of social mobility.

[2] Malthus, op. cit. ii. 257.

each, and the proportion which they bear to each other, may be so altered as greatly to improve the harmony and beauty of the whole.[1]

It has often been remarked that Malthus is more full of contradictions than almost any other writer of his fame. He constantly nullifies in a footnote what has previously taken six pages to explain. The passage just quoted is a good example in this respect. On one hand there is a picture of mankind with strong moral tendencies, improving itself constantly—a society on a 'ladder'. (This may be taken to mean either the individuals within the society—a familiar political simile—or the society as a whole.)[2] On the other hand we have the allusion to the principle of population, the subject of the weighty volumes to which these phrases form a conclusion—a principle which appears to condemn mankind to misery and vice unless it can make prodigious efforts. About these efforts Malthus himself was always sceptical, as is shown in the correspondence with Senior. Again, he considers the class structure to be rigid, but he saves himself by saying that we might alter the proportions of proprietors to labourers. This can only mean that a number of labourers must eventually pass into the ranks of proprietors. (Unless he meant that labourers through moral restraint should diminish their numbers considerably, and proprietors increase theirs by prolific breeding and consequent subdivision. He can hardly have meant that—there would have been nobody to do the hard work for all these extra gentlemen.)

We can only conclude that Malthus was at least as much aware as his contemporaries that here was a powerful check indeed—but he could not afford to accord it the prominence it deserved, for it would have destroyed much of the force of his main argument.

We have already quoted Senior's description of the man who postpones marriage in the hope of rising in the 'unencumbered state', and who sees ever new goals on the horizon as he ascends. Elsewhere he spoke of the hope of acquiring, by the accumulation of a longer celibacy, the means of purchasing the decencies which give a higher social rank.[3] The hope of rising is closely connected with the ambition to do so, although they are not the same thing. Several writers noticed that although in a vague way many people would hope to improve their lot one day, the lower orders in particular did not seem to possess the

[1] Ibid. ii. 261–2.

[2] In the first edition of the *Essay* (p. 65) he used 'ladder' in the sense of a definite series of steps in the ascent of the individual, but here it *might* mean the progress of society.

[3] Senior, *An Outline of the Science of Political Economy*, p. 38.

driving ambition to do so—a much more active sentiment, strong enough to exercise the necessary check on marriage. '. . . the labouring classes should have a taste for comforts and enjoyments, and . . . should be stimulated by all legal means in their exertions to procure them' wrote David Ricardo.[1]

We have already referred to T. R. Edmonds's *An Enquiry into the Principles of Population*, published in 1832, which saw in the hopelessness of the poor population the chief threat of excessive fertility. Part of the author's elaborate system of removing this threat consisted, naturally, of new avenues along which the labourer might confidently march into comfort and prudence. Chapter VIII is devoted to the 'Means of enabling the Labourers to shape out work for themselves without Detriment to others'. This contains sections on the widening of channels of employment, enabling ingenious operatives to become master manufacturers, and providing skilled jobs for others.[2] Later parts deal with the provision of education through Mechanics Institutions, and even provincial universities. All this was designed to make the ascent in the social scale the *normally attainable goal of the working man.* Ambition, hopes, and the means of fulfilling them became one vast social system of upward movement.

W. F. Lloyd put the matter clearly:

> One great point with respect to the preventive check is a motive for procrastination, and this can only be looked for in the assured prospect of an advance in circumstances with the advance in age. A curate, who is without hopes of further advancement . . . marries at once upon his curacy. But if he has reasonable expectation of preferment, he is apt to feed himself with hope, and . . . to postpone his marriage. . . . The same principles are calculated equally to operate throughout all ranks of society.[3]

The practical question arose whether the industrial system of England was in fact fulfilling the required conditions. We have seen that most of the eighteenth-century French writers regarded their class division as fixed. The authors we have quoted so far in this section

[1] D. Ricardo, *Principles of Political Economy and Taxation* (London, 1821; 1895 ed.), p. 77.

[2] [T. R. Edmonds], *An Enquiry into the Principles of Population* . . . (London, 1832), pp. 169 ff.

[3] W. F. Lloyd, *Two Lectures on the Checks to Population, Delivered Before the University of Oxford in Michaelmas Term, 1832* (Oxford, 1833), lecture i, p. 62. Lloyd thought that emulation, the desire to imitate the example of others, lay at the back of much effort, (ibid., p. 74). We have seen that Alison expressed similar ideas. Further examples in Rickards, op. cit., p. 248: 'Not . . . fear of . . . distress; but . . . stimulus of social emulation.'

seemed to assume that in England mobility of this sort was an accomplished fact. The younger Samuel Laing cast some doubts on this. Having said that the only way of stopping the poor from increasing too fast was to raise their standard of living, he went on to ask why, for instance, the industrial system of Lancashire failed to produce this check. He came to the conclusion that under the old domestic system, a man might still have risen to be a manufacturer; but the factory system, with its requirement of starting capital, blocked this road.[1] Moreover, like Lloyd, he recognized the fact that trade fluctuations under the factory system removed the sense of security which had been the cause of stability in the social system, and thus further undermined the prudence which was already thin on account of the diminished prospect. We now know Laing to have been wrong; the factory system did not prevent small men from becoming masters, and trade fluctuations were not the only cause of instability work; had never been obtainable in a smooth and even flow even before the Industrial Revolution. But the ideas he put forward about the institutional framework of the rise, and the importance of a sense of security, are recognized as fundamental in the more elaborate systems which we shall outline later.

We have quoted Richard Jones's sanguine description of a civilized society at the beginning of this section. He certainly had no doubts as to the fact that the upward process was continuing: 'the multiplication of the newly risen, or rising, is a phenomenon which meets us on every side'.[2] Everywhere he noticed the habit of waiting for a better opening to secure the means to purchase ever higher orders of commodities. But he saw that the strength of this sentiment was not everywhere equally strong. Given a certain increase in the rate of wages, for instance, it could not be determined without reference to a large number of criteria, whether the effect would be what Malthus claimed, i.e. an increase in numbers, or a change in habits of consumption which in due course would lead to a reduction of population. One of the most important of these criteria was the question whether the social system of the country facilitated or impeded the free movement between classes.[3] Only where the chances of rising were good, could the refining effects of wage increase operate. In fact it was his constant assertion that the desire to postpone marriage was rarely an isolated phenomenon.

[1] S. Laing (the younger), *National Distress: Its Causes and Remedies* (London, 1844), p. 77.

[2] Jones, op. cit., p. 104.

[3] Ibid., p. 171.

With it went a general refinement of spirit and manners, a taste for the better things of life—we would now say, in the modern jargon, that the sex instinct could be sublimated. Hence the conclusion that the effects of postponement were cumulative—the longer a man abstained from marriage, the more he cultivated habits which were not easily forgone for the sake of a wife. But unless the primary conditions were fulfilled—that men should be able to satisfy secondary wants with the proceeds of higher wages, and that there should be a prospect of further advancement—these happy results would not follow.

In France and Germany the ideas which we have outlined are mostly to be found in the more complex theories which will form the subject of the next section. A number of writers were aware of the powerful effect of the prospect and desire for advancement in its own right. Robert v. Mohl, who obtained much of his stimulus from writers like Alison, added the urge to work oneself up into a higher class of society as an equal partner to the fear of falling from a given level, in the work of checking the expansion of population.[1] This laid a clear duty upon the state to do everything to facilitate, by economic and legal conditions, maximum production and free movement to attain it.

In France L. Passy noticed as early as 1831 in Normandy, before industrial changes took place, that the aim of parents was to restrict the number of children so that they could not only maintain the parental standard, but, if possible, advance to a higher level still. Ambition was the cause of depopulation. The city labourer could not aspire to anything—he could not buy a house however hard he saved. But the country labourer watches the sales of ever-smaller parcels of properties —he can by saving one day put himself or his children into a higher social position.[2]

By the end of the nineteenth century the importance of ambition was widely recognized. At least one French author, P. Leroy-Beaulieu, elevated *l'arrivisme* to a key position in his system. This is the desire

[1] R. v. Mohl, *Die Polizeiwissenschaft nach den Grundsätzen des Rechtsstaates* (Tübingen, 1866, 3 vols.), i. 93 ff.: 'Der Drang danach, sich in höhere Klassen der bürgerlichen Gesellschaft emporzuarbeiten.' He did not believe that this solved all population problems—he was well aware of the dangers of over-population and wished to regulate marriage accordingly. But this must be understood to apply in a society where the above-mentioned check was not yet operating strongly enough.

[2] L. Passy, in *Journal des économistes* (2nd ser., 1862), xxxvi. 425–7. Quoted in J. J. Spengler, *France Faces Depopulation* (Durham, North Carolina, 1938), p. 162. Spengler thinks that Passy is the best predecessor of Dumont. He quotes some eighteenth-century examples, ibid., pp. 46–48, showing ambition as a check to marriage. In England, by 1831, the idea was, of course, widespread.

to get to the highest possible position as fast as it can be done. It precludes children until one has 'arrived', and it means that the number of children will be limited so that they do not impair the success attained.[1] In Germany Paul Mombert elaborated on the effect of the possibility of advancing in the social scale in his *Bevölkerungslehre* (1929). In all these recent authors, the hope of rising becomes but one of many psychological factors operating in a given social framework.

We shall now turn, therefore, to the history of the institutional conception in which ambition and hope function: that of social capillarity.

3. SOCIAL CAPILLARITY AND VERTICAL MOBILITY

The ideas which we shall discuss in this section are commonly associated with the name of Arsène Dumont and other Frenchmen, and the state of French society at the end of the nineteenth century, which they described. Yet, in essence, a number of earlier writers had drawn attention to the idea.

The analogy is from the physical world: under the force of capillarity, liquids will rise in a very thin tube. Oil rises in a wick, and sap in trees in the spring. Under the same irresistible urge, families rise in the social scale. The process as such has already been described in this book. What is new here is the idea that it forms an autonomous principle in modern democratic (and capitalist) society. Capillarity is an inevitable law of nature—given the liquid, and the channel, and an outlet at the top, the process will automatically take place. As long as the tree is alive, nothing will stop the sap from rising. The notion of a self-destroying aristocracy or oligarchy fits in well with this concept—there is always room at the top, and those least encumbered with unnecessary luggage will rise fastest, all along the ladder, to take up the vacancies. Alternatively, we may picture a society in a state of continuous economic expansion. Income structure will be in the shape of the conventional pyramid, but as prosperity increases, so the upper sections of the pyramid will be larger, as more people come into those categories, and new layers will be added at the top. At the same time, what had previously been the lowest layer will shrink and disappear as those who composed it are promoted to a higher group. In this case we need not even assume that the top layers will consist of moribund

[1] P. Leroy-Beaulieu, *La Question de la population* (3e éd., Paris, 1913), p. 403. Similar ideas appear in many French writers, notably Gonnard and Landry. We shall not pursue the variants into the twentieth century.

families, though there is, of course, the constant threat to their position through excessive division of wealth amongst heirs. In a society such as we have described, the hope of rising, and the ambition to do so, will be well-nigh universal. Then the effects described by Dumont and others will be evident—the intense preoccupation with the possibility of advancement; the *arrivisme* of Leroy-Beaulieu.

The later periods of Greek and Roman history already provide abundant evidence of the existence of such movements, but only a scholar intimately acquainted with both classical literature and the concept itself could say with certainty whether it was recognized as such.[1] The manumission of slaves, the enfranchisement of aliens, the promotion of citizens within their different orders, the failure of noble families to reproduce themselves, and the astonishing career of some of the later Roman emperors are all parts of the process of rapid movement through the ranks of society which alone could give rise to the hopes and ambitions we have postulated as prerequisites.[2] Perhaps it reached its climax at the end of the second century of our era, when L. Septimius Severus became emperor of Rome—a man descended from African stock, and married to a Syrian wife, without connexions among the traditional Roman families.[3] Tacitus, the uncompromising aristocrat, condemning descendants of emperors for marrying (or not marrying!) commoners, is our witness for the opposite movement. The old divisions were no longer. But those who wrote about these events regretted them, and did not make a new social system out of them.

It will be seen that a democratic political system forms an integral part of the situation where capillarity operates.[4] To this extent we may say

[1] See the passage from Tacitus cited above (Ch. II, section 3) relating to the importance of freedom under conditions of political liberty.

[2] For modern descriptions see (Greece) W. W. Tarn, *Hellenistic Civilisation* (London, 1927), pp. 86 ff.; (Rome) O. Seeck, *Geschichte des Untergangs der antiken Welt* (Stuttgart, 1920–2, 6 vols.), i. 351; and M. I. Rostovtzeff, *The Social and Economic History of the Roman Empire* (Oxford, 1926), pp. 175–7 (promotion of equestrian orders), pp. 311–13 (manumissions). J. Beloch, 'Die Griechen bis auf Alexander den Großen', *Weltgeschichte: I, Geschichte des Altertums* (J. v. Pflugk-Harttung, ed., Berlin, 1910), pp. 301 ff., draws attention to the rise of the ex-tradesman in Athenian society in the fourth century—tanners and potters became great politicians.

[3] R. v. Pöhlmann, 'Römische Kaiserzeit und Untergang der antiken Welt', *Weltgeschichte: I, Geschichte des Altertums* (J. v. Pflugk-Harttung, ed., Berlin, 1910), p. 544, calls this the true end of the Augustan constitutional tradition.

[4] Dumont thought it essential. P. Sorokin does not consider that 'vertical mobility' is confined to democracies: op. cit., p. 138. Moreover, democratic societies may also be highly stratified.

that those writers who showed that an extension of political democracy tended to reduce fertility were forerunners of the whole notion. These will be treated below (Chapter V). Meanwhile we shall mention only those authors who may be said to have established a system of social mobility in which fertility declines.

Perhaps the earliest mention of this effect is to be found in the French writer, C. F. J. Auxiron. In an orderly account of political science, perhaps not quite as divorced from moral judgements as his title suggests,[1] he considered the question of an optimum population and came to ask himself how over-population might be prevented. Here he makes his significant suggestion, which is worth quoting in spite of the fact that it is rather an isolated instance of the thought and refers to what was then held to be an unlikely contingency: 'Les voies les plus naturelles et les plus douces que l'on puisse prendre sur cet objet (de prévenir l'excès de population) c'est d'inviter au célibat par des commodités, de favoriser le mouvement des classes. . . .'[2]

The way upwards lay through the *Collèges*, he thought, whereby many members of the working classes entered the higher professions, notably the priesthood, which was mostly recruited in this way. Auxiron clearly thought that the process had already gone a little too far: the superior classes suffered from excessive competition, the working class was enfeebled, unless its members were swelled again by those who had to descend from above as a result of the ascent of the others, since total wealth was fixed. But those families which were threatened with descent usually died out. His conclusion was that it would be best if manual workers did not go to college quite so much—let them stick to their fathers' trades. In the end, Auxiron seems to have been carried away a little by the prospect of social mobility, for he does not refer again to the point from which he started—that it was a useful check to over-population.

In Scotland we have James Grahame, whose *An Inquiry into the Principle of Population* appeared in 1816 in Edinburgh, a book at once stigmatized by Malthus as 'a slight work without any very distinct object in view'.[3] Grahame was essentially an optimist—like so many of Malthus's opponents, he neither believed that population would outrun subsistence, nor that any special steps should be taken to encourage a reduction of fertility. There was a process of elimination,

[1] Auxiron, op. cit. (for full title see p. 105, note 4). [2] Ibid. ii. 307 ff.

[3] Malthus, op. cit. (5th ed.), iii, Appendix, p. 388. It might be noted here that Grahame was a Scot, as of course was Alison; Jarrold, though English, was educated at Edinburgh.

he agreed, but it was part of a good design, for it weeded out the weak.[1] After an introduction dealing mostly with Malthus's ideas and other writers, his first chapter dealt with the structure of society in general.

> The population of a great state is, and ought to be, mainly replenished by the marriages of the lowest ranks; and it is essential to the moral and political prosperity of a country that the lower ranks should be always full.[2]

This is necessary, for the rich and the great have always failed to propagate themselves. So the upward movement from that great base of the pyramid is needed: 'The natural order of things is, that the higher ranks should be frequently and extensively recruited from the lower.'[3] In this way, national improvement and happiness will always be found to be in a progressive state. But if the lower orders are thinned out, movement might be the other way, with detrimental results. In his recapitulation, Grahame asserted that it was the mark of the crude state that aristocracies were fruitful and permanent—but in a commercial state like England mobility and progress went together: new upper classes were constantly recruited from below.[4]

Thomas Jarrold's *Dissertations on Man* appeared ten years earlier than Grahame's book, but his picture of society is not as complete as Grahame's. He adds, however, an important constituent part of our theory. A doctor practising in industrial Lancashire, he came to the conclusion that the very fact that men could rise and fall in society had an adverse effect on their nervous systems and hence on their powers of reproduction. It is easy to dismiss his diagnosis as nonsensical. But if one interprets his theories as meaning that those whose minds are most preoccupied with their fears and ambitions in this respect, have fewest children, we have a fair anticipation of the later propositions.

The anxiety state which he describes is very similar to that which was described by Leroy-Beaulieu more than a hundred years later. Honest men, he thought, did not become parents in the year in which they were adjudged bankrupts. The man who has climbed a few steps up on the ladder is filled with dread when he looks down. Descent is a 'forbidden path'. An educated person can never attune his mind to the

[1] J. Grahame, *An Inquiry into the Principle of Population: Including an Exposition of the Causes and the Advantages of a Tendency to Exuberance of Numbers in Society, a Defence of the Poor-Laws, and a Critical and Historical View of the Doctrines and Projects of the Most Celebrated Legislators and Writers, Relative to Population, the Poor, and Charitable Establishments* (Edinburgh and London, 1816), p. 166.

[2] Ibid., p. 96.

[3] Ibid., p. 97.

[4] Ibid., pp. 276 ff.

lot of a peasant. If he fails, therefore, he becomes a mere outcast. Like Grahame, Jarrold asserted that commercial aristocracies were infertile, but in his case the reason was precisely this preoccupation with their own insecurity.[1] We could not imagine the same fears having so strong an effect in any society not founded on the principle of rapid mobility described by Jarrold.

Archibald Alison has already been quoted several times for his opinion on social attitudes in a changing world. Arguing always from his own observations, he saw that the continuous influx of people from the lower classes into the 'middling ranks of society' was a fundamental law of nature:

> It is the continual pressure *from below* which occasions the excessive competition in every profession and business of life. Ask the physician, the lawyer, the tradesman, or the merchant, to what cause the difficulty which they experience in making their way in the world is to be ascribed, and they will all answer that it is the influx of persons into their professions from an *inferior rank* which creates the competition. If their numbers were to be recruited only from the descendants of their *own class* in society, comparatively little difficulty would be experienced. It is the constant wish of such classes, by positive or prohibitory regulations, to secure themselves from the effects of a competition which is felt to be so distressing. A vain attempt, to expect by human institutions to prevent the operation of the most important law which Nature has provided for the regulation of the numbers of mankind![2]

Here again we have an interesting anticipation of writers like Leroy-Beaulieu, especially with reference to the idea of intense competition in professional and commercial occupations. Doctors and lawyers were singled out by many authors, both because it was one of the favourite ambitions of poor young men to be one or the other (particularly in Scotland!) and because the time of highest earnings was not likely to be reached till middle age.[3]

What strikes the reader at once, when he turns to Jarrold or Alison after the French writers of the eighteenth century, is that the society they describe has been revolutionized. Quite obviously the professional and business people of their time depended on their own efforts for their position in life. Their anxiety concerned the success of their hard

[1] T. Jarrold, *Dissertations on Man* . . . (London, 1806), pp. 255–7, 262–9. See Leroy-Beaulieu, op. cit., esp. pp. 262–3. Many other writers have commented on the general characteristics of an advanced economic civilization.

[2] Alison, op. cit. i. 112.

[3] Leroy-Beaulieu, op. cit., pp. 220 ff., 263. Also: A. Dumont, *Dépopulation et civilisation. Étude démographique* (Paris, 1890), pp. 245 ff.—'Apreté de la concurrence illimitée'.

work. What a different world from that of the young James Boswell when he first arrived in London! No breakfasts with personages of consequence—rather, early rising and late study determined their reward. True, commissions could still be purchased in the army. The Civil Service reforms, and entry by examination were still to come. Many back doors still stood open. But while it was true that the path to advancement was not barred to the incompetent and vicious younger son, it was, on almost equal terms, open to ambition and talent. It depends on one's general outlook whether one thinks of early Victorian society as the almost unclouded paradise of the old ruling classes, or whether one is lost in admiration at the careers of the many newcomers. On one hand there are the aristocratic bishops, on the other hand there is Isaac Milner, Dean of Carlisle. There can be no doubt about the impression the situation created on contemporary writers. Was not Peel himself the grandson of a weaver? Robert Owen, the ex-apprentice of a Stamford draper, George Hudson, the upstart lion of society until he fell, the countless bag-of-oatmeal heroes of Samuel Smiles's widely read books—were they not evidence enough that the rise to the very top was possible for the young man of parts, and a rise of some sort almost inevitable? In short, what counts in the system of social mobility is the atmosphere, the spirit of the times, rather than the statistical evidence of the antecedents of those who eventually got to the top.

Since it was a systematizing age, it is not surprising to find that the common observation was elevated into a general law of nature by a good many writers, with far-reaching consequences. Thus, A. H. Moreton described a social pyramid of which he whole-heartedly approved. Himself the offspring of a noble family, and a Member of Parliament for his county, he was aware of the general tendencies of aristocracies and the infertility of the wealthy.[1] His book attempted to place fertility in relation to the status and occupation of human beings. His search was for 'a cause which retards the rate of increase in a greater proportion than the diminution of mortality quickens it'.[2]

The diminution of mortality, of course, was in itself the result of physical advance. But for the arrest of growth, we must look to the origin of the class structure at any given time.

[1] His own family did not die out. The Moretons became Earls of Ducie in 1837, and the line continues. The first Earl was a famous agriculturalist.

[2] A. H. Moreton, *Civilization, or, a Brief Analysis of the Natural Laws that Regulate the Numbers and Conditions of Mankind* (London, 1836), ch. vii, p. 129, on the effects of civilization upon the health, longevity, and increase of mankind.

If we look through the different grades of society, with the exception of the lowest, we shall find, that, in the majority of instances, the individuals who compose them derive their origin from families of a station below that which they at present hold.[1]

In one sense the observation is merely a truism, since only the most ancient and royal families could trace back their descent to persons of equal status for more than a few hundred years. But in its contemporary setting the statement has meaning. There were the countless new peerages, the yeomen's sons describing themselves correctly as gentlemen, the new iron and cotton masters. *John Halifax, Gentleman*, and *Pride and Prejudice*, were amongst the most popular books of the age. Not all could find security, but all could hope, and those who hoped helped to check population.

The result is the constant fear of losing status and the hope of rising further. (He quoted Grahame with approval on that point.) Not only marriages, but births would be reduced. Was this to be deprecated? By no means:

An inattentive observer . . . might think the facts of a differential birth-rate exceptions to the benevolence of Providence; yet they appear to have contributed more than any other cause to the happiness of mankind.

The gradual diminution of the numbers of the higher orders, without lessening their own enjoyment, leaves an access to wealth and honours open to all beneath them. Thus every man, by his own exertions, may hope to elevate himself to a state above that in which he was born. The son may raise himself another step.[2]

The writers we have quoted (and to them we could add most of those who were, in general, aware of the effects of ambition) may be said to have established a pattern of social change as being both natural and beneficial. Two developments follow. The one leads us to Darwin. For if in the development of the pyramid (or ladder), some only rise, others are weeded out. As Grahame pointed out, there is a period for the individual of 'probation of that noviciate of infancy—a rehearsal for roles in the after life'[3]—so that many must die before they reach adult age. Those who succeed, it is universally implied, must be the fittest for the social struggle ahead. None of the writers concerned, unfortunately, seems to have faced very clearly the problem of selection. How was it to be determined who were to be the lucky ones who moved up? Malthus himself had to some extent posed the question,

[1] Ibid., pp. 135–6. [2] Ibid., pp. 143–4.
[3] Grahame, op. cit., pp. 167–8.

but failed to answer it. Yet it is out of the discussion on the movements of human population that work on evolution, and eugenics, eventually arose.[1]

The other development was towards more closely reasoned explanations of fertility changes in human society. These were developed in France, and to a lesser extent in Germany, but, significantly, not in England. The essential difference between these new theories and the older ones is that they treat the same processes as if they were evils. The reason for this lies in the fact that the arrest of population increase in France was beginning to have unfavourable results for the country. Since the outcome was to be deprecated, the causes inherited the epithets originally applied to the results. It is the process of the eighteenth century reversed: what had been evidence of deterioration to the moralists, became virtues in the eyes of a world imbued with Malthusianism. Now the new-found virtues became vices. Jones's 'cheerful ascent' becomes a desperate struggle to advance. Where the English liberals had been glad to see the efforts of the individual, able to make his way by his own ability, Dumont deplored the cult of the individual at the expense of social solidarity.[2]

Arsène Dumont was a crusader—a man passionately interested in exposing the reasons for the decline of the French nation; anxious to introduce practical remedies to arrest it. But the explanation he devised was to have universal application. He based his work on very detailed statistical observations in various parts of France over a period of years. The results, nevertheless, were formed into a scheme extending over the whole of history and pre-history, and all human society. This meant that a great many of his conclusions had no foundations of fact at all. Thus his views on the relations between the occupations of fathers and sons are very different from those of writers who confined their theories to those which lent themselves to some statistical proof.[3]

Dumont's principal ideas which interest us here are those which follow from the views we have already outlined in England. His first

[1] For a discussion of this aspect see J. A. Field, *Essays on Population and Other Papers* (H. F. Hohman, ed. and comp., Chicago, 1931), pp. 71–76.

[2] This question will occupy us again in Ch. VII, when we discuss Spencer and other 'biological' theories.

[3] For a recent assessment of Dumont's work, with biographical details, see J. Sutter, 'Un Démographe engagé: Arsène Dumont, 1849–1902', *Population* (Jan.–Mar. 1953), viii, no. 1, pp. 79 ff. Further accounts of his and related theories in Spengler, *France Faces Depopulation*, pp. 156 ff.

proposition was that: 'Le progrès de la natalité est en raison inverse de la capillarité sociale.'[1] This is only an extension of the earlier observation, that men will limit their children in proportion to their prospects in life. The second proposition claimed that the higher the individual climbed on the social and economic ladder, the greater the sense of his own value and the greater his enjoyment of his advantages. The third then said that the more this individual progress went on, the less the nation benefited in numbers.[2] Fourthly, if there is a centre of culture, it will act as an attraction—social capillarity will have the effect of channelling the right people in that direction; the centre will gain in brilliance, and its attraction will increase. This proposition is in accord with the age-old belief that large towns—especially the seat of courts—are graves of population. Perhaps the Montmartre which Dumont had in mind was the equivalent of the Versailles of the eighteenth century.[3]

The fifth proposition concerns the relative influence of the pull of capillarity on those who are already somewhere near the top, and those who are far removed from it. The more distant the goal (and this can only happen in a democracy), the greater the effort made to get there, and the more devastating the effect on the individual. These are the 'rules of capillarity'. Dumont elaborated the system, the 'human form of the universal tendency to progress':

> Guidée par un instinct infaillible et fatal, chaque molécule sociale s'efforce avec toute l'énergie qui peut lui rester disponible . . . à monter sans cesse vers un idéal lumineux . . . comme l'huile monte dans la mèche de la lampe.[4]

The whole thing results in the break-up of the family—unlike the Chinese situation, where the denial of the individual results in enormous fertility (compare Cantillon's explanation of the same facts). Whatever obstacles there may be, democracy does away with them. In the democratic state (see Alison's model) knowledge and ambition filter down rapidly from above. New classes enter political life and thus add to the spheres where men may reach the highest goals. In the economic world,

[1] The 'propositions' will be found in Dumont, op. cit., p. 130.

[2] Spengler, *France Faces Depopulation*, p. 158, mistranslates the third proposition. There is no mention of 'rationality' in it (the word is meaningless in any case); the French version is 'en nombre *est* en raison inverse', not '*et* en raison'.

[3] Spengler's inference (by the use of the word *hinterland*) that Dumont meant a geographical centralization only, is unnecessary. The *foyer de culture* of the original may well refer to a centre of activity within a given locality. The analogy is from the physical world: 'un point où convergent les rayons lumineux après réflexion ou réfraction' (*Larousse*).

[4] Dumont, op. cit., p. 106.

where wealth signifies individual superiority, all legal obstacles have long been removed. In the intellectual world the same thing applies.

Dumont had much to say on the influence of religion and philosophy in their effect on the character and ambition of the individual. There is no opportunity here to discuss these theories in detail, though we shall return to some of them under other headings. Many of them were so wildly wide of the mark when compared to the facts (e.g. his differential fertility of religions) that it is not surprising that Dumont has been so largely ignored or vilified.[1] At least he had this merit: that he drew attention to the need for investigating individual attitudes in their social context in order to determine national population trends. At a time when many scholars (notably in Germany) were still floundering in discussions of potential fertility and agricultural productivity, Dumont firmly steered thought towards social psychology.

His compatriot, P. Leroy-Beaulieu, starting from the idea of 'civilization', expressed very similar views in relation to the effects of a system where the individual could normally expect to rise, and consequently had ever larger ambitions.[2]

> L'absence de toute résignation à rester dans la condition où l'on a été placé par le sort, ainsi que l'effroyable concurrence dans toutes les professions intellectuelles, accrue et développée avec soin par les stupides encouragements de l'État moderne, retarde, d'ailleurs, de plus en plus l'âge des mariages, presqu'en tout pays, ce qui affaiblit . . . la fécondité matrimoniale.[3]

> Ce qui nous semble distinguer les départements les plus improlifiques de France, c'est un trait différent de caractère, c'est un trait opposé, à savoir, en employant un terme nouveau qui mérite d'être retenu parce qu'il est expressif, c'est *l'arrivisme*, l'esprit *arriviste*, la tendance à se pousser le plus haut possible et l'idée que d'une part, il ne faut pas s'embarrasser d'enfants pour arriver soi-même haut et rapidement et que, d'autre part, si l'on veut que sa progéniture arrive haut et vite, il convient de concentrer les efforts et la fortune sur une ou deux têtes seulement, plutôt même sur une que sur deux.[4]

Here we have the whole disease of French society analysed—yet once again we see that the sentiment is extremely old—Polybius is close to

[1] But some authors, notably Dr. Enid Charles, give him his due.

[2] Leroy-Beaulieu, op. cit., esp. p. 220. For a review, see Spengler, *France Faces Depopulation*, pp. 163 ff. and *passim*.

[3] Leroy-Beaulieu, op. cit., pp. 262–3. In a footnote to the above passage, he says that state encouragement is not surprising, seeing that politicians form, with certain exceptions, 'une des classes les plus viles et les plus bornées de sycophantes et de courtisans qu'ait jamais été connues à l'humanité'—i.e. social climbers *par excellence*.

[4] Ibid., p. 403.

Leroy-Beaulieu.[1] In some form or other, these considerations were to be mentioned by many authors after 1900. It may perhaps be appropriate to mention one other author who introduced a new term into the discussion, and at the same time contrived to reunite the two developments of the old argument which we described—the Darwinist, and the Dumontian. This was K. A. Wieth-Knudsen, a Dane, whose work was published in 1908.[2] For him, society became ever more like the 'struggle for existence' as the division of labour progressed—a social progress of selection takes place in which individuals try to improve their position by such doubtful expedients as saving. There is no such thing as certain 'progress', as the result of this process. But there is present all the time, despite the possibility of simultaneous degeneration, a constant social force which he calls *opdrift* (German *Auftrieb*), upward or rising drift or tendency. Wieth-Knudsen introduces a long series of works where the social and biological explanations are intermarried, and which fall beyond the scope of this essay.[3]

In this chapter we have tried to trace the history of the idea of a developing society, through the individual's prospect of a rising standard of living, and the hope of rising in the world, to the stage where such notions are elevated into complete social systems—explanations of the progress of society as such. In the following chapters we shall attempt to work out the history of preconditions for the operation of a prudential check—notably the political and social characteristics of such mobile societies.

[1] For the modern French ideal of a two-child family, see E. de Goncourt, *Renée Mauperin*, quoted by P. Ariès, *Histoire des populations françaises et de leurs attitudes devant la vie depuis le XVIIIe siècle* (Paris, 1948), p. 482. 'Elle s'avait arrangée pour avoir deux enfants.' The third was too much; it interfered with the fortune of the others.

[2] K. A. Wieth-Knudsen, 'Formerelse og Fremskridt, økonomisk-demografisk-biologisk Syntese . . .'. See *Politisch-anthropologische Revue* (Hildburghausen, 8. Jahrgang, 1909–10), pp. 150–1, from which this summary is taken.

[3] See G. Mackenroth, *Bevölkerungslehre; Theorie, Soziologie und Statistik der Bevölkerung* (Enzyklopädie der Rechts- und Staatswissenschaft. Abteilung Staatswissenschaft, Berlin, 1953), ch. iii, esp. pp. 239 ff. 'Siebungs- und Auslesevorgänge.'

V

THE POLITICAL AND SOCIAL BASIS OF VOLUNTARY RESTRAINT

I. THE DIFFUSION OF PROPERTY AND EQUALITY OF INCOME

ARSÈNE DUMONT consciously connected the race to attain economic goals with the existence of political and social systems in which such movements could alone take place. In this he was not the first. We have already shown a number of writers who assumed, or expressly postulated, a high degree of mobility amongst the classes. Thus two arguments are closely connected: that the possibility of economic advancement acts as a check to population; and that the diffusion of property, an increase in equality and democracy, will act in the same way. In the first case, the existence of the necessary political institutions is tacitly assumed; in the second, it is supposed that certain economic movements will follow, which in turn lead to the checks already discussed.

Yet we have here no mere variant upon the old theme. For in describing the importance of matters which relate to the state and its laws, we also re-enter the field of policy from which all population theory once began. In a totalitarian state, it is open to governments to advance selected individuals out of each class and thus create the hopes which may check the progeny of their fellows. But then in such an arbitrary system children may not be a handicap—on the contrary, we have numerous examples of just such promotion being reserved for those with large families. Rarely have bachelors been favoured by official intent. In a society, however, where governments seek to achieve their end by more indirect means of intervention, the only policy open to the state which wishes to put a term to the rapid expansion of the property-less and hopeless classes, is to achieve those conditions of equality and opportunity which will have the effects already described. Conversely, those who were alarmed at the fall of the birth-rate during the last century were not slow to attribute this fall to an excess of enthusiasm for the ideals of the French Revolution. It is only a short step from this reflection to the demand for a less egalitarian society, free from the dangers of national degeneracy. The movement reached its climax in the Nazi state with its insistent demand for 'more children for the Führer' and the complete denial of individual rights to those outside the party hierarchy.[1]

It must be stated at the outset that at any rate until the end of the eighteenth century, it was almost universally believed that concentration of property in few hands led to depopulation, and that a greater measure of distribution would lead to more marriages and births. We have already seen that the notion that the 'have-nots' were particularly prolific emerges in a clear form in the industrializing phase. In France in particular, where by far the most trenchant criticism of inequality was born, the idea was universal that redistribution of property would lead to greater fertility. Since most writers considered these matters as part of a moral system, it was natural that they should sweepingly condemn together the two evils of inequality and depopulation. With these they associated many other social and political ills.

There is a temptation, therefore, to ascribe the change in the prevailing view of the effects of greater equality, which occurred in the Malthusian period, to mere opportunism: equality was desirable; therefore in the age of fears of depopulation it is offered as a remedy for that evil, and in the next age confidently advertised as the cure for the opposite ill. But this view is superficial. It would be much more correct to say that the majority of the early writers had no means of testing their theories. They accurately observed societies composed of a few wealthy landowners and large numbers of land-starved or landless labourers, ranging from a state of absolute serfdom to a precarious independence of *metayage* or copyhold and cottage. In the towns they also saw a property-less mass of wretches, and such were the uncertainties of the lives of these masses that the population did not increase very rapidly (though much more rapidly than most of the writers believed). Since contraception did not form part of their world, and since in fact in rural societies the custom of marrying as soon as one could get a cottage or holding was widespread, their deduction that additional tenancies would help the birth-rate was quite logical.

Moreover, what we know about the population increase of the

[1] For a good example of this attitude, see T. Valentiner, 'Die seelischen Ursachen des Geburtenrückganges', *Politische Biologie, Schriften für naturgesetzliche Politik und Wissenschaft* (München–Berlin, 1937), Heft 2, p. 57 (speaking of the 'kinderverneinender Liberalismus'): 'Unter Liberalismus verstehe ich die Geisteshaltung, die dem Einzelnen das Recht zugesteht, sich sein Leben so einzurichten, wie es ihm paßt, ohne Rücksichtnahme auf die Nächsten und die Volksgemeinschaft.' Valentiner is one of the many who quote Polybius to chastise social conditions they dislike and to advocate stronger remedies.

period of the Industrial Revolution in England lends a good deal of support to the older theory. Many authorities have advanced the view that in rural areas the decline of the system of servants living-in, and the spread of cottages, and in urban areas the decline of apprenticeship, helped to foster earlier marriage and also increased the total proportion of people marrying. If the lack of a place to live, or the difficulty of obtaining a situation in trade, were obstacles to marriage, then the altering economic system did cause an increase in population, as well as being one of its consequences. Many writers have pointed to the fact that one of the easiest ways of starting a family was to go to the United States, obtain a homestead, and then produce as many children as possible, since they were an asset on the holding. If one hears little in the United States about the harmful effects of ownership on the birth-rate, it was presumably because each son who wanted a holding of his own could get one, without subdivision of the parental farm.

The diffusion of property in the nineteenth century, however, was the result of different forces, and took place against the background of a different social structure. Essentially, the reformist writers had called for a living, a minimum subsistence, some elementary security for the oppressed masses. But the demand of the nineteenth century was not for a minimum—that had been provided by the Speenhamland system and proved disastrous to self-respect and order. What was required now was a standard of decencies, to use the Senior phrase. Equality in the respectable age meant the chance for every man to become respectable, too. From this, caution about marriage and offspring followed quite naturally. It could be expected that the advocates of greater equality should put it forward as one of the points in its favour that it would help to ward off the Malthusian menace. This is no *volte-face*; it is a justified expectation. And once again the facts bore out their contentions—France, where peasant proprietorship and petty bourgeois decencies were most widespread, first saw the arrest of population growth. In England and Germany the break came later—but then only a very small minority of families in either country could be said to have benefited from economic expansion in any sense other than that the idea of an acceptable minimum changed with time.

Before the eighteenth century the connexion between the distribution of property and the numbers of men had only been given scant attention. Aristotle had criticized Plato's *Laws*, in which it was proposed to have a fixed and indivisible number of estates, each held by a citizen. Since no provision could thus be made for any number of children in excess of those who could be found a vacancy officially through the death of their father or a childless citizen, it would be necessary to limit the number of children. The implication here is the one which thinkers accepted until recent times: the number of holdings varies directly with the marriage- and birth-rates.[1] It does not seem to have occurred to Plato or Aristotle that under such a system men would wish to restrict the number of children even without governmental edict, to spare them the shame of poverty. That poverty, vice, and disorders would result, Aristotle did not doubt, and from this Malthus later concluded that the Stagirite would have agreed with his theories, particularly with regard to the proposition that systems of equality cannot succeed unless accompanied by strict control of population.[2]

Hume and Wallace were at least agreed in their acceptance of this idea, that equality was favourable to population. Hume thought that a man with a large estate would be in a more precarious situation, and therefore less likely to marry, than a man with a small but secure property.[3] Wallace concurred, and said that for the same reason he was in favour of the equal division of property amongst a man's children. This is in line with his condemnation of the system of primogeniture, which we have already described.[4]

Most French writers of the period contributed germs of the later notions of the effects of equality—without ever doubting, however, that the immediate effect of redistribution of property would be an increase in population.[5] Claude Helvetius (1715–71),

[1] Aristotle, *Politics*, bk. ii, ch. vi. A solitary early example of the realization that equal division of property leads to depopulation is William Temple, the Trowbridge clothier, previously quoted. In *A Vindication of Commerce and the Arts* (1768; reprinted in *A Select Collection of Scarce and Valuable Tracts on Commerce* (J. McCulloch, ed., London, 1859)), p. 510, he censured the institutions of Lycurgus, precisely because they had depopulated Sparta. Unfortunately he does not make it clear why he thinks so, but the context leads one to suppose that he saw the point which Aristotle missed.

[2] How far Aristotle anticipated Malthus has been discussed widely. See L. v. Bortkiewicz, 'War Aristoteles Malthusianer?', *Zeitschrift für die gesamte Staatswissenschaft* (June 1906), lxii. 383.

[3] D. Hume, 'Of the Populousness of Ancient Nations', *Essays and Treatises on Several Subjects* (1752; new ed., Edinburgh, 1825, 2 vols.), i. 393–4.

[4] R. Wallace, *A Dissertation on the Numbers of Mankind, in Ancient and Modern Times* (Edinburgh, 1809), Appendix, p. 168. Also pp. 17–18.

[5] J. J. Spengler, *French Predecessors of Malthus* (Durham, North Carolina, 1942), p. 73 (Argenson); p. 84 (Danguel); p. 101 (Moheau); p. 252 (D'Holbach); p. 258 (Saint-Pierre); p. 273 (Forbonnais), &c. Moheau ingeniously suggested that emulation was possible only where inequality prevailed—we will not be prudent to keep up with the Jones's unless the Jones's are better off than we are. Alison later used precisely the same point to advocate greater diffusion of property! Amongst Italian writers, both Beccaria

a materialist philosopher of education and a forerunner of Marx, demanded an increase in the number of proprietors by redistributing land to the property-less labourers, whose low wages and misery made it difficult for them to marry.[1] Yet the contrast he draws between the large masses of the labourers and the small number of exploiting proprietors seems to suggest that something other than the normally assumed relationship between property and fertility might exist. Certainly Malthus, for all his belief in the positive correlation between income and fertility, thought of the acquisition of property as leading to greater prudence. But on the whole the pre-revolutionary demand for greater equality and an end to exploitation was designed to increase the population, and the reiteration of the demand for precisely the opposite purpose did not come till later.[2]

Condorcet (1743–94), one of the two utopian writers who provoked Malthus's first *Essay*, provides us with the transitional view on the connexion between equality and fertility. Under conditions of moral and physical progress, he thought, human life would be prolonged, and this would eventually result in a diminution of the desire to propagate the species. Eventually, rational Man would come to count happiness as more important than existence.[3] This state of affairs strikes us as being very different from the sort of economic calculations with which we became familiar. Under Condorcet's system, it is an unselfish concern for the general well-being of society, not a preoccupation with one's own or one's children's fortunes, which dictates restraint. For the nearest cousin to this noble sentiment, we must look to the man whose wrath Condorcet aroused—Malthus himself. Naturally, Malthus would have condemned the loose sexual conduct which Condorcet envisaged. But the idea of a society based on mutual regard and prudent conduct as a result is surely arch-Malthusian! In the very counterblast to Condorcet, the first *Essay*, Malthus conceded something of Condorcet's preconditions: where he spoke of the fear of a descent in society, which would keep a man from marrying without proper means, he followed

and Filangieri (d. 1787) believed that population would increase through redistribution. (See C. E. Stangeland, *Pre-Malthusian Doctrines of Population; a Study in the History of Economic Theory* (New York, 1904), pp. 294–5, 333.)

1 Spengler, op. cit., pp. 245–9.

2 Ibid., pp. 323, 337 (Necker and Linguet).

3 M.-J.-A.-N. de Caritat, Marquis de Condorcet, *Sketch for a Historical Picture of the Progress of the Human Mind* (1795; J. Barraclough trans., London, 1955), pp. 173 ff., esp. pp. 181–9.

this statement of fact with a warning: 'If society be held desirable, it surely must be free, equal, and reciprocal society, where benefits are conferred as well as received; and not such as the dependent finds with his patron, or the poor with the rich.'[1]

William Godwin also believed that the new order of equality would lead to a change in habits of reproduction. This does not mean that he was in favour of giving property to all to hold. In one sense he still leans heavily on the former view: property, being at the root of inequality, is a check on the indefinite expansion of population. It means that the resources of the earth are not fully used. But where the earlier writers then envisaged the desired increase in population following from redistribution, Godwin's abolition of the old form of private property was to lead to an increase only in the short run, and eventually to a stationary population. In his first consideration of the question, in his *Political Justice*, he may be said to stand near to Condorcet's position. He believed that the check to unlimited expansion of population was a natural principle which would operate in the dim distant future when the world should be full—he was much taken with Benjamin Franklin's idea that mind could become omnipotent over matter, and that procreation, like pain and sleep, was a conquerable human foible. Malthus having described the absurdity of this proposition in the *First Essay*, Godwin promptly changed his ground, and as we have seen in his reply to Parr's *Spital Sermon*, used the usual arguments concerning the prudence of enlightened man—a sentiment which might be anything from moral virtue to mere pride.

To Malthus's particular objection to a system of equality—that it would lead to selfish people throwing their extra children as a burden on the community—he replied that in the society which he envisaged the universal atmosphere of benevolence towards others would lead individuals to reason differently. Godwin made the best of both worlds; whether it was from motives of individual concern, or from moral causes, the just society would never suffer from excessive population. Godwin stands, in a way, at an important cross-roads—the utopian socialists, and later some of the Marxists, relied upon a new attitude to society to prevent the indefinite growth of population. The economists, on the other hand, came to emphasize the advantages of self-regarding prudence. In the first tradition, Godwin is a link with the idealists of the French Revolution. In the second, he is the man who argued with

[1] T. R. Malthus, *An Essay on the Principles of Population* (Everyman ed., 1914, 2 vols.), i. 236.

Malthus, in the main-stream of English social and economic thought. The gap which separates the protagonists is not so great.[1]

In France in the nineteenth century a new turn was given to the development of views on the effects of property by the provisions of the *Code Civil* (since 1804) which removed the old testamentary freedom and made an equal division of landed property amongst all heirs compulsory. The result was soon seen to be an increased anxiety, on the part of landholders, to avoid minute subdivisions by reducing the number of possible heirs. Two lines of thought follow. One concerns the new type of family associated with this system. This was developed by Le Play and will be discussed later. The other idea is the simpler one that in all societies those who hold property are prudent, and that hence the diffusion of property would arrest population increase. To some extent such arguments apply universally, even where there is no legal division of heritable property—we have already seen that many eighteenth-century writers equally attacked the right of primogeniture as being unfavourable to population, in view of the difficulties of placing younger sons in suitable employments. In other words—those who hold land will seek to keep it intact and unencumbered. The threat may come either from the duty to divide such land on death, or from the custom of charging the estate to provide settlements for younger children.[2] As A. Legoyt wrote in 1847:

> It is, besides, the anticipated consequence of our civil and social institutions which, in bringing about each day a greater sub-division of the territorial and personal fortunes of France, develop in the breast of the population instincts of conservation and well-being. With a more equal distribution of wealth . . . due to our civil laws . . . the spirit of order and conservation tends to propagate itself.[3]

[1] Godwin's place in the controversy is discussed in C. Brinkmann, ed., *William Godwin—Robert Malthus* (Stuttgart, 1948). For the views of other English socialists on the growth of prudence in an enlightened society, see for instance W. Thompson, *An Inquiry into the Principles of the Distribution of Wealth Most Conducive to Human Happiness; Applied to the Newly Proposed System of Voluntary Equality of Wealth* (London, 1824), p. 536. But he was not convinced that it would work without artificial aids.

[2] The whole question is discussed in J. J. Spengler, *France Faces Depopulation* (Durham, North Carolina, 1938), pp. 148 ff. He quotes there some early views on the effects of forcible distribution of property. It is open to doubt whether the *Code Civil* aggravated an existing problem, or merely perpetuated it. The intense desire for land always meant a tendency to produce bidders for small plots, and then a grim fight to keep them intact or possibly to augment them. A low birth-rate would solve the contradiction involved. A. France (according to Spengler, ibid., p. 153) quoted Rabelais as saying that parents place children in monasteries, &c., to avoid splitting up the property.

[3] A. Legoyt, in *Journal des économistes* (1st ser., 1847), xvii. 174 ff., 190. Quoted in Spengler, *France Faces Depopulation*, pp. 110–11.

The observation was made elsewhere. Sir Francis d'Ivernois had described the low birth-rate of certain areas in French-speaking Switzerland and had attributed it to moral restraint. But the elder Laing had criticized this view:

> Is it not more reasonable to suppose that the possession of property has given to the whole population the habits of caution and prudence, and the use of gratifications of civilised life, which necessarily postpone marriages until a later period of life, and until a property is acquired adequate to the higher standard of living introduced by this universal diffusion of property?[1]

The conclusion is obvious:

> Give the poor property, as a class, by abrogating the feudal law of succession, and all other impediments to the widest diffusion of property through society, and the moral and economic restraints arising from property . . . would postpone their marriage age. . . .

Laing went on to assert boldly that he thought the reason for the declining number of births in France was to be found in the expanding class of small proprietors.[2]

The same policy was advocated by a number of writers, often to express opposition to Malthus's demand for a reduction of cottages and his defence of existing distribution of property.[3] Amongst the English writers who suggested smallholdings was W. T. Thornton (1813–86), a widely travelled man who saw service with the East India Company and later at the India Office. Like so many people in his age, he was seriously perturbed about the spectacle of continuing poverty in the midst of an expanding economy, and refused to accept the simple Malthusian wage-fund theory that the remedy lay in the labourer's own hands—that if they refrained from marriage and procreation, their

[1] S. Laing (the elder), *Notes of a Traveller on the Social and Political State of France, Prussia, Switzerland, Italy, and Other Parts of Europe, During the Present Century* (London, 1842), p. 347. The reference is to Sir F. d'Ivernois, *Enquête sur les causes patentes ou occultes de la faible proportion des naissances à Montreux* (Geneva, 1837).

[2] Ibid., pp. 349–50. In an earlier chapter on France, Laing had stated that Arthur Young's prediction, that France would become a 'pauper warren' through subdivision, had not come true. Laing's explanation of the observed fall in the birth-rate is certainly among the earliest on record. See also ibid., p. 46. In a later work, *Observations on the Social and Political State of the European People in 1848 and 1849* (in *Notes of a Traveller* (ser. 2, London, 1850)), Laing lost some of his enthusiasm for small property.

[3] For his opinions on cottages in his evidence to the Emigration Commissioners, see K. Smith, *The Malthusian Controversy* (London, 1951), p. 313. His views on private property, and its superiority over common or equally divided land, are most concisely stated in *A Summary View of the Principle of Population* (London, 1830; reprinted in *Introduction to Malthus* (D. V. Glass, ed., London, 1953)), pp. 143–9.

incomes would rise. Instead, he pointed out, as others had done, that it was the hopelessness of the situation of the masses that caused their apparent recklessness, and so, in his two books on *Overpopulation and Its Remedy*, and the *Plea for Peasant Proprietors*, campaigned for a well-organized system of allotments and smallholdings which were to create pride and prudence amongst the many.[1] If the world were inhabited only by people of property, he wrote, it would probably soon become depopulated by natural failure of the species.[2]

Thornton wielded great influence on thought mainly through his intimate friendship with John Stuart Mill, and was the instrument of Mill's conversion away from the wage-fund theory.[3] Mill had, as is widely known, taken a lively interest in Malthusian problems throughout his life, and may, like Thornton and others, be called a modified follower of the Malthusian doctrine. But on this point of the importance of property Mill differs from Malthus. He admits that a mere redistribution would accomplish nothing in the long run.

> If all instruments of production were held in joint property by the whole people, and the produce divided with perfect equality among them, . . . there would be enough to make all the existing population extremely comfortable; but when that population had doubled itself, as, with the existing habits of the people, under such an encouragement, it undoubtedly would in little more than twenty years, what would then be their condition?[4]

But he believed, more than Malthus, that the existing habits could be modified—by raising the standard of living. If they could be given the means of earning a higher income, this change might be induced.[5] Thornton's suggestions thus found an echo in Mill. Had not Malthus himself praised the habits of peasant communities in Norway and Switzerland?[6]

Thornton had taken some of his best examples of the prosperity of smallholders from the Channel Islands, and Mill warmly recommended his readers to investigate the happy system of proprietorship prevailing

[1] W. T. Thornton, *Over-population and Its Remedy; or, An Inquiry into the Extent and Causes of the Distress Prevailing among the Labouring Classes of the British Islands, and into the Means of Remedying It* (London, 1846). And: *A Plea for Peasant Proprietors, with the Outlines of a Plan for Their Establishment in Ireland* (London, 1848).

[2] Thornton, *Over-population and Its Remedy* . . ., p. 119.

[3] Sir L. Stephen, *The English Utilitarians* (London, 1900, 3 vols.), iii. 203 ff.

[4] J. S. Mill, *Principles of Political Economy* (6th ed., London, 1902), part i, bk. 1, ch. xiii, para. 2, p. 118.

[5] On this, see Stephen, op. cit. iii. 184.

[6] See Malthus, *Essay on Population* . . . (Everyman ed.), i, bk. 2, chs. i and iv.

in these islands.[1] He believed that to be a small proprietor was a form of education in itself, and thus fulfilled another requirement for the acquisition of prudent habits. But the main result was the emergence of 'prudence, temperance, and self-control'.[2] The outcome must be clear: a check on population. True, other writers had thought exactly the opposite was correct. Not only the French writers, but McCulloch and even the sagacious Richard Jones had mistaken the effects. Mill attacked them heavily—he believed their error might be due to observations in cases where peasants had enough land only for a low standard of living. There, of course, the checks would not operate. But if the peasant is in a comfortable position, he knows that subdivision will yield an insufficient living for his children: thus he will endeavour to preserve the holding intact, and, if possible, to augment it. Mill quoted approvingly from Laing's book:

> It is the depending on chance, where judgment has nothing clearly set before it, that causes reckless, improvident marriages in the lower, as in the higher classes, and produces among us the evils of over-population; . . . as it is, where certain subsistence is, by our distribution of property, the lot of but a small portion instead of about two-thirds of the people.[3]

Mill was evidently familiar with the earliest statistical investigations of the connexion between property and fertility, for he quotes Legoyt and Léonce de Lavergne in his later editions (as did Thornton).[4] And so he concludes:

> As the result of this enquiry . . . I conceive it to be established, that there is no necessary connexion between this form of landed property and an imperfect state of the arts of production; . . . [and] that no other existing state of agricultural economy has so beneficial an effect on the industry, the intelligence, the frugality, and prudence of the population, nor tends on the whole so much to discourage an improvident increase of their numbers; . . .[5]

The Malthusian in Mill had found a satisfactory remedy for the great evil. But there was also the socialist in Mill—the man who wanted something done at once to accomplish the reform he had in mind. Did not all this involve redistribution (for landowners would not willingly

[1] See Thornton, *A Plea for Peasant Proprietors* . . ., pp. 99–104, and J. S. Mill, op. cit., pp. 167–8. Like Thornton, Mill warned against excessively small properties (ibid., p. 171).

[2] Mill, op. cit., p. 173.

[3] Ibid., p. 175, quoting from Laing, *Notes of a Traveller*. . . .

[4] Legoyt's article appeared in 1847, and de Lavergne's work from 1855 onwards. For details, see Spengler, *France Faces Depopulation*, pp. 110–13.

[5] Mill, op. cit., p. 182.

raise a class of peasant competitors to disfigure the countryside), great systems of education, the colonization of new lands? We cannot here discuss what this conflict involved, or how far Mill solved it. But no other author on the connexion described here conveys so exactly what underlies the economic checks—a political system within which they are free to operate.

The doctrine of Mill was taken up in literary form by Charles Kingsley—whose burning Christian zeal against the deadly teaching of Malthus formed a proper counterpart to Mill's measured thinking. The answer to wretchedness is in part soberness and prudence, he admits, but it is also organization and reform, whether through Chartism or otherwise. That was the message of *Alton Locke*. But it is more in the novel in which he deals with rural economy, *Yeast* (first published in 1848), that Kingsley clearly describes how a man may be saved from folly by property. It is when the hero, Lancelot, contemplates the fate of the poacher, Grawy, that he comes to think of the difference ten acres of farmland might have made to him earlier in life. It was the system of landlords who took all the available farms into their own hands and then failed to make the most of them, that created a discontented agricultural proletariat and at the same time kept the country short of food—were the landlords efficient, they could compete with foreign corn; as it is, they must exclude it by heavy duties if they can (but the Corn Laws had just been repealed).[1]

Sismondi, too, had recommended the remedy of property. Under systems where the father had property, and the law made him divide it equally amongst his sons:

> he sees the limit beyond which this division would make them descend from the rank which he has himself filled, and a just family pride, . . . makes him abstain from summoning into life, children for whom he cannot properly provide.[2]

Policy, in England at any rate, was beginning to be formed. The Allotments movement in England gained force. Even the semi-Malthusian Poor Law of 1834 made provision for them. In 1843 a Select Committee was appointed and gave some impetus to voluntary action. But it was not until the end of the century, when Malthus had lost much

[1] For an account of Kingsley's views, see H. A. Boner, *Hungry Generations; the Nineteenth Century Case Against Malthusianism* (New York, 1955), pp. 162 ff.

[2] Mill, op. cit. i, bk. ii, ch. vii, para. 4, quoting from J. C. L. S. Sismondi, *Les Nouveaux Principes d'économie politique ou de la richesse dans ses rapports avec la population* (2nd ed., Paris, 1827), vol. i, bk. iii, ch. iii, p. 171.

of his influence, that the movement gained anything like national significance. By then it was no longer necessary to recommend it on the grounds that it would keep down population.[1]

Sir Archibald Alison advocated the division of land amongst numerous proprietors with the same ends in view as Laing and Thornton had done, but the means whereby the desirable result was to be accomplished were more indirect. If there were but one very large proprietor in each district, labourers could not hope to attain his rank, and would not therefore seek to imitate his refined habits. Prudence is impossible under these circumstances. But if there are many proprietors (and they must, above all, be resident on their estates to achieve this), the tenantry may well emulate them. He did not advocate that all should have equal holdings: on the contrary it would be better for some to have quite small holdings, so that their moderate comforts might be the more easily seen to be within the reach of their people. Ireland, he thought, suffered particularly from the fact that most of its landlords were absentees, and he vigorously opposed McCulloch, who thought that this state of affairs did no great harm.[2]

Abroad, Sismondi was, as we have seen, amongst those who sought to remedy the over-rapid increase of workers by the creation of a pre-capitalist peasant proprietor class. The French socialists similarly sought in some new system of landownership and tillage a basis for new attitudes which would either check population or restrict its growth to the pace of the growth of subsistence.[3] Decisive statements of the connexion between property-holding and population trend were made by French demographers starting with the elder Bertillon, who began his observations in 1855 and in 1874 published his article 'Natalité' in the *Dictionnaire encyclopédique des sciences médicales*.[4] Following his lead, detailed statistics were published showing the extent of the distribution of land in France, and the small size of the average peasant's family. Notably Bertillon, Leroy-Beaulieu, and, of course, Dumont, stressed the importance of this factor. But amongst these later writers, the mentality of the proprietor as such is no longer seen in isolation.

[1] See Sir J. H. Clapham, *An Economic History of Modern Britain* (Cambridge, 1926–38, 3 vols.), i. 472–4.

[2] Sir A. Alison, *The Principles of Population and Their Connection with Human Happiness* (Edinburgh, 1840, 2 vols.), i. 107–8. See also Jones's system of gradation, below, sect. 2.

[3] See J. J. Spengler, 'French Population Theory since 1800', *Journal of Political Economy* (1936), xliv. 749–53, on Fourier and others.

[4] The acknowledgement of this origin is in his son's book, J. Bertillon, *La Dépopulation de la France* (Paris, 1911), p. 128.

Whether, as with Dumont, the desire to acquire and preserve land is part of a wider 'social capillarity', or, as with Leroy-Beaulieu, it is the *arrivisme* typical of the spread of civilization, we are faced everywhere with a complex mental process which was only dimly seen amongst the earlier writers.[1]

Some authors eventually went so far as to advocate a reversal of the trend in ownership so as to arrest the decline in births,[2] and no doubt the Soviet collective farm and the suppression of the *kulak* may in themselves be taken as expressions of the belief that individual property leads to anti-social attitudes, of which the refusal to produce children for the state is just one. The trouble is that although the writers quoted made out a fairly good case for their view that property leads to a careful attitude towards marriage and children, it could not be assumed that people would increase their fertility if, *ceteris paribus*, they were deprived of personal ownership. It was found that such problems could not be studied in isolation, and that there were other factors, both social and economic, to be taken into account.

A middle-of-the-road view was taken by the Italian sociologist and reformer F. S. Nitti (1868–1953), who to some extent reconciled the opinions of the eighteenth and nineteenth centuries in his theory that under a system of fair division of wealth, the birth-rate will eventually settle down to an 'appropriate' level, without the dangers of either under- or over-population. Instead, as in Plato's state ideal, there will be one family for each holding and a steady pattern of reproduction will emerge.[3] In this idea we recognize echoes of Muret's and Malthus's Switzerland, and Thornton's Channel Islands, and are also provided with a link forward to the optimum theories of population. At the end of the nineteenth century the movement which had started as a demand for allotments merged in the larger demand for land reform, and this took many different forms. The redistribution of property was one of the chief planks in the platform of the non-Marxist socialists. One of the foremost amongst these was Nitti's master, Achille Loria (1857–1943), who also attributed over-population to the maldistribution of landed property. Wealth in the hands of the few, he thought, led to a failure to develop productive resources, whilst the hopeless situation of the

[1] For a full account of these writers, see Spengler, *France Faces Depopulation*, notably ch. vii.

[2] See also P. Lafitte, quoted ibid., p. 161.

[3] F. S. Nitti, *Population and the Social System* (London, 1894), quoted in United Nations, *The Determinants and Consequences of Population Trends* (New York, 1953), pp. 33–34.

masses of the property-less workers led to their reckless propagation. A balanced increase in subsistence and population was only possible under some system of co-operation and the removal of inequality.[1] The movement founded by Loria and Nitti was to have great practical importance in Italy, where the contrasts of living-standards between property-owners and landless proletariat were possibly greater than anywhere else in western Europe, and the break-up of the large estates, especially in southern Italy, became one of the principal aims of all reformist movements.

When one recalls Archdeacon Paley's remarks about the salutary effects of persuading the Indians to eat meat, one is driven to consider, in connexion with the ideas here quoted, what their authors would have thought of the great land-giving movement of Vinova Bhave in the 1950's. Although undoubtedly the foundations of this crusade are in the first place ethical, one may see this particular attempt to raise the standard of life of the landless masses, by a measure of redistribution, in the light of this widespread observation that peasant property creates the wish to limit families. One wonders if the Indian government's campaign to popularize contraception may not be helped by the land movement.

2. DEMOCRACY AND CIVIL LIBERTY

The supposed effects of the diffusion of property on the equalization of incomes, the subject of the last section, might be observed, at least in theory, under almost any form of government where individual property was recognized. But the right to hold property, and to transmit it to an heir, is not a necessary proof of the existence of a democratic state. Under the system of landholding which was most common in England until the days of enclosure and the agrarian revolution, the individual copyholder was entirely deprived of political rights, and his chances of rising above the class of his origin were exceedingly small. Yet he had usually the right to pass on his land to an heir on the payment of a suitable heriot. In France, individual proprietorship was also quite usual before the Revolution. But the concern of the philosophers in France, Great Britain, and America at the end of the eighteenth century was with political rights in the first place and economic equality only afterwards—or not at all. Some thought, as the Chartists did later, that

[1] A. Loria, *La Legge di popolazione ed il sistema sociale* (Siena, 1887), and *Analisi della proprietà capitalista* (Turin, 1889), i, ch. v, quoted in Nitti, op. cit., pp. 132 ff

the cure for economic ills would follow easily from the reorganization of government so as to give the masses a voice in the affairs of the nation.

As in the case of property, those who considered the effects of political rights on population mostly assumed that an increase would follow. As long ago as 1699 Charles D'Avenant wrote: 'Securing the Liberties of a Nation, may be laid down as a Fundamental for increasing the Numbers of its People.'[1] Other writers agreed with him, except Wallace, who was committed to the belief that the world was best peopled when a slave economy prevailed. Montesquieu was more specific:

> The propagation of the species is wonderfully aided by a mild government. All republics are a standing proof of this; especially Switzerland and Holland, which, with regard to the nature of the land, are the two worst countries in Europe, and which are yet the most populous.[2]

Once again the problem comes to our notice which already occupied us in the last section. Was logic made to turn turtle so that democracy might now serve the cause of Malthus? It does not seem likely. The old call for good government had been prompted by abuses which were truly depopulating, simply because under that régime the minimum conditions for existence were not fulfilled. But democracy,[3] participation, self-government—these things in the context of post-revolutionary Europe meant a good deal more than the minimum of existence. An enlightened despot could govern well and multiply his subjects by avoiding costly wars, liberating serfs, and emptying the prisons. The constitutional monarch was asked to provide a framework in which the

[1] C. D'Avenant, *An Essay upon the Probable Methods of Making a People Gainers in the Ballance of Trade* (London, 1699), p. 32, quoted in R. R. Kuczynski, 'British Demographers' Opinions on Fertility, 1660–1760', *Political Arithmetic; a Symposium of Population Studies* (L. T. Hogben, ed., London, 1938), p. 310, where references to Short, Hume, Tucker, and Bell will also be found.

[2] C.-L. de Secondat, Baron de la Brède et de Montesquieu, *Lettres persanes* (J. Davidson, ed. and trans., London, 1922), Letter cxxiii, p. 224. On the other hand, Montesquieu seems to have blamed the decline of Rome partially on its form of government. W. E. Hickson, *Malthus; an Essay on the Principle of Population, in Refutation of the Theory of the Rev. T. R. Malthus* (London, 1849), p. 46, cites Edward Gibbon: 'The long peace and the uniform government of the Romans had introduced a slow and secret poison into the vitals of the empire'—and states that Montesquieu was the originator of the thought.

[3] We do not here distinguish between Dumont's 'Caesarian' and 'Republican' Democracy (A. Dumont, *Dépopulation et civilisation, Étude démographique* (Paris, 1890), p. 129)—since the former is hardly connected with the ideals with which we have been dealing.

least of his subjects could, and within a comparatively short time did, aspire to be his Prime Minister.

But again the change in observed habits was, to say the least, opportune for the advocates of democracy. It had not been part of the case of the *philosophes* that complete social mobility would promote population—indeed, most of them did not demand it. When the democratic countries were in fact the first to notice a slackening of population pressure, the blame was not, at first, laid on good government as such, but on the results which inevitably followed from the granting of greater personal rights and opportunities. Of these the eighteenth century had not dreamt—yet some of its far-sighted writers could divine something of the possible results of the new order.

Moheau was amongst the first to doubt the efficacy of democratic government for increasing population. He agreed that this rule was nearest to the natural order, but had not Greece, a republic, been rent by strife, until Alexander united it? Was not the Roman republic full of troubles? Contemporary democracies, he thought, were in the same situation. On some estates there were more people in a semi-servile situation than there would be in conditions of freedom. (But this he thought no argument in favour of slavery.)[1] His reasoning does not seem very clear on the subject—but there is no doubt that democracy meant something to him not so far removed from Dumont's later conception—a turbulent, free-for-all state, contrasted with the orderly progression of a more autocratic government.

The authors of the nineteenth century, however, did not think of mob-rule republics when they spoke of the effects of government on population. Rather, it was constitutional and peaceable rule which they felt to be the precondition for the emergence of prudence—where Moheau had felt uncertainty to be characteristic of democracy, his successors pointed to the definite expectations of the subject. But in both cases the result would be the same—a reduction of fertility.

Amongst the clearest statements of this position at the beginning of the nineteenth century are Malthus's own. In the Appendix to the fifth edition (1817) he considered not only the objections which some of his known enemies had made, but he even set up some imaginary ones of his own, which he proceeded to demolish. One of these was the argument that one ought not to risk the promulgation of any new opinions which may alarm the prejudices of the poor, but instead quietly initiate

[1] M. Moheau, *Recherches et considérations sur la population de la France* (Paris, 1778), part ii, pp. 57–64.

policies which will raise their education and status.[1] The reference was, presumably, to his plan to withhold all aid from the poor—which had aroused the prejudices, to say the least, of the poor and some of their friends.

> It may be said that, according to my own reasonings and the facts stated in my work, it appears that the diminished proportion of births, which I consider absolutely necessary to the permanent improvement of the condition of the poor, invariably follows an improved government... we have only to proceed in improving our civil polity, conferring the benefits of education upon all, and removing every obstacle to the general extension of all those privileges and advantages which may be enjoyed in common; and we may be quite sure that the effect, to which I look forward, and which can alone render these advantages permanent, will follow.[2]

He decided against reliance on this course on the grounds that more would have to be known on the exact way in which this method worked, and meanwhile it would be better to break the truth as gently as possible to the poor at large—not to do so would be to be afraid to spread the truth (which consisted of his own theories), and once truth was suppressed, who knows what fate might befall knowledge and virtue.

He came back to the importance of good government in his *Principles of Political Economy*, first published in 1820. There he attributed the failure of the English population to rise in the period 1720–50, when cheaper food increased real wages, to the fact that good government prevailed, and that the people enjoyed 'all the advantages of civil and political liberty in an unusual degree'. The law and the higher orders respected them, and so they took advantage of the price fall to bring about 'a decided elevation in the standard of their comforts and conveniences'.[3] As it happens, he was probably wrong, in the sense that modern research has shown the period after 1730 to have been one of rapidly rising population after the stagnation of the first part of the century. But it does not affect the argument. Malthus, in his customary manner, concedes his main position in an aside.

Ten years later, in the *Summary View of the Principle of Population*, he repeated all those elements of his theory which, after a third of a century of controversy, he thought most important, and there he

[1] Malthus, *Essay*... (5th ed., 1817), iii, Appendix, pp. 374–5.

[2] Ibid. The passage was cited with approval in *The Progress of Society* (London, 1830), p. 352, by Robert Hamilton, F.R.S., Professor of Mathematics at Aberdeen. The context is a plea for a general extension of art and civilization as a means of checking population.

[3] Malthus, *Principles of Political Economy*... (London, 1820), pp. 228–9.

quoted fully some further passages from the *Principles*. The argument ran thus: high wages may lead to two results—either a rapid increase of population, because the extra money is spent on rearing larger families, or a higher standard of living. The choice is determined by general habits, and these in turn by outward circumstances. The first result will follow from a preference for present gratification and little respectability, generated on the whole by 'despotism, oppression and ignorance', the second from civil and political liberty, and education, which produce beings given to 'looking before and after', who cannot:

acquiesce patiently in the thought of depriving themselves and their children of the means of being respectable, virtuous and happy.[1]

Of all the causes [he continues] which tend to generate prudential habits among the lower classes of society, the most essential is unquestionably civil liberty. No people can be much accustomed to form plans for the future, who do not feel assured that their industrious exertions, while fair and honourable, will be allowed to have free scope; and that the property which they either possess, or may acquire, will be secured to them by a known code of just laws impartially administered. But it has been found by experience, that civil liberty cannot be permanently secured without political liberty. Consequently, political liberty becomes almost equally essential; and in addition to its being necessary in this point of view, its obvious tendency to teach the lower classes of society to respect themselves by obliging the higher classes to respect them, must contribute greatly to all the good effects of civil liberty.

What Malthus meant by political liberty, and what institutions would oblige the higher classes to respect the lower, is not quite clear. One can only imagine him in the act of placing on a pedestal some sober farm labourer, a bachelor, spending half of his eighteenpence a day on food and necessaries, and the rest on books of an improving nature. Certainly he did not mean that his class should have to woo universally the mob that was the terror of candidates in Westminster.[2] But we must admit that this vague generalization constituted a new direction—and one that came to be adopted more widely during the nineteenth century. But so anxious were some of Malthus's opponents to discredit everything

[1] Ibid., p. 250, as quoted in *A Summary View of the Principle of Population*, in *Introduction to Malthus* (D. V. Glass, ed., London, 1953), pp. 155–6.

[2] At least Frances Place, who accepted Malthus's arguments on the whole, had no doubts about the political preconditions of prudence. See F. Place, *Illustrations and Proofs of the Principle of Population, Including an Examination of the Proposed Remedies of Mr. Malthus and a Reply to the Objections of Mr. Godwin and Others* (1822; N. Himes, ed., London, 1930), pp. 152–3, 168–72.

he said, that many of them did not take up this point at all, but continued to assert that better government meant a greater population.[1]

Alison, as we would expect, was concerned with the conditions under which his specific, Emulation, would be fostered. In 'feudal or barbarous ages', where there were great differences between the nobility in their castles and their tenantry, there was no hope for any individual aspiring to copy the manners of his lords and masters. In the East, the people still lived as they had done in the days of Cyrus or Alexander, thanks to the continuation of the feudal system. He did not specifically lay down the characteristic of the system he had in mind—opponent of reform that he was, we could not expect him to advocate the vote as a means to genteel living. But the implication of the mobility of occupation which we have quoted earlier is clearly a society where most forms of privilege have been abolished.[2]

George Rickards was more specific. He had gone farther than Malthus in describing the machinery of improvement which must be put at the disposal of the lower orders. Where Malthus had only stressed the need for security of property, Rickards added the rights of labour. A political and social system was required which 'as in our own country, opposes no barrier to energy and perseverance, but makes the rewards and honours of the state accessible to the talents and virtues of the humblest citizen'.[3]

The same idea was expressed by most of those who advocated greater economic mobility—Laing (the younger), Moreton, and others. Richard Jones stressed the need for civil liberty, the absence of 'impassable barriers between the aristocracy and the peasantry' and unjust laws which prevented the ascent of the body of the people. Like Alison, he thought that the absence of intermediate orders, as in Poland, prevented the creation of hope in the minds of the lower orders; fortunate a country like England with numerous classes of people between the highest and the lowest. Wherever a system of castes or other limited privileges is perpetuated, he claimed, no progress could be expected. The state must constantly watch out for laws restricting competition, such as gilds and craft regulations, which prevent economic advancement.[4] This assertion, like Rickards's demand, is naturally to be taken

[1] e.g. G. Ensor, *An Inquiry Concerning the Population of Nations: Containing a Refutation of Mr. Malthus' 'Essay on Population'* (London, 1818).

[2] Alison, op. cit. i. 105.

[3] Sir G. Rickards, *Population and Capital: Being a Course of Lectures Delivered before the University of Oxford in 1853–54* (London, 1854), p. 253.

[4] R. Jones, *Literary Remains, Consisting of Lectures and Tracts on Political Economy*

as part of the general liberal philosophy in the spirit of Adam Smith. Just as in the previous century equality and civil liberty had been invoked as sure remedies for the dearth of population, so now they served their purpose equally well to help to lay the Malthusian spectre and to advance the cause of Reform and Free Trade.

With the second half of the nineteenth century the concept of a democratic state became more refined. It was no longer merely a question of opportunity. The individual, it was considered, behaves differently altogether in a democratic society. He is encouraged to think of himself as a person who matters, and equal to the best, the highest, the richest in the land. As a result, his selfishness, his concern for his own advancement, and for his children (if any) becomes more pronounced.

These ideas were mostly developed in France, but they owe much to the sociological work of Herbert Spencer. This will be outlined in a later chapter. Already Le Play's 'Unstable Family' was seen to be the outcome of the French Revolution—not only because of the inheritance provisions but because of the decreased dependence of the child on the family in general. The break-up of the 'Authoritarian Family', due to the loss of identity of the homestead as a centre of activity, led the children into the towns. Many who have not accepted the Le Play thesis have nevertheless diagnosed the same restless spirit in the new state. Jacques Bertillon traced the influence of the Revolution through a decline in the influence of religion, the *Code Civil*, individualism, and the 'democratic spirit' in general: 'il inspire à chaque homme le désir de s'élever . . .'.[1]

In Dumont's work the disparagement of democracy reached its climax. Seeking for an explanation of the decline in births which he believed to be peculiar to France, he found it in the unique nature of French democracy. Switzerland and the United States were also democracies—but they were federal in character, Protestant, and realist. The French state was centralized, Catholic and idealist. But it was not on the influence of the Church or idealism that he laid most of the blame—there were other countries where these were strong and births were still numerous—but on democracy:

Nous sommes une démocratie. Par une lente évolution accomplie pendant la durée de plusieurs siècles aux dépens de la royauté et de l'aristocratie, le

(W. Whewell and Cazenove, eds., London, 1859), p. 249 (Circumstances which govern the effect of wages on population), and pp. 493–506 (Text of Haileybury Lectures), lecture vii, sections 4 and 5, 'Intermediate Classes' and 'Civil Liberty and Power of Advancing'.

[1] Bertillon, op. cit., p. 124.

Français, d'abord serf et sujet, s'est élevé à la dignité de citoyen et de souverain. La forme politique a donc changé du tout au tout.[1]

There was a legacy, however, bequeathed to the new democratic state by the *ancien régime*. Centralism, idealism, and Catholicism, those were the creeds which were still current in France. To each now the epithet 'democratic' was applied, but there remained an inherent contradiction in terms, which could destroy society:

> Trois fois l'epithète jure contre son sujet . . . L'absence totale d'harmonie dans les différentes sphères de notre activité mentale et la disparition de la paix intime qui en serait le resultat, voilà un trait qui est spécial à la France contemporaine . . .

The implication is that democracy has been superimposed on traditional characteristics and values, and that the restless, split mind which results will disrupt the state. Similar arguments were to become familiar in Germany in the Nazi period. The people there were spared the conflict between Nordic mythology and democracy.

Dumont stressed that the advent of democracy did not mean greater equality in fact: it only meant that everyone saw himself free to aim at the highest position and greatest fortune. From this follows the capillary ascent:

> . . . des circonstances spéciales à la France du XIXe siècle ont fait grandir parallèlement l'égalité en droit et l'inégalité en fait; du progrès de ces deux termes antithétiques est résulté un attrait immense et général vers la richesse devenue le seul moyen d'influence et de considération; et cette passion ayant . . . trouvé moins aisément à se satisfaire par le travail et l'esprit d'initiative que par l'économie, la compression de tous les désirs et la diminution des charges de famille ont contribué par une large part à la diminution volontaire du nombre des naissances.[2]

We need not follow Dumont into the ramifications of his theory. But the broad conclusions (if not the remedy)[3] were accepted by many of his contemporaries and in some form are incorporated into most modern texts.

Later, R. Gonnard and others took up the antithesis between poli-

[1] Dumont, op. cit., p. 100.

[2] Ibid., p. 258.

[3] His proposals were socialist in character. Given greater equality of income and property, the ascensional urge would be lessened. Decentralization, secularization, and the creation of a new social mythology of hard work and fruitfulness would then achieve the desired result; ibid., ch. xx. The essence of the system was the subordination of the individual to the state.

tical equality and economic inequality.[1] Dumont's idea of bureaucratic centralization, which made the generally ill-paid but theoretically unlimited career of the *fonctionnaire* as desirable as it undoubtedly still is, was taken up by a number of writers, including J. Jung and H. Clément. Modern sociologists have investigated the peculiar demographic behaviour of civil servants' families.[2]

Even those who did not accept that economic inequality was necessarily a cause for the emergence of this spirit, frequently blamed the democratic system. Thus Leroy-Beaulieu characterized the 'civilization' which he used as his basic explanation as being particularly democratic —its benefit were felt by all ranks in society. In other words, everyone had a larger or smaller slice of the cake, and believed themselves to be equal, even if they were not so in fact.[3] It may be remarked that Dumont's contention that Switzerland and the United States did not show the reduction of fertility because they were federal states, was not accepted by other demographers. Men like E. Levasseur, who sought to present objective statements on population trends rather than political theses, were disturbed by the correlation of democracy and a low birth-rate.[4]

By the beginning of the twentieth century it was no longer possible to isolate the effects of democratic government or the diffusion of property. Industrialization had begun in most countries of the West; the powers of land-owning aristocrats were waning everywhere. Countries with large surplus labour forces were decanting them rapidly into the United States. Finally the war obliterated many old national and social distinctions. Henceforth only extremists would seek to blame the decline in births on one particular cause. Instead, thought turned more and more to the general question of the role of the individual and the family in society, and the development of human society as such.

A long-term pattern suggests itself as a result of these researches into opinion about government and population. The mercantilists and similar schools obviously believed in strong state action to foster population—action which might be of a repressive character. The reformers suggest that a liberal and democratic order might produce

[1] See Spengler, *France Faces Depopulation*, pp. 162 ff. This section contains numerous further references from which the following quotations are also taken.

[2] For references, see United Nations, *Determinants and Consequences* . . ., pp. 87–88.

[3] P. Leroy-Beaulieu, *La Question de la population* (3e éd., Paris, 1913), pp. 184, 186, 220.

[4] E. Levasseur, *La Population française* (Paris, 1892), iii. 492. References to Switzerland as below average fertility in Europe and the north-eastern United States.

better results. But when population does grow and the alarm is sounded, writers are happy to find that after all the powers of democratic organization to raise families have been over-rated, and that in fact prudence follows democracy. But there are some who do not wish to promote democracy even if it does curb population, and so there occur the curious episodes of the official repression of marriage in Austria and the German states which early in the nineteenth century made Malthus such a hated figure.[1] This stage passes, and then suddenly democracy falls from grace and is roundly blamed for the danger arising to the state from depopulation. The demand is heard once more for firm state action, even if it is anti-democratic, and the fostering of population in the twentieth century reached its absurd climax in the Nazi state. But democracy, not to be outdone, began to devise ways of its own to increase the birth-rate—even if that included the punitive taxation of bachelors. Thus population theory merges into population policy.

3. THE ROLE OF EDUCATION

We must now turn to two particular aspects of the theory of the democratic state which are often found as examples of the changes which are supposed to occur, typically, when the framework of society assumes an altered political complexion. Education is both the foundation and the end-result of democracy, and the higher status of women in society is a concomitant of the general move towards greater equality.

In this case, the fertility effect was supposed to arise in two forms: either as a simple correlation of education and infertility, or in the Malthusian guise as a means of leading the poor to an appreciation of the means of their own salvation. For the most part, the moral demand for more education has been happily joined with an answer to the over-population spectre. As with democracy, equality, and women's rights, it was fortunate that the policies of enlightened reformers in the social sphere were seen to be also valuable specifics for economic and political ills. If, on the other hand, the danger was thought to be that of depopulation, education was either ignored or deliberately played down. At least the suggestion that more education would lead to a greater population does not seem to have appeared,[2] and in this respect this particular argument differs from some of the others already discussed.

[1] For this period, see D. V. Glass, ed., *Introduction to Malthus* (London, 1953), p. 39.

[2] Except in the sense of bringing up orphans and others to a useful trade and preventing them from falling into idleness and immorality. See Spengler, *French Predecessors . . .*, p. 22 (on Bossuet); p. 54 (Melon); p. 93 (Jaubert), who appears to have suggested that foundlings be 'educated slightly'.

At the end of the eighteenth century French philosophers began to think in terms of a new world. In almost every case this involved the creation of a new race of men—different in their outlook and organized in a new social relation. This in turn meant education for all to play their part in the new society. Men everywhere began to believe that the natural forces could be subordinated to human reason. But the process of reasoning is one which may be instilled even in the short run, whereas the biological changes of which other writers expected great things could only be made in the long period.

Thus we find a whole group of men pointing to the hope for progress through education. The general principles were stated clearly by Rousseau. 'The art of forming man' knows no limits to what may be achieved.[1] Saint-Pierre and Helvetius saw a prospect of new institutions created by legislation and men educated to fit into the new pattern. Condorcet, above all, had great faith in the possibilities of re-forming human nature. As each person became more educated, so inequalities would gradually lessen. Since the characteristics of educated men could be inherited, the movement would be progressive. With ever greater knowledge of the techniques of production, human life would be prolonged and at the same time a spirit of concern for the community would develop which in time would limit procreation. Happiness would matter more than numbers, and this insight would conquer thoughtless selfishness.[2] Godwin shared much of Condorcet's optimism regarding the 'educability' of mankind. Higher enjoyments, he believed, might one day replace much of the present sexual preoccupation. Malthus did not agree. Even allowing the occasional case where 'great intellectual exertions tend to diminish this empire of passion over man',[3] he did not believe that this meant any real diminution of 'the passion between the sexes'. Even given some probability of this, he thought the chances of the lower classes attaining any 'high degree of intellectual improvement' were exceedingly slim.

But as we know, Malthus's scepticism regarding these far-reaching

[1] J.-J. Rousseau, *Émile*, Preface. It is interesting to note that Rousseau drew attention to a factor which limits the frequency of marriage: in primitive society mating is indiscriminate; in civilized nations people have to mate according to individual tastes and preferences, in accordance with custom and public opinion. The educated find it difficult to choose exactly the right partner (quoted in W. Boyd, *The Education Theory of Jean-Jacques Rousseau* (London, 1911), pp. 202–9).

[2] See Spengler, *French Predecessors* . . ., pp. 261–3, and note on Condorcet above.

[3] Malthus, *Essay* . . . (1st ed., 1798), p. 217. Unfortunately Malthus, according to his own evidence, had a bad toothache when he answered this point, and was therefore even less able than usual to appreciate the power of mind over matter.

notions did not prevent him from becoming the first serious advocate of educational measures to increase the chances of voluntary restraint amongst the masses. Nothing was said about this in the first *Essay*, but in the later work there is every evidence that he believed in the possibility of fundamental changes. Amongst the higher ranks of society, he thought, pride and independence were sufficiently encouraged by education to make marriage habits consistent with prudence.[1] But amongst the lower classes we must try to infuse 'a portion of that knowledge and foresight, which so much facilitates the attainment of this object in the educated part of the community'. He recommends a system of parochial education 'upon a plan similar to that proposed by Adam Smith'. To the usual syllabus he would add instruction in the principles of population, and of political economy.[2] It is easy to dismiss such precepts by saying that this was part of a grand design to keep the poor-rates down and the poor from grumbling. But this would not be fair, for Malthus was anxious to stress that marriage was desirable, if only it could be contracted under conditions of tolerable comfort. It was just the absence of a taste for comforts which seemed so characteristic of the poor. True, he thought the condition of Scotland happy because there the peasants were kept from tumultuous behaviour by their system of education, despite their great poverty. But this he thought was due to their inferior soils, and at least they exercised a degree of prudence and foresight which kept their conditions from getting worse. So education is added to good government as a precondition of prudence:

In an attempt to better the condition of the labouring classes of society our object should be to raise this standard as high as possible, by cultivating a spirit of independence, a decent pride, and a taste for cleanliness and comfort. The effect of a good government in increasing the prudential habits and personal respectability of the lower classes of society has already been insisted on; but certainly this effect will always be incomplete without a good system

[1] Malthus, op. cit. ii. 210. Alfred Marshall later thought that the taste for comforts came in already early in the eighteenth century, with the adoption of wheat as a staple food, and that this began to check the rate of increase: *Principles of Economics* (8th ed., London, 1930), p. 175. See Ch. IX below.

[2] Amongst French writers, Count Pellegrino Rossi, Professor at the Collège de France, and editor of the best-known French version of Malthus, advocated instruction in political economy as a remedy—*Cours d'économie politique* (Brussels, 1840–2), i. 200–56, quoted in Spengler, 'French Population Theory since 1800', *Journal of Political Economy* (1936), xliv. 586. This article also contains references to other French writers of the period who believed strongly in the efficacy of educational methods. See extracts from F. X. J. Droz and E. Buret, ibid., pp. 746–7.

of education; and, indeed, it may be said that no government can approach to perfection that does not provide for the instruction of the people. The benefits derived from education are among those which may be enjoyed without restriction of numbers; and, as it is the power of governments to confer these benefits, it is undoubtedly their duty to do it.[1]

In the *Summary View* of 1830 he again quoted from the *Principles of Political Economy* the view that education is a necessary complement to civil and political liberty.[2]

As he did in the case of liberty and equality, Malthus here again mounted a violent attack on the authors of views which he himself had come to hold quite strongly. The society which he advocated bore, in several important characteristics, a strong resemblance to that of the visionaries. Whatever the immediate practical application of his theories, his thoughts were always fixed on a society without poverty or ignorance, based on the free association of equal individuals conducting themselves as social beings.

Yet to quote Malthus at length on this point, and to show how much he agreed with his adversaries on the need for education, is not to parade him as an enlightened and progressive thinker. By 1800, and even more strongly so by the end of Malthus's life, education played a role in public thinking which made it almost impossible to write a work on moral philosophy or economics without avowing oneself to be an ardent educationist. The motives of the advocates of education, naturally, were mixed.

Fervour was almost universal—the demand came from the Utilitarians and the Socialists, the Evangelicals and the Oxford Movement, Young England and the Manchester School. Some thought it was a way of saving the soul of heathen England, others thought it would dispel all superstitions including Christianity. Some believed it would teach the poor to be obedient and more productive, thus securing higher profits to their masters, others thought it would teach them to revolt at once. It was a sure way to reform, and a substitute for it. A few voices were heard counselling restriction of education to rudiments sufficient to secure Bible-reading and good manners (even Hannah More once excused her activities to her bishop on the score that she confined herself to those objects). But in general, education was the battle-cry of all the 'progressive' elements in Regency England, and had become the slogan of the die-hards in the early days of Victoria and Albert.

[1] Malthus, *Essay* . . . (Everyman ed., 1914), ii. 215.

[2] Malthus, *A Summary View of the Principle of Population*, pp. 156–7.

This universality poses a new problem in the history of these theories. One detects a change in the usual order of events. In the case of the extension of democracy and equality, their supposed effects on population acted, as it were, as a selling point: 'However much you may dislike these things', the reformers seem to say, 'you must grant that they are a good specific for over-population, so you must join us in our demand for them.' In the case of education, such an approach appears superfluous. If, then, education and fertility are often linked, it is because the desire for the better instruction of the people was widespread, and the appeal to the relationship, therefore, forms a convenient axiomatic starting-point for the attack on Malthus. This is the impression one has, for instance, in the case of T. R. Edmonds. At any rate the association between education and low fertility seems to date from this time, long before statistical investigations confirmed what had once been a great hope, and in time was to be a great fear.

The need for education, then, was stressed by every writer of the era of controversy—the Malthusians followed their master in advocating it as a remedial measure; his opponents pointed to the same means as being sure to prevent the onset of the evil. So closely were both sides agreed on policy, that on any topic like that of popular education, it is impossible to tell the two apart. For an example of the one side, we may take Dr. Thomas Chalmers, the Glasgow minister who became Professor of Philosophy at St. Andrews and later held the chair of Theology at Edinburgh. He had taken a lively interest in social questions since his days as a parish priest, and was a popular writer and preacher on economic subjects. Like many others in his time, he found it easier to secure the society he desired by limiting the population than by enlarging the resources of mankind.

> But the only way of rightly accomplishing this, is through the medium of a higher self-respect, and higher taste for the comforts and decencies of life among the people themselves. It is only moral and voluntary restraint that should be aimed at, or that can be at all effectual. . . . This is evidently not the achievement of a day, but the slow product of education working . . . on the habits and inclinations of the common people. . . .[1]

He declared the aim of 'every enlightened philanthropist and patriot' to be the raising of the standard of enjoyment, even at some cost to himself—but he did not think that it could be accomplished by legislation or repressive measures. The 'narrowing of society' was to be

[1] T. Chalmers, *On Political Economy in Connexion with the Moral State and Moral Prospects of Society* (2nd ed., Glasgow, 1832), p. 552.

accomplished by the self-interest of the labouring classes, who could then secure a larger share of the total product.

Critics of Malthus expressed themselves in much the same way. T. R. Edmonds placed education at the head of the chapter on the 'Means of strengthening the feeling of self-respect in the labourer'. Nobody, he wrote, could now check the progress of education; it had begun, and we could only steer it in the right direction.[1] The best policy was not to encourage utopian notions of a perfect society, but to proceed to the practical improvements now possible. 'Is any mode so desirable or efficacious, as solid, judicious, and comprehensive education?' Knowledge was an artificial want, and must therefore be encouraged. Nothing will be more important to a young man anxious to improve himself than the purchase of books. What could be better to prevent marriage?

After discussing the various plans for the organization of education (including the continuation of moral instruction up to the age of twenty-one, when it is most needed!) he stressed that it must not be gratuitous—otherwise it is not an artificial want. The labourers must be taught prudence by the very cost of gaining knowledge. We will not follow the rest of his arguments for payment, which are a little absurd. But we note that he observed that education was becoming more and more necessary for the attainment of a higher wage. In this connexion he notes mechanics' institutions which 'have sprung up in all the large towns'. They fulfilled a double purpose: again as artificial wants, and as wholesome organized diversions for the working classes analogous to the clubs and theatres frequented by their employers.[2]

There is an interesting echo of Edmonds's account of pastimes amongst various classes in Thorstein Veblen's writings seventy years later. In *Imperial Germany*, the Icelandic-American sociologist (1857–1929), contrasted England and Germany before the First World War —the Germans were supposed to use the equivalent of mechanics' institutions, and the British workman indulged in the 'systematic diversions' which, according to Edmonds, were then still the privilege of the employing classes.[3] In another work, Veblen called the habits of conspicuous consumption in towns the 'most effectual of the Malthusian

[1] [T. R. Edmonds], *An Enquiry into the Principles of Population* ... (London, 1832), p. 200.

[2] Ibid., pp. 201–8.

[3] T. Veblen, *Imperial Germany and the Industrial Revolution* (new ed., London, 1939), p. 197.

checks' and thought they acted most strongly amongst the scholarly classes because they had less income and most appearance to maintain.[1]

Edmonds did not say how young people of eighteen were to find the time for moral instruction—presumably he meant evenings and Sundays. But other writers were serious enough to propose shorter working hours as a means of obtaining the necessary degree of education, and in the controversies surrounding the Bills to reduce the length of the working day, the Malthusian (or anti-Malthusian) argument was not infrequently used.[2] We have already seen Rickards's observation that the introduction of machinery demanded a more educated working man, who would be expected to use his mind more than his muscles. John Stuart Mill thought that one of the effects of increasing organization and power of trade unions amongst skilled workers would be depopulation in the Malthusian sense: knowing that the maintenance of their power (and therefore their wages) depended on the entry into their crafts, they might be inclined to begin by restricting their own families.[3] But Lujo Brentano was surely misinterpreting Mill a little when quoting this chapter and speaking about the reduced fertility of skilled workers as such. Brentano himself certainly believed that the educational work of the new trade unions was helping to keep down the numbers of the working classes.[4] He also observed that the ever-increasing demands for the training of skilled workers would automatically postpone marriage, even in the absence of psychological effects. The same point was made by many British social historians. Education was therefore in the employer's interest in every sense; he needed more competent workmen, and if education meant refinement, he would have less trouble from them. The country would benefit because of their increased prudence. How harmonious were the population laws of the industrializing period!

The English authors quoted so far, though convinced that education reduced the birth-rate among the lower classes, had not yet made any

[1] T. Veblen, *Theory of the Leisure Class* (1899; London, 1949), p. 113.

[2] See W. F. Lloyd, *Two Lectures on the Checks to Population, Delivered Before the University of Oxford in Michaelmas Term, 1832* (Oxford, 1833), pp. 47 ff. Prudence depends on the reasoning faculty, which can be improved by education and experience. Constant labour at an early age is a bar to this.

[3] Mill, op. cit., p. 243.

[4] The quotation is in 'Die malthusische Lehre und die Bevölkerungsbewegung der letzten Dezennien', *Abhandlungen der historischen Klasse der Königlich Bayerischen Akademie der Wissenschaften* (Munich, 1909), xxiv. 585 ff. The other statement was made in his inaugural address at Berlin as early as 1871. Brentano was probably the most knowledgeable German of his time in the field of British economic history and therefore well qualified to make judgements on the impact of industrial organization on the country.

statistical observations on the connexion between education and fertility. It would have been difficult to do so in England; for the most educated classes in the country at the time had a record of high fertility indeed. The clerics, if we may take the Rev. Amos Barton or Mr. Quiverful as examples, were not exempt from this rule. Karl Marx poured out his venom on the parsons who wrote so sanctimoniously about the need to restrict population, and themselves contributed to its increase to a quite unbecoming extent.[1] That enthusiastic band of quasi-Malthusians, Francis Place, James Mill, and Edward Gibbon Wakefield, intellectuals all, had a bad record: 'rare fellows we to teach restraint', Place commented, after discovering that between them they probably had no less than thirty-six children.[2]

But in France the matter stood differently, and there statistical evidence could be provided earlier than in England. Almost the first definite statement that could be made was on the connexion between illiteracy and high fertility.[3] The reasons for this connexion were not made clear by the writers, but we may assume that the very poor were also the illiterate, and that the correlation was connected with economic rather than intellectual status. But a number of writers claimed that the more intelligent or literate youths would tend to leave the village and migrate to towns, where fertility was lower in any case, leaving behind the illiterate and those without initiative.[4] This at once raises the larger issues of the general effects of migration, especially emigration. These lie outside the scope of the present work, but it may be noted that many of the factors already described (e.g. ambition, desire not to lose status) may easily result in depopulation by driving the most vigorous and fertile young people out of the country.[5]

The second line of approach concerned the ever-increasing cost of rearing children, and the fact that longer periods of compulsory education deprived parents of their children's services as wage-earners. As regards the first part of this argument, we have already mentioned some of its antecedents in the section on children in Chapter III. It would

[1] K. Marx, *Das Kapital,* (1867 ed.), i, quoted in R. L. Meek ed., *Marx and Engels on Malthus* (London, 1953), p. 83.

[2] Place, op. cit., p. 10.

[3] Spengler, *France Faces Depopulation*, p. 74. The first reference is to Fayet in 1858.

[4] Ibid., note 17. Cauderlier's theory. Cauderlier, who was a Belgian, blamed cities in general and believed in a decline of fecundity. His work, *Les Lois de la population en France,* was published in Paris in 1902.

[5] The Webbs blamed emigration for the lack of leadership in trade unionism. Later writers believed that a high proportion of emigrants was furnished by shiftless folk, lured by tales of easy money. The same criticism would apply to Cauderlier's migration theory.

hardly apply to the working classes. But the fact that children began to be uneconomic was noted in the second half of the century.[1] This movement was in turn the result of another—the reforming crusade which stopped child labour in the industrializing countries. In agrarian regions, the children had been of use as helpers, but they did not bring in a cash wage as they did in cotton areas, for instance. It is this loss of net monetary income which may be decisive in the long run. But the spirit which produced the legislation was the same which accorded a higher consideration to the value of the child altogether—the spirit of which Ariès said that it made the child a tyrant in the nineteenth century. How far we need to blame this effect on education is therefore an academic question: new values produced a desire for education, and that education in turn gave wider currency to the new ideas.[2]

A third effect of education, closely allied perhaps to the migration theory, concerns the ideas which it implants in young people. This effect, also noticed in France by Bertillon and Leroy-Beaulieu, would be shown in the postponement of the age of marriage, a larger requirement of minimum income before marriage, and perhaps an aesthetic dislike for a frequent process of child-bearing. This negative effect led some writers to turn their wrath on education just as they had done in the case of democracy.[3]

Dumont's particular explanation of infertility lay in the fact that education, especially on the French model, increased the delusion of equality. Children of all classes imbibed the same ideals and aspirations under the universal system of schools. No such observation could have been made in England![4] Moreover, education inculcated the spirit of Truth, and Truth is the enemy of procreation:

> . . . l'attraction que la vérité exerce sur l'homme se trouve encore constituer une cause très active de diminution de la natalité. A force de recherches et d'observations patientes, l'homme est arrivé à amasser une telle quantité de vérités scientifiques que peu à peu elles ont pris toute la place occupée jadis par les systèmes de théologie ou de métaphysique.[5]

All this scientific curiosity helps to upset the old order; it creates

[1] Spengler, *France Faces Depopulation*, p. 169.

[2] For the importance of the economic factor in this connexion, see S. H. Coontz, *Population Theories and the Economic Interpretation* (London, 1957), pp. 145 ff., and Ch. IX below.

[3] e.g. Leroy-Beaulieu, op. cit., p. 220. 'Les enfants ne sont plus rémunérateurs!' Later he advocated a reduction of schooling and the inculcation of a new spirit of contentedness with one's lot in the best Malthusian manner, to achieve the opposite effect. (See Spengler, *France Faces Depopulation*, p. 170, note 96.)

[4] Dumont, op. cit., p. 246.

[5] Ibid., pp. 259–60.

conflicts and contradictions. One can imagine Dumont sighing for the superstitious days before the great enlightenment. The individual then had counted for little, but our anthropocentric sciences (as well as the doctrine of individual salvation preached by the Catholic Church) had combined with lavish education to produce selfish personalities.

At least one of these ideas finds an echo elsewhere. The scientific universe is a well-ordered regular mechanism, the industrial state is a planned state. In both every individual has his proper place. From this springs a general 'sense of order' in which indiscriminate breeding is impossible. This had already been remarked by Legoyt in 1847.[1]

The concept was developed much later by the German Julius Wolf, who attributed this rising sense of order to the effects of widespread education for the masses.[2] A very considerable change had taken place since the death of Malthus. More was known about the French universal system of education. In Germany an appreciable part of the population was receiving university or higher technical training. In England a mild form of state support for voluntary systems had been replaced by universal compulsory elementary education, and in 1902 secondary education had been put on a firmer basis. In the days of Richard Jones, London and Durham had been the only places of higher education which made any contribution to the advancement of people outside the restricted circle of Oxford and Cambridge—by the date of Wolf's book six provincial universities had been added. If the early nineteenth century aroused most commonly the observation that it was easy for a man to rise in the world by early rising and great thrift, the age of Wells and Webb was much more inclined to point to the ladder provided by education. Perhaps the economic difficulties of the period 1873–96 gave a shock to the bag-of-oatmeal theory from which it never quite recovered. For a short time, the ethos of the early Labour movement restored to fashion the career of the man who started as a half-timer at eleven in the mill, but even this was shortly to be replaced by emphasis on the propriety of rising via the eleven-plus examination. If the means were different, the effect was exactly the same: marriage was out of the question for the son of a tradesman seeking to qualify as a doctor, for just as long a period as it had been for the son of a weaver seeking to amass capital to start a cotton mill.

[1] *Journal des économistes* (1847), xvii. 174 ff., quoted by Spengler, *France Faces Depopulation*, p. 110.

[2] J. Wolf, *Der Geburtenrückgang. Die Rationalisierung des Sexuallebens in unserer Zeit* (Jena, 1912), p. 41.

Thus education came to be at once the most important step in the ladder which led to the top, and the most widespread obstacle to early marriage. By the time Wolf wrote, a number of accurate statistical investigations had been made. Fahlbeck had studied the aristocracy and professional classes in Sweden, and del Vecchio the connexion between illiteracy and fertility in Italy.[1] After the First World War the decline in the income of the middle classes produced again the problem of the rising cost of education of children according to their tradition. The Second World War completed the process of redistribution of incomes and thus new studies were produced on the relation of education and the birth-rate.[2] But as with other factors, the educational process has become so merged with other significant social, economic, and political changes, that a positive correlation between attainment in that sphere and variations in the birth-rate becomes more and more difficult to establish. Besides, no two authorities seem agreed even as to the best hypothesis, supposing it to be capable of proof, of the exact sequence of effects of better education on the attitude towards reproduction. Most of them think, however, that some sort of connexion exists. Perhaps once again we are faced with a thesis which many know intuitively to be true, though proof is difficult. The sociologists especially have a tendency to explain the behaviour of educated Western man in such complicated abstractions that the matter is taken out of the realms of mathematical proof—it is all a question of the *Grundgesinnung*. At this stage the historian has little to contribute.[3]

4. THE STATUS OF WOMEN

When we discussed the position of children in the family, we did not differentiate between boys and girls. In fact, many of the expenses

[1] P. E. Fahlbeck, *Der Adel Schwedens (und Finlands). Eine demographische Studie* (Jena, 1903). G. S. del Vecchio, *Gli Analfabeti e le nascite nelle varie parti d'Italia* (1894). All quoted by Wolf, op. cit. See also Steinmetz, 'Der Nachwuchs der Begabten', *Zeitschrift für Sozialwissenschaft* (1904), quoted by P. Mombert, *Studien zur Bevölkerungsbewegung in Deutschland* (Karlsruhe, 1907), p. 143. The conclusion is that especially those successful in intellectual careers fail to reproduce themselves as fully as their parents did. See also Ch. VI, section 2.

[2] For sources, see United Nations, *The Determinants and Consequences of Population Trends*, pp. 81, 89. Those who believe in the theory that refinement produces sterility would no doubt explain the reversal, in recent years, of the fertility trends of the professional classes in some countries by the absence of domestic servants.

[3] Except perhaps to record an old German proverb:

'Lehrers Kind und Pfarrers Vieh,
Gedeihen selten oder nie.'

usually listed by writers who lamented the prohibitive cost of bringing up offspring applied to girls—such as instruction in the arts dictated by fashion, dowries, and the process of 'bringing out'. In this sense only we may say that excessive regard for the position of women was already a bar to marriage in the eighteenth century. We recall Ange de Goudar's saying: 'on trouve mal-honnête de ne pouvoir faire paroître une femme dans le monde avec un certain éclat . . .'.[1] This theme appears frequently in Western writers, but it really constitutes merely a variant of the old theory that it is the maintenance of a given standard which limits fertility—it does not matter in this case whether it is one's own tastes or the supposed needs of a woman.[2]

A different picture, however, emerges from eighteenth-century France if we consider the institution of the 'salon'. For here we definitely have the woman possessing individual status. In a matriarchal society women also have status—but this is of necessity linked with the expectation that they will bear children. In a patriarchal society women did not attain until lately any position where they might refuse to bear children until they could perform some role independently of their husbands. This provokes the question of whether nineteenth-century European society was patriarchal—opinions differ.

There is a third role for a married woman which may give her status—that of wage-earner by necessity. This is a comparatively recent phenomenon, and even in England, where it was supposed to be most common, it was in practice confined to textile districts until the war of 1914–18, and the rise of light engineering industries.[3] When the habit did become widespread, women were accorded very different treatment from that brought to light by the Royal Commissions of the 1840's, or portrayed by Zola in *Germinal.* When women were able to take time off to have their babies, infant mortality dropped. There is again, here, a fundamental relationship between falling birth- and death-rates.

In this way the question of the development of birth-control is strongly linked with the movement for women's rights; quite apart from any economic considerations which may persuade the husband to

[1] A. de Goudar, *Les Intérêts de la France mal entendus* (Amsterdam, 1757, 3 vols.), i. 184.

[2] See G. Mackenroth, *Bevölkerungslehre; Theorie, Soziologie und Statistik der Bevölkerung* (Enzyklopädie der Rechts- und Staatswissenschaft. Abteilung Staatswissenschaft, Berlin, 1953), p. 408. 'Die Frau wird gewissermaßen selbst Mittel der Aufwandskonkurrenz.' He draws attention to the 'Babbitt' type whose wife's expenditure has to conform to the norm he expects.

[3] For an extended discussion of this question, see Coontz, op. cit., pp. 153 ff., and Ch. IX below.

practice abstinence, there is the woman's demand to 'have her body to herself'. Since she cannot, however, refuse her husband access to her, it is only with contraception that she may hope to accomplish her aim.[1]

The main demands for women's rights, and the forecast of a reduction in the birth-rate in consequence, has come from socialist writers. Their attitude stems, of course, from a general concern for the welfare of the individual and the family. This was the approach, for example, of William Thompson (1755–1833), who was one of the most important early English socialists, the group which provided the link between the revolutionary period and Marx on one hand and democratic socialism on the other. Thompson's interests were mainly in the direction of co-operation and the rights of women. Marriage, he thought, had become a squalid affair—it served the satisfaction of instincts, and produced misery. How much more noble it could be if it were a free union between equals! If women could have rights to property, and votes, how much more easily would families be controlled!

> Where women are brought up and treated like rational beings, and enjoy in all respects equal advantages with men, they will not, like ripe fruit or bales of cloth, be fought for; their opinions will be of some trifling weight in the disposal of their persons and happiness for life.[2]

Thompson naturally was an advocate of some form of birth-control, although he does not seem to have been very specific about the means to be employed.[3]

John Stuart Mill may be noted both as one of the earliest propagandists of the birth-control movement and the best-known advocate of women's rights in his time. In the *Principles*, book iv, chapter vii is devoted to the 'probable futurity of the labouring classes'. In this he advocated the adoption of policies which would make the labouring people of the country less dependent on the upper classes; more self-reliant, educated, and politically responsible. The most important consequence which he foresaw was that of more provident modes of conduct 'and that population . . . will bear a gradually diminishing ratio

[1] It might be suggested that the husband's economic restraint would also depend on the existence of contraceptives. But as we have shown, the idea that the man might practise continence within marriage was widespread long before any general spread of contraceptive knowledge.

[2] W. Thompson, *An Inquiry into the Principles of the Distribution of Wealth* (London, 1824), p. 558, quoted in K. Smith, *The Malthusian Controversy*, p. 169.

[3] See J. A. Field, *Essays on Population and Other Papers* (H. F. Hohman, ed. and comp., Chicago, 1931), p. 95. Details in N. E. Himes, *Medical History of Contraception* (Baltimore, 1936); Thompson, op. cit., pp. 547–50. See also R. K. P. Pankhurst, *William Thompson, 1775–1833; Britain's Pioneer Socialist, Feminist, and Co-operator* (London, 1954).

to capital and employment'. This most desirable result would be accelerated by another change, which lies in the direct line of the best tendencies of the times: the opening of industrial occupations freely to both sexes.

The same reasons which make it no longer necessary that the poor should depend on the rich, make it equally unnecessary that women should depend on men, and the least which justice requires is that law and custom should not enforce dependence (when the correlative protection has become superfluous) by ordaining that a woman, who does not happen to have a provision by inheritance, shall have scarcely any means open to her of gaining a livelihood, except as a wife and mother. Let women who prefer that occupation, adopt it; but that there should be no option, no other career possible for the great majority of women, except in the humbler departments of life, is a flagrant social injustice. The ideas and institutions by which the accident of sex is made the groundwork of an inequality of legal rights and a forced dissimilarity of social functions, must ere long be recognised as the greatest hindrance to moral, social, and even intellectual improvement. On the present occasion I shall only indicate, among the probable consequences of the industrial and social independence of women, a great diminution of the evil of over-population. It is by devoting one-half of the human species to that exclusive function, by making it fill the entire life of one sex, and interweave itself with almost all the objects of the other, that the animal instinct in question is nursed into the disproportionate preponderance which it has hitherto exercised in human life.[1]

We have quoted this passage in full because it contains the essence of our argument. Rapidly changing economic conditions are closely allied with the social problems of justice. Once again the remedy for an abuse in the structure of society is held to be an efficient means also for the attack on a major economic evil. In the best utilitarian tradition, the instinctive response to the demand for a remedy for a flagrant abuse is shown to have all the correct implications necessary to commend it to the practical politician. The individual is elevated and the community benefits. In the middle classes women will lose their state of utter dependence on the male. Those of the lower orders will at least be able to choose, rather than be forced into, one career or the other. The content of marriage is raised above the animal level.

We cannot deal here with Mill's general campaign on behalf of women. But it may be said that the logic he provided did much to fight those who saw in Malthus's doctrine an immutable law. It was widely held, for instance, that the restriction of women to the duties of wife

[1] Mill, op. cit., bk. iv, ch. vii, para. 3, p. 459.

and mother was a natural law, which reinforced the law of population—inasmuch as it was necessary for Malthus's purpose that the sexual instinct should remain exactly as it was. Mill exploded this myth, in *The Subjection of Women*, when he pointed out that if child-bearing was woman's natural function, it was curious that if they had freedom to do anything else, there almost certainly would not be enough of them for this task to ensure the perpetuity of the race. What the moralists really meant, he thought, was that society needed women as child-producers, and that it must therefore compel them to act as such, much as the Navy press-ganged sailors.[1]

Other writers of the time expressed themselves less clearly than Mill. Nevertheless, the idea was widespread. It often took the form of the suggestion that physiological changes would follow from a change in women's status or occupation. In Fourier's *nouveau monde industriel et sociétaire*, women would work, and their new robustness would render them less capable of bearing children, apart from a postponement of puberty, through exercises.[2] While these notions were fairly widely adopted, his suggestion of Free Love, although also part of the movement for women's rights, found little favour: 'La pluralité d'amants est évidemment un obstacle à la fécondité.'[3]

Proudhon's explanation of the changes was more subtle. In the new society there would be such changes in organization and occupation that there would come a time when

> cohabitation is less sweet, more painful, than continence; and this moment comes the more quickly the more they devote themselves to labor, to study, to Justice and her works. The woman above all, to the extent that she participates in the social and intellectual life, loses her aptitude for maternity: when the finer instincts blossom, the amorous inclination cools. . . . Love of children purges conjugal affection of eroticism. . . .[4]

This hope is, of course, typical of all the utopian socialist writers, and Proudhon's hope of a 'sublimation' of sexual urges merely repeats Godwin's and Condorcet's vision.

[1] J. S. Mill, *The Subjection of Women* (2nd ed., London, 1869), pp. 49–50.

[2] Summary from Spengler, 'French Population Theory since 1800', *Journal of Political Economy* (1936), xliv. 749, and L. Elster, 'Bevölkerungswesen', *Handwörterbuch der Staatswissenschaften* (4th ed., Jena, 1924), ii. 775.

[3] F. M. C. Fourier, *Le Nouveau Monde industriel et sociétaire* (Paris, 1829; Brussels, 1840), quoted in Elster, loc. cit.

[4] P. J. Proudhon, *De la Justice dans la révolution et dans l'église* (Paris, 1858), i. 347, quoted by Spengler, 'French Population Theory . . .', op. cit., pp. 752–3. I have followed his translation except for a different rendering of 'vertu prolifique' and 'à mesure'.

But these flights of fancy amongst the more intellectual socialists were not, after all, so very far removed from the firm promises to women by more realistic political thinkers like August Bebel (1840–1913), whose major work, *Die Frau und der Sozialismus*, went through at least fifty editions after its publication in 1883. Bebel, the first great parliamentary leader of German social democracy, shrewdly made his appeal to the women of the working classes by showing them that only under socialism would they have a chance to fulfil themselves. He was, like most of his political friends, an anti-Malthusian, but not yet a neo-Malthusian. He subscribed to Laing's thesis (and Marx's approval of this) that hopeless poverty produced large families and foresaw a time when social justice, and the emancipation of women, would lead to smaller families.[1] His theme was continued, in rather more forceful form, by a number of other German socialists. The most extreme logical conclusion of the wage-fund theory, as derived from Mill, is to be found in the idea that one could combine an alleviation of the lot of working-class women with an upward movement in wages by means of a 'birth-strike' (*Gebärstreik*). Amongst the advocates of this was Dr. E. Bernstein, who called the limitation of births 'a revolutionary weapon'.[2]

A more sophisticated attitude was that of the Marxist Karl Kautsky (1854–1938), in his second, more mature, work on population, written in 1910 after his break with the official movement, *Vermehrung und Entwicklung in Natur und Gesellschaft*.[3] In this he did not confine himself to some simple contrasts between the prolific, hopelessly poor woman under capitalism, and the honoured, equal, career-woman under socialism with her relative infertility. Nor did he accept the thesis that women would be sterile simply because they worked hard, or that increasing prosperity produced barrenness. He did see the importance, however, of the increased need for female factory-workers, which coincided with the rapid spread of contraceptive knowledge after 1880, and the urbanization trend, which reduced the possibility of bringing up children. Here then it is the economic emancipation of the woman within a general system of exploitation, which is combined with birth-control to produce a new status for women. Kautsky was well satisfied

[1] A. Bebel, *Die Frau und der Sozialismus* (1883; Stuttgart, 1911), pp. 494, 503 ff.

[2] For an account of this see the essay 'Bevölkerungsprobleme als Weltanschauungsfragen', by the Catholic conservative Max Scheler, in *Moralia* (Leipzig, 1924, 3 vols.), iii, part ii, pp. 161–3.

[3] Published Stuttgart, 1910. The earlier work was *Der Einfluß der Volksvermehrung auf den Fortschritt der Gesellschaft* (Vienna, 1880). This was frankly neo-Malthusian.

with this explanation,[1] because it dispensed with any admission that the observed tendency for the birth-rate to fall was due to any rising standard of living. Moreover, it enabled him to reject the thesis that under the increase in well-being which socialism would produce, the population would shrink even more rapidly. He specifically investigated the question whether the increased intellectual activity of women, given equal status everywhere, would lead to infertility, as, he said, Spencer had claimed. His answer was that this result would only follow from the prevailing unhygienic and soul-stunting method of education for women. If this were changed, they would develop a sound attitude towards their progeny, and towards society. With this, they would be able to do what was required, both if under-population or if over-population was threatened; in the latter case, Kautsky had no objections to birth-control. It was only under the existing system, when moral restraint would benefit only the rich, not the workers,[2] that he deprecated it. In this thought he is, of course, a follower of Lassalle, not of Mill. This more complicated theory does not in any way detract from the fact that Kautsky believed as much as did Mill or Bebel that the equality of women would lead to some form of control over fertility—it is immaterial in this case whether the result is slow increase, standstill, or reduction.[3]

Turning to non-Marxist writers, we also find some recognition, *ex post* rather than *ex ante*, of the connexion between the status of women and fertility. Naturally those who accepted Spencer's reasoning would see in any extension of education or responsibility to women an increased possibility of a reduced birth-rate.[4] This was the opinion of Walter Bagehot. His exposition is interesting because of his notion of a cyclical development of human fertility, which places him to some extent amongst those who saw some analogy between the life-cycles of human beings and societies:

> Probably of all causes which regulate . . . population, the nervous state of the woman is the most important, and it seems to have a kind of cyclical

[1] Kautsky, *Vermehrung und Entwicklung* . . ., pp. 187, 192 ff.

[2] Ibid., ch. xvi, pp. 242 ff., 256 ff.

[3] The socialist attitude towards population awaits fresh analysis. For bibliography see Ch. IX, section 3. Kautsky's theory of women at work and contraception would not hold water once it was seen statistically that the fall in the birth-rate was not greatest in the classes where women went out to factory work.

[4] Perhaps it should be stressed that Spencer also believed hard physical work in women to be detrimental to fertility. Not only his flat-chested blue-stockings but women of the labouring classes reduce their powers of child-bearing. See *System of Synthetic Philosophy. Principles of Biology* (London, 1899 ed., 2 vols.), ii. 511, para. 367.

course as society advances. [In the primitive stage hard work and scanty food keep down fertility, then better conditions increase it.] After that, not only the luxury of which [Adam Smith] speaks, but education and the habit of using the mind, tend almost certainly to diminish the producing power. There is only a certain quantity of force in the female frame, and if that force is invested . . . in one way, it cannot be used in another.[1]

The exact role which women came to play in modern communities was analysed by a great number of writers round the turn of the century. Paul Leroy-Beaulieu in France thought the feminist movement had developed farthest in the Anglo-Saxon countries, but was spreading fast to France:

Elles s'insinuent dans la médecine; elles commencent à se faufiler, en quelques pays, dans les professions juridiques.... La masculinisation de la femme est, à tous les points de vue, un des grands périls de la civilisation contemporaine. C'est un facteur desséchant et stérilisant.[2]

If Bagehot and Kautsky mark the intermediate stage, when the feminist movement has ceased to be the hope of those who feared overpopulation, Leroy-Beaulieu is typical of the new age which saw in it a threat to their civilization. Dumont thought that in a society which had achieved a high moral standard, women followed or at most accompanied men—in a disintegrating society they vied with the male, and tried to overtake him.[3] So, too, moans Spengler, the High Priest of Decay:

The arch-woman, the peasant woman, is a Mother. Her whole destiny desired from childhood, lies in this world. But now there is the Ibsen-woman, the comrade-wife, heroine of cosmopolitan literature from nordic drama to Parisian novel. She has mental conflicts instead of children, marriage is a problem in Arts and Crafts, the main thing is 'to understand one another'. It does not matter whether an American lady cannot find sufficient reasons for having children, because she does not want to miss a single 'season', a Parisienne, because she fears her lover will leave her, or an Ibsen heroine, because 'her body belongs to herself'. They all belong to themselves, and are all infertile.[4]

More dispassionate observers noticed the same tendencies. Brentano described how the emancipation of women, starting in the upper classes,

[1] W. Bagehot, *Economic Studies* (R. H. Hutton, ed., London, 1888), p. 141.

[2] Leroy-Beaulieu, op. cit., pp. 270 ff., 273. For other writers in France of the same period, see Spengler, *France Faces Depopulation*, pp. 169–70.

[3] Dumont, op. cit., p. 481.

[4] O. Spengler, *Der Untergang des Abendlandes, Umrisse einer Morphologie der Weltgeschichte* (Munich, 1924), ii. 124.

gradually spread downwards. Women made social demands—they did not wish to be put out of circulation for the best years of their youth. Women's education removed any notion that they were men's inferiors, they wished to share their work and recreation. As a result, more educated women remained spinsters (the stigma of the single state gradually disappeared), and within marriage, once contracted, the same factors operated: the competition of other enjoyments became stronger. Couples began to calculate the marginal utilities of different ways of gratifying their desires—the process of creating children (even supposing this not to be divorced from sexual intercourse by contraception) and the joy of seeing them grow, has to be set against inconvenience and pain in bearing them, the risk of illness for them and the mother, and the possibility of indigence for parents and children alike.[1]

cost of children

It will be seen that in the case of this argument again there is a continual awareness of trends in a changing society—no matter whether the explanation tends towards a physical effect leading to barrenness, or a psychological process reducing the will to have children, and facilitating the application of contraception.

[1] Brentano, op. cit., pp. 505 ff. Also J. Wolf, *Die neue Sexualmoral und das Geburtenproblem unserer Tage* (Jena, 1928), p. 31, and works cited in United Nations, *Determinants and Consequences* . . ., pp. 76, 78, 79. It should also be noted that many books and pamphlets advocating birth-control make some reference to the enhanced status due to women in modern society.

VI

SOME SPECIAL VARIANTS

IN earlier chapters we had occasion to note that the borderline between a belief in the physiological effects of certain factors, and in their psychological effect on voluntary action, was never clearly drawn. Many writers refused to be precise, and simply noted that a particular mode of living, or development, was usually accompanied by a decline in the birth-rate, or in marriages. In most cases these habits or policies were the subject of treatises advocating or denouncing them, with their sterilizing effects sometimes as an additional reason for the author's attitude, or indeed as the main argument in favour or against. Much of this type of writing may be classed as unorthodox or even dismissed as simple lunacy. But the attitudes revealed often struck a chord in contemporary feeling. From our point of view, they are worth investigating chiefly because in one sense or another, almost all the relationships described may be seen as part of the general changes associated with a higher standard of living, with industrialization, democracy, and enlightenment.

Two types of argument here presented, those relating to eating habits and those concerned with the effect of religious beliefs, are particularly interesting because they are amongst the most violently contested doctrines of population. Any general account of the history of population theories would need to show equally the view that religion was favourable to the birth-rate and the opposite belief; the idea that more food means more people; and that the converse is true. But here we need to show chiefly those writers who stressed the depopulating influences of better feeding and less praying, since in this context alone they may be seen as part of the development of a more general argument.

I. FOOD THEORIES AND RELATED TOPICS

Luxury in general was always held to lead to sterility, primitive life to prolific offspring. Originally, the condemnation of over-eating was part of the widespread onslaught on all forms of bodily indulgence. In time, as scientific pretensions came to be more popular than moralizing, the attack switched from the general to the particular, and writers singled out different aspects of easy living as the particular causes of sterility. Nevertheless, this type of argument has always remained a favourite with moralists and writers of social satire. Explanations vary from one writer to another. The picture presented to the reader is usually that of the spent, lethargic, and fat *bon viveur*, incapable of enjoying his surfeit of pleasures and doomed to a slow and inglorious death. The argument on the connexion between sterility and overeating originally appeared rarely in isolation, but it is curious to note how it survived even when other strictures on gross indulgence fell into the background. At first, only the rich food of the wealthy was mentioned, but later on it was noted that abundance could be found even amongst the lower orders—like Temple's porter who could be viciously luxurious with a herring.

The propounders of this theory were on safe ground. Gluttony was condemned in the Old Testament and in the New, frugality was preached by most philosophers and all the saints; fasting was practised by many religions and even secularists recommended vegetarian diets. Most people believed that the worst consequences could result from overeating and drinking. The ancient world seems to have known the connexion between diet and fertility. Interpretations differ, but according to Michael Sadler, Hippocrates was said to have condemned soft habits, especially in women. He particularly opposed a sedentary life as leading to muscular laxity.[1] Amongst Roman writers the elder Pliny, in his *Natural History*, devoted much time to the study of the causes of fertility. Most of what he said may be dismissed under the heading of superstition, but Doubleday also quotes him as saying that fat people, whether men or women, are altogether barren.[2] Lucretius also said that 'it matters much on what diet life is supported' when we consider fertility: he did not tell us what we should eat, but perhaps it would be just to infer from the context, where he advocates highly naturalistic behaviour, that he referred to simple food rather than fasting.[3]

[1] M. T. Sadler, *The Law of Population: a Treatise, in Six Books; in Disproof of the Super-fecundity of Human Beings, and Developing the Real Principle of Their Increase* (London, 1830, 2 vols.), i. 577. His translations from Latin and Greek often violate the original. In this case, Hippocrates' *De aëre, locis et aquis* simply describes soft climates as infertile, at any rate in the passage cited.

[2] 'Steriliora cuncta pinguia et in maribus et in feminis.' G. Plinius Secundus, *Naturalis historia*, xi. 212. The passage deals with animal fertility. Quoted by T. Doubleday, *The True Law of Population Shewn To Be Connected with the Food of the People* (London, 1842; 3rd ed., 1853), p. 28.

[3] T. Lucretius Carus, *De natura rerum*, bk. iv, lines 1260 ff.

Hippocrates had a facetious disciple in François Rabelais, whose *Gargantua and Pantagruel* contains a fine collection of what are probably popular jokes about fertility. In the third book, Rondibilis the physician is called in to advise Panurge on the subject of his marriage, and tells him what things are likely to reduce his sexual capacity. The first amongst these is excessive wine-drinking—moderate drinking is useful ('Master Priapus was the son of Bacchus and Venus'), but intemperance leads to a 'dissipation of the generative seed'.[1] Amongst the other causes of impotence are hard work and fervent study—on the former cause he cites Hippocrates, who was obviously a friend of moderation—since not only soft living caused infertility, but also over-hard work, as he thought the Scythians performed.

Michael Sadler, who was a fervent believer in the capacity of advanced societies to solve their population problems, had a habit of quoting ancient authorities for his opinions. Unfortunately, as we already saw in connexion with the Bible, he would often twist the sense to fit in with his schemes where the quotation is easily verified, and where his reference is vague it has to be taken with more than a grain of salt. So he quotes, on the question of diet, the universal provider of opinions on all subjects, Francis Bacon, and a reference to the original gives only a slight hint that the philosopher may have followed the classical line. Speaking of generation,[2] Bacon allows that the condition of the parents is important, but, like Lucretius, he does not say exactly what are the vital conditions: '. . . some are begotten of fathers immediately after repletion, or when they are drunk; others after sleeping, or in the morning'. But he is sure that: 'all things in moderation . . . are best . . . a state of body not too lusty or full . . .'.[3] This Sadler construes to mean that repletion is an enemy to generation! However, Bacon thought that if there were anything remarkable about the number or strength of the children of the Spartans (which he doubted), that would be due to the parsimony of their diet. Sadler is therefore undoubtedly right in numbering Bacon amongst those who, on the whole, favoured moderate eating. Whether from the ancients or Bacon, the idea certainly passed into common usage.

The eighteenth century provides many examples. Thomas Short had much to say on the physiological conditions of fertility, and though he

[1] F. Rabelais, *The Histories of Gargantua and Pantagruel* (J. M. Cohen, trans., London, 1955), pp. 373 ff.

[2] F. Bacon, *Works* (B. Montagu, ed., London, 1834, 15 vols.), xiv. 349. 'History of Life and Death', misquoted and with wrong reference, in Sadler, loc. cit.

[3] Bacon, op. cit., p. 350.

condemned a 'thin, watery diet' he was equally sure that 'high stimulant Food, Drinks or Sauces' were no promoters of progeny. Nor were idleness, night-revelling, and unseasonable hours—except in that they increased the number of illegitimate children.[1] Dr. William Buchan, a Scots physician, was the author of one of the most popular medical guides of the time—his *Domestic Medicine* (originally published 1763) ran into many editions. The book is full of good rules, as well as the usual superstitions and folk remedies. His style is vigorous:

> Would the rich use the same sort of food and exercise as the better sort of peasants, they would seldom have cause to envy their poor vassals and dependants the blessing of a numerous and healthy offspring, while they pine in sorrow for the want of even a single heir to their extensive domains.[2]

Obviously the poorer peasants had not enough to eat, and were infertile on that score. Not until the twentieth century did it become clear that even people actually starving might be prolific.

Although one of the most famous precursors of the modern standard-of-living theory, Archdeacon Paley, could be quoted as saying that the conversion of the Indians to meat-eating would soon stop them from increasing, it has to be clearly understood that he did not thereby imply any physical effects of their diet. The argument, as we have seen, was purely psychological: the more complicated the customary diet, the greater the measure of voluntary restraint. Considering the refinement which population theory had reached in the days of Ferguson and Paley, it is perhaps a little surprising to find the food argument coming back into favour in the post-Malthusian period. Yet it is understandable that this should be so. In a sense, this may be taken as a natural consequence of the observation that the poor were prolific—if it is true that the starving wretches can still breed like rabbits, then lack of nourishment is no obstacle but an abundance may well be. To isolate this aspect of poverty and wealth is not quite such a stupid procedure as it may sound. At a time when, as it was widely believed, by far the greatest item of expenditure in the budget of the majority of the families of the country was the purchase of bread, and when

[1] T. Short, *New Observations, Natural, Moral, Civil, Political, and Medical on City, Town, and Country Bills of Mortality* (London, 1750), pp. 143–9. Quoted in R. R. Kuczynski, 'British Demographers' Opinions on Fertility, 1660–1760', *Political Arithmetic; a Symposium of Population Studies* (L. T. Hogben, ed., London, 1938). Kuczynski quotes Graunt (1662) and Gregory King (1696) for the same general opinion, and Corbyn Morris for similar opinions on drinking: op. cit., pp. 296–9.

[2] W. Buchan, *Domestic Medicine; or, a Treatise on the Prevention and Cure of Diseases, by Regimen and Simple Medicines* . . . (1763; new ed., London, 1880), p. 365.

bread formed the basis of the scale of poor relief, it could very properly be inferred that the social gradations, at any rate up to the middle classes, were largely gradations of food.

But there was an even more cogent reason for the importance of the food argument at this time. If Malthus said that increased subsistence produced more population, the shortest answer obviously was to say that it produced the opposite effect: that abundance reduced fertility. This saved a great deal of wrangling about the ratios, or about the significance of any of Malthus's historical material.

The first author to base a part of his answer to Malthus on this simple argument was Simon Gray, author of a tract, *The Happiness of States*, published in 1815 (it had been written in 1804), and a more elaborate work *Gray versus Malthus*,[1] published in 1818 under the pseudonym of George Purves, and purporting to be a comparison of the validity of the arguments of Gray and Malthus.[2] Gray made much of the fact that, in general, larger populations were better able to supply their wants, through the division of labour. But he recognized (and by this time failure to do so was the hallmark of only the least intelligent opponents of Malthus) that even when progress in the field of supply had been made to the utmost capacity of human ingenuity, there might one day be too many people, and it was therefore necessary to say clearly why he thought the danger of over-population did not exist even in the long run. For this reason he produced the notion again that 'superabundance reduces fecundity and population'. In chapter vii he specifically rejected the idealistic view that good government alone will mean a lessening of fertility, but he agreed with Jarrold that man could rise to a higher stage of civilization where reproduction would occupy a less important place in his scheme of things. The central point, however, is the general rise in the standard of living. With that easier life comes the abundance of food which is so inimical to fertility, as the stationary population of China clearly shows.

It is worth considering for a moment, at this stage, the part played by the poor Chinese in these arguments, since the variety of interpretations advanced help us to understand some of the basic confusions of the debate. For Cantillon, as we saw, they were an example of a population geared to very few wants, but kept in equilibrium at that

[1] G. Purves (Simon Gray), *Gray versus Malthus. The Principles of Population and Production Investigated, and the Question: Does Population Regulate Subsistence, or Subsistence Population? . . . etc., Discussed* (London and Edinburgh, 1818).

[2] On this part of the controversy, see K. Smith, *The Malthusian Controversy* (London, 1951), pp. 217 ff.

level. Malthus interpreted the same relationship of people and subsistence as meaning that their numbers were kept down by the constant operation of the positive check. For Gray (possibly misled by pictures of fat mandarins) they were a people kept infertile by excessively soft living and rich food. Archdeacon Paley thought that the Chinese population was excessive, and this was supposed to be due to the fact that 'the species of food to which custom hath reconciled the desires and inclinations of the inhabitants, is that which, of all others, is procured in the greatest abundance, with the most ease, and stands in need of the least preparation'.[1]

Doubleday, as we shall see in a moment, thought the Chinese amongst the most prolific races due to the very poor diet to which they were accustomed.

Apart from the disagreement about facts, there is also the inability common to these writers to apply logical analysis to such facts as they had. They seem to assume that there are no gradations of income, and therefore they do not see any need for a threshold position—some point above which foresight is exercised (or physiological infertility begins). However few the wants, in Cantillon's scheme, there must always be some people who cannot satisfy even these, and must therefore either die of starvation or fail to marry. Malthus makes a different mistake in saying that their numbers are kept 'down' without having any population figures at all. Gray is simply absurd, and Paley does not tell us why the population does not keep on growing if food is so easy to grow and prepare.

Lest it be thought that such confusions were only possible in those early days of economic work, it should be pointed out that even the great Alfred Marshall could make judgements of this kind without thinking the matter out. He might be cited as a subscriber to the 'food' theory because he spoke of the check to population occasioned by the adoption of wheat as the staple food of Englishmen in the first half of the eighteenth century. But this was clearly an uncomplicated standard-of-living argument—people will not marry if they cannot do so at their 'customary' level. The passages in question[2] show Marshall in a

[1] W. Paley, *The Principles of Moral and Political Philosophy* (9th ed., London, 1793, 2 vols.), ii. 354–5.

[2] A. Marshall, *Principles of Economics* (8th ed., London, 1930), bk. iv, ch. iv, sections 1 and 6, quoting Eden as one of his authorities. Marshall firmly believed in the standard-of-living theory, as well as the mental strains on fecundity (see section 2, and Ch. IX). For a full account of Marshall's views on population, see J. J. Spengler, 'Marshall on Population', *Population Studies* (1955), viii. 264, and ix. 56.

bad light as an historian. Firstly, like the five authors on China, he leaves unanswered the most important question: why could the Englishman insist on wheaten bread when all other nations were kept on a standard of rye, or even peas, or oats, or rice? In other words, is it really of much use to talk about some simple mathematical relationship between available subsistence and the size of population without inquiring into the origins of the particular standard at which equilibrium must be obtained? Secondly, he was wrong in his facts, as were his less profound predecessors, for the retardation of the rate of increase did not follow until more than a hundred years after the adoption of the wheat standard in the south of England, and the slow growth of population in the early part of the eighteenth century was not due to any reluctance to marry.

In the case of such theories, therefore, we must be even more sceptical than usual about the author's ability to distinguish fact from fiction, to place his thesis in a proper conceptual framework, and to rid his mind of general prejudices. Nevertheless, the idea recurs with persistence and is worth following up since it fits into the general pattern.

The credit for elevating the question of diet to the highest position it reached must go to Thomas Doubleday, a Newcastle man, with a manufacturing background, and a prolific writer on a wide variety of subjects. His political affiliations were Radical, and opposition to Malthus would be bred in a man of his stamp long before he could think of an effective answer. He was an opponent of the new Malthusian Poor Law and this may have led him to a study of the conditions under which the poor lived. His main work was *The True Law of Population*, first published in 1842.[1] His law was bold and simple: 'the *plethoric* state invariably checks it [the population] and the *deplethoric* state invariably developes it.'[2] The proof was simple: the poorly fed Irish and Scots, living on potatoes and fish respectively, were prolific, and so were the starving Chinese and Indians, and indeed the poor everywhere. He quoted Pliny's remark which appears earlier in this chapter: fat people, whether men or women, are always rather barren. On the other hand, the Pitcairn islanders, living on yams, multiplied tenfold in forty years.[3] In France, where many fat peasants are found, fertility was low, but in England, amongst Chadwick's urban slums, life abounded. In fact, everywhere great prosperity, privilege, and exclusiveness produce a decline in numbers, and poverty the opposite

[1] Doubleday, op. cit. [2] Ibid., p. 20. [3] Ibid., p. 78.

effect. He contrasted the proud and rich merchants of Geneva, or the Quakers, with the expropriated Catholics of Ireland. Apart from food, he was particularly interested in the question of social stratification as an obstacle to marriage (see above, Chap. Two, section on aristocracies), but he was sure in his own mind that the different diets to which these various groups were accustomed were the real clue to the mystery.

His book was possibly the most popular of the anti-Malthusian writings of the nineteenth century. This was partly due to the simplicity of the argument, and its outward plausibility, and partly due to the appeal of the theory of abundance at the time when the Corn Law agitation was at its height. If it were true that plentiful provision of cheap food was a sure specific against over-population, then this constituted a splendid argument for the Free Traders. It is ironical, of course, that it was precisely over the failure of the potato crop in Ireland that the last duties on corn were repealed: the pro-genitive tuber having given out, the ruling classes of England were forced to permit the free importation of anti-genitive corn.

Modern research has shown Doubleday's thoughts on the potato standard to be somewhere near the truth, but for the wrong reasons. As Dr. Salaman demonstrated,[1] the potato diet was balanced and had all the necessary nourishment for healthy survival. What made the potato-eating Irish so prolific was not the poverty of their diet, but the smallness of the plot of land which would support a family, and the associated readiness to marry early, and without capital, and absence of worry about the number of children. In other words, it was their low standard which ensured their survival—as Cantillon had said of the Chinese.[2]

Doubleday's book, which ran through at least three editions, aroused a great deal of comment, much of it sceptical and hostile. But he had at least one devoted follower in William Hickson (1803–70), the London shoe manufacturer who became a noted educationalist and reformer. It is possible that he became interested in Doubleday through the fact that it was during his editorship of the *Westminster Review* that a critical review of the book (by William King-Noel, first Earl Lovelace) appeared in its columns. Hickson's *Malthus: an Essay on the Principle of Population* was first published in the *Review* and then in book form in 1849. In general, he was something of a utopian of the school of Condorcet and Godwin, but in the short run

[1] R. N. Salaman, *The History and Social Influence of the Potato* (Cambridge, 1949).
[2] See also K. H. Connell, *The Population of Ireland, 1750–1845* (Oxford, 1950).

he based his anti-Malthusian optimism not on the ultimate fading of interest in sexual activity, but Doubleday's food effect. This he quotes at great length.[1] His main conclusion regarding the effect of food and soft living on population was that they would act both by reducing the parents' powers of reproduction, and by enfeebling the offspring. It should be noted that he refers frequently to animal food—he did not think the people of Great Britain would die out as a result of the repeal of the Corn Laws, a cause for which he worked for long. Indeed, he had enough knowledge of the conditions under which the majority of his fellow countrymen lived to have no fear of the immediate consequences of the food effect. But he believed in it sufficiently to keep it as a long-term safety factor. It meant, as it did to many of his contemporaries, that contrary to Malthus's opinion, every effort should be made to procure more plentiful food for the labouring population. Conscience dictated this course, and intelligence recommended it.

Outside England the food theory does not seem to have gained much of a foothold. A solitary exponent is the French utopian socialist Ch. Fourier (1772–1837), who seems to have anticipated Doubleday by a few years—but then, as we have seen, the idea was an old one. In Fourier's 'societary state' population was to be held in bounds by four checks—all of them aspects of a more advanced form of living. One of these was the greater physical vigour of the women, which would render them less fertile; another a species of polygamy and polyandry which he called 'phanerogamic customs', which reduced fertility presumably just as others claimed prostitutes became sterile; thirdly he hoped puberty would occur later in life if young people were given other interests in life than sex in the early stages of their education, and became absorbed in them; and lastly the more refined and plentiful food available in his society would reduce fecundity.[2] Amongst his followers who accepted his thesis were H. Renaud and T. Fix—these two both writing after Doubleday's book had become known in France.[3] But by the time these ideas came to the attention of Frenchmen the problem of a stationary population was already upon them, and however attractive the *gastrosophie* might be to them as a means of limiting population, many of them could see that their misfortunes were due to less pleasant causes.

[1] W. E. Hickson, *Malthus; an Essay on the Principle of Population, in Refutation of the Theory of the Rev. T. R. Malthus* (London, 1849), pp. 47, 73.

[2] J. J. Spengler, 'French Population Theory since 1800', *Journal of Political Economy* (1936), xliv. 749. The ideas were taken from works by Fourier published in the 1820's.

[3] For sources, see Spengler, ibid., p. 750.

Thus the Doubleday theory seems to have died a natural death in the second half of the nineteenth century—mainly because it became increasingly difficult to separate better food from other aspects of increased comfort. As food cheapened, so an ever greater part of total income was devoted to the consumption of goods and services.

Yet it was to suffer a resurrection in our own time. One curiously inspired guess came from a well-known German observer of the British scene, G. v. Schulze-Gävernitz, whose knowledge of English literature was sufficiently large to make it quite possible that he knew of Doubleday or Hickson. In his book on British imperialism he put forward the view that the decline of fertility observed in Australia may have been due to their habit of eating vast quantities of meat.[1] On the other hand, the observation that hunger and fertility went together came to be made with increasing frequency. René Gonnard, writing in 1923, was disinclined to brush aside the Doubleday theory, as had become the fashion; he could see that the poor and vegetarian people were prolific, while the carnivorous nations were suffering a rapid reduction of fertility.[2]

Although by this time 'psychological' theories of population were available by the dozen, there have emerged again in our own time authors who would blame physical causes for the evident decline in the birth-rate. Unwilling to accept the evidence for the spread of contraceptive methods, they argued that changing modes of life must be held responsible. Some of these authors would describe practices which were quite obviously harmful to general health, others found modern life brought people into contact with injurious substances.[3] Lastly, a Latin-American author, Josué de Castro, familiar with the background of his material, evolved a complete theory of the effect of diet and fertility in his book *Geography of Hunger*.[4] He listed countries according to the protein content of their diet, and showed that those who ate most

[1] G. v. Schulze-Gävernitz, *Britischer Imperialismus und englischer Freihandel zu Beginn des zwanzigsten Jahrhunderts* (Leipzig, 1906), p. 196, quoted in K. Oldenburg, 'Über den Rückgang der Geburten- und Sterbeziffer', *Archiv für Sozialwissenschaft und Sozialpolitik* (1911), xxxii. 319 ff. This article examines critically some of the assumptions of the standard-of-living school.

[2] R. Gonnard, *Histoire des doctrines de la population* (Paris, 1923), p. 313.

[3] For details, see United Nations, *The Determinants and Consequences of Population Trends* (New York, 1953), p. 75. These include Professor Hogben's theory that women reduce their fertility by frequent bathing, since soap is a spermicide. 'Alcoholism' is an obvious refinement of our age on older forms of drunkenness.

[4] J. de Castro, *Geography of Hunger* (Paris, 1949; Eng. trans., London, 1952), esp. pp. 70–72.

protein had the lowest fertility, and vice versa, and tried to give some reasons for this curious correlation. He has been attacked by many writers, partly because his statistics omit a good many countries which do not fit conveniently into his ascending and descending series, and partly because he does not appear to give sufficient weight to other circumstances of the life of poverty which is symbolized by staple diets of rice or coarse grain.

In sum, discussions of the validity or otherwise of the food theory have now almost become irrelevant. What is widely accepted today is the theory that if the standard of living of backward countries is raised their population problems may be solved. But if the success of this policy is dependent on the conversion of Hindus to beef-eating, rather than other manifestations of material prosperity, it may well be doomed to failure.

2. INTELLECTUAL ACTIVITY

In the section on the effects of education we related the supposed connexion between learning and low fertility to several major causes which fitted in with the context: these associated education with refinement, the knowledge of the higher wants, and an understanding of political economy in general and the works of Malthus in particular. There was also the high cost of education and the possibility of a career leading to a higher position in society. All these causes operate clearly on the psychological plane. But there is also another view, that intellectual activity has the effect of producing sterility in its devotees, and that this is a characteristic feature of the complicated life which many people, especially those with responsibilities, lead in modern society. As we shall see, a further extension of this idea is to be found in the socio-biological fertility schemes of Herbert Spencer and his associates. While the Spencerian theory operates at a social level, and makes for comparisons between one society and another, both the educational and the intellectual idea, on different planes, are concerned with differential fertility within one society.

In its origins the idea is probably medieval. Scholarship was associated with monastic life. Even those who were not in orders usually remained single if they wished to devote their lives to study. In England the fellowships of the colleges were, until very recently, the preserve of single men. The studious man (women did not enter into the picture) was one whose inclinations, income, and surroundings made him unfit to be a husband and father. It is worth quoting the Rabelaisian nonsense which is probably quite representative of what many people thought. The passage is part of the advice of the physician Rondibilis, on how infertility may be avoided. Study is one of its causes:

Fourthly, by fervent study. For by this means the spirits are so dissolved that not enough is left to impel this generative secretion to its destined place, and so to inflate the cavernous nerve whose office is to ejaculate it for the propagation of humankind. To prove this to yourself, contemplate the form of a man intent on some study. You will see all the arteries of his brain stretched like the string of a cross-bow . . . [here follow strange anatomical details]. So in such a studious person you will see all the natural faculties suspended, all the external senses blocked. In short, you will judge him not to be living in himself but to be ecstatically transported out of himself. For philosophy is nothing else but the contemplation of death. Possibly that is why Democritus blinded himself, preferring the loss of his sight to the reduction of his contemplations, which he left to be interrupted by the straying of his eyes. That is why Pallas, the goddess of wisdom and protectress of scholars, is said to be a virgin; that is why the Muses are virgins; that is why the Graces remain perpetually chaste . . . [even Cupid avoided attacking the Muses].[1]

Towards the end of this passage he also quotes Hippocrates as saying that a great part of the material of reproduction springs from the brain and spinal column.

So too Ange de Goudar, in the eighteenth century, lists excessive mental occupation amongst the causes of sterility: 'L'humeur, le génie, les préjugés, l'esprit de société, la délicatesse . . . l'esprit philosophique. . . .'[2]

Malthus seems to have felt that there was a connexion. In the first *Essay* he tries to dispose of the notion that man might one day be less addicted to sexual activity (as Godwin had suggested) when he had developed into a higher species of being. The highest form known to Malthus, naturally, was the intellectual, and so he examined him—and found him wanting, since:

some men of the highest mental powers, have been addicted not only to a moderate, but even to an immoderate indulgence in the pleasures of sensual love.

[1] Rabelais, op. cit., p. 375.

[2] A. de Goudar, *Les Intérêts de la France mal entendus . . . etc.* (Amsterdam, 1757, 3 vols.), i. 172.

But he felt it necessary to allow

> that great intellectual exertions tend to diminish the empire of this passion over man.[1]

Yet he could not hope much from that, since there was no prospect of the mass of mankind surpassing those few 'brightest ornaments of the species'. What Malthus here considers, of course, is the sexual inclination as opposed to sexual effectiveness—but no doubt this distinction did not yet enter the scheme of things. At any rate the young Malthus was undoubtedly impressed by the tales of the adventures of the eighteenth-century *littérateurs*. At a later stage he seems to have become less sure of the truth of his objection, for the passage just quoted is one of the few totally omitted from later editions.

As we would expect, Malthus's opponents brought the theory forward in connexion with their attempts to show that a better society would be less prolific. John Weyland, an East Anglian author, Member of the last unreformed Parliament, and Fellow of the Royal Society, was one of the chief sponsors of the idea that progress in civilization provided automatic checks to population. Intellectual activity was part of this progress, and its effects were held to be both physical and moral.

> ... in proportion to the continued necessity of mental exertion or abstraction, many, who could well afford to rear a family, are placed in situations and pursuits where a voluntary abstinence from marriage, and the incapacity and indisposition to rear large families, becomes very general. . . .
>
> [In the later stages of progress] many of the people will be also lifted above the rank of the lower orders, and be affected by those artificial arrangements of society, which, though they universally produce high mental cultivation, do very much diminish the natural powers of increase in mankind.[2]

He ends his book with a panegyric on the sterile part of the population: it is upon these ranks that the task of mental thought for the whole society often devolves. These are precisely the men who are least likely to become the fathers of large families—a condition, if they fulfil the duties of it, that must evidently tend to subtract from their public utility.[3]

A variant on this theme was the theory of Thomas Jarrold, who

[1] T. R. Malthus, *An Essay on the Principle of Population* (London, 1798), p. 217.

[2] J. Weyland, jnr., *The Principles of Population and Production, as They Are Affected by the Progress of Society; with a View to Moral and Political Consequences* (London, 1816), pp. 63–65. He refers in the last passage to the views of Dr. Trotter for an account of the effect of civilization on physical powers.

[3] Ibid., p. 427.

believed that the strain of worrying about one's position in society had adverse effects on fertility. In general, it was man's lot to rise ever further above the animal state, and as various faculties were brought into use in that process—most of them mental powers—so the powers of reproduction diminished. Those overburdened with anxieties do not produce at all.[1] Later on, he contrasts the fast increase of the American farmers with that of other people who were philosophers, or shone in literature or science.[2] Here again it is hard to separate intellectual activity from the other attributes of civilization: but the old prejudices against the sexual powers of the scholar stand out as an important component part of the whole edifice.

The Spencerians made much of this aspect. Spencer himself felt it to be a prime cause:

> ... absolute or relative infertility is commonly produced in women by mental labour carried to excess. . . . This diminution of reproductive power is not shown only by the greater frequency of absolute sterility; nor is it shown only in the earlier cessation of childbearing; but it is also shown in the very frequent inability of such women to suckle their infants.[3]

Elsewhere he points out the apparent connexion between high cerebral development and prolonged delay of sexual maturity, exceptional fertility in connexion with a sluggish mind, and sterility due to excessive mental strain during the process of education.[4] In fact it is precisely this train of circumstances which provides the core of the whole theory of the antithesis of individuation and genesis.

The enthusiasm with which many writers took up this point again prompts some reflections on the spirit of the times. The mid-Victorians were prolific, and at any rate in the middle classes, proud of it. The normal family portrait of Father surrounded by his numerous family leaves no doubt about this. This age of increasing prosperity coupled with cheap servants, and the advent of certain technical aids to domestic life (such as hot-water systems and water closets), made this a period when children were less of a burden than they had been, and were to be again a few decades later.

Now Spencer was a critic of this family—especially of the values of the educational system that went with it. Besides, he disliked the

[1] T. Jarrold, *Dissertations on Man Philosophical, Physiological and Political; in Answer to Mr. Malthus' 'Essay on the Principle of Population'* (London, 1806), pp. 249–56.

[2] Ibid., p. 281.

[3] H. Spencer, *System of Synthetic Philosophy. Principles of Biology* (London, 1899 ed., 11 vols.), ii, part vi, ch. xii, pp. 512–13, para. 367.

[4] Ibid., paras. 346, 366.

smugness of the satisfied *paterfamilias*—perhaps even the pride in something which they had no right to claim as their own merit. The theory which he propounded could be seen as a slightly malicious attack on the prevailing ethos—you, the proud ones, are near-animals; I, the intellectual, the advanced being, have a right to glory in my barrenness. It would be highly instructive to see how many predecessors and followers of Spencer were infertile.[1] He provided them with a rationalization, and a highly flattering one at that. Beatrice Webb was an early worshipper at the Spencerian shrine, but she could hardly have seen in herself the frail, flat-chested blue-stocking of Spencer's description, who had, by education, been made useless for motherhood.

Amongst the followers of Spencer in this respect were the American Henry Carey[2] and the English economist Walter Bagehot. The latter, like anyone else concerned with the future organization of society under a better form of government, found it necessary to make his peace with the Malthusian bogy—no one could hope, in the nineteenth century, and few could today, to speak about the coming millennium without first settling the question of how the progress of population was to be checked. Bagehot called on Spencer to provide the answer: 'This means that men who have to live an intellectual life, or who can be induced to lead one, will be likely not to have so many children as they would otherwise have had.'[3] He calls this statement a philosophical doctrine and alleges that the best philosophers subscribe to it. London, he believes, is such a hot-bed of intellectual activity that the constitutions of men and women are much affected. 'There is only a certain *quantum* of power in each of our race; if it goes in one way it is spent, and cannot go in another.'

With Spencer and Bagehot we enter that period of discussions on population which is overshadowed by the impact of Darwin rather than of Malthus. Already in the eighteenth century, Joseph Townshend, in his celebrated example of the goats of Juan Fernandez, had demonstrated the necessity for the survival of the fittest; Malthus had implied it with his examples of positive checks bearing most heavily on the less-refined forms of human life. To these ideas Darwin had declared

[1] The ascertainable score is as follows: Rabelais—possibly one natural son. John Weyland—married, o.s.p. Thomas Jarrold—two children. Spencer and Carey—unmarried, no children known. Bagehot—married, o.s.p. Alfred Marshall—married late, o.s.p.

[2] H. C. Carey, *Principles of Social Science* (Philadelphia, 1858–60, 3 vols.), iii, ch. xlvi.

[3] W. Bagehot, *Physics and Politics, or Thoughts on the Application of the Principles of 'Natural Selection' and 'Inheritance' to Political Society* (new ed., London, 1885), p. 199.

himself indebted. But the establishment of the principle of natural selection as a major law of nature inevitably brought forward the eugenic question—would the fittest to survive be also the best? Many writers raised the bogy of a conscienceless proletariat multiplying itself rapidly, while the more prudent better classes restricted their offspring. Soon, it was feared, it would be a question of the survival of the unfittest people, in the social sense. That was the problem the 'culture optimists' faced. The failure of the best brains to reproduce themselves was only part of their perplexities. If, as Alison and others had pointed out earlier, the withering away of the upper layer was a perfectly natural phenomenon, and not to be feared if only the upward path was smooth to those who had to rise to replace it, then in this particular context the question of popular education was of the greatest importance. The solution of the dilemma created by Malthus and Darwin on one hand, and Spencer on the other, was found in the spirit of Matthew Arnold.

Many of Spencer's followers in France, already quoted, laid stress on the effect of concentration of energies in studies. Their view was shared by some of the socialists of the middle of the century, who, like their predecessors fifty years earlier, saw mankind in such a rosy haze of virtue in coming ages that the eradication of the sex instinct was almost a necessity. The earlier writers had mostly stressed the elevating effect of just government as such. Now men like Proudhon described in detail those aspects of life which would help men to overcome their more primitive instincts. Under the old régime, he claimed, enforced idleness and emptiness of mind had caused rapid population increases. But if mankind were only organized so as to devote themselves to labour and study, the position would be reversed. 'Men of meditation, energetic thinkers, all great workers, are of mediocre capacity in the service of love.'[1] As we saw in the section on the status of women, Proudhon expected a great check to increase to arise from their equal status in society—and one of the signs that they had achieved this was fuller feminine participation in social and intellectual life. Everywhere writers make it clear that the studious life reduces both the inclination and the capacity for successful sexual activity. Yet, with more elaborate statistics becoming available to the population theorists, the sterilizing effect of intellectual activity by itself lost favour. By the end of the nineteenth century the idea was fully merged into the more general theories. An echo of it appeared in the writings of Alfred Marshall.

[1] Quoted in Spengler, 'French Population Theory . . .', op. cit., p. 752.

In the section of the *Principles* which dealt with the standard of living and its effect on population he also thought that fecundity was diminished

> by severe mental strain; that is to say, given the natural strength of the parents, their expectation of a large family is diminished by a great increase in mental strain. Of course those who do high mental work, have as a class more than the average of constitutional and nervous strength; and Galton has shown that they are not as a class unprolific. But they commonly marry late.[1]

Poor Marshall, he married late, he married as pure an intellectual as he himself was, and they had no children. The passage is, as usual, complete with its own neutralizer, but it may have given him satisfaction to have such an alibi, which our later generation does not think at all necessary.

But as with so many other theories deeply rooted in popular prejudice, a recent scientific revival may be noted. In medical literature dealing with the causes of infertility in married couples, nervous tension due to a variety of causes figures prominently, and that this is found amongst men and women of high intellectual attainment seems to be confirmed by experience. Statistics of differential fertility, of course, do not deal with fecundity, but it is a fair assumption, in view of the medical findings, that not all the difference in family size between manual labourers and intellectuals is due to voluntary restraint. This, however, is outside the scope of our considerations.

3. RELIGION AND ENLIGHTENMENT

In the nature of things the question whether the increase or decrease of membership of a particular church, or of religious feeling in general, have made any contribution, positive or negative, to fertility patterns, is one likely to arouse deep partisan feelings. No agreement exists amongst demographers about the effect of particular beliefs on fertility. It often happens that a particular group, like the French-Canadian Catholics, have a distinct pattern—but there is no evidence that this is solely connected with the religious beliefs they hold. Nevertheless, there have been sufficient writers who have claimed that the decline of religion (which they equate with the spread of enlightenment and civilization in general) has had much to do with the decline in fertility, to warrant inclusion of this factor in our list.

[1] Marshall, op. cit., bk. iv, ch. iv, section 5, p. 185.

At the same time the weight of opinion the other way is such that it is only fair to quote what others have said to prove the opposite point. The most widespread of all statements amongst the demographers of the pre-Malthusian period, next to the assertions about luxury, was that the Roman Catholic religion was inimical to population, since it kept many men and women in enforced singleness and made a virtue out of virginity. Many writers advocated the suppression of monastic houses for that reason alone. Needless to say, they were mostly Protestants or agnostics.[1]

But equally the charge was made that Protestantism led to infertility, since it meant the relaxation of that strict code of behaviour (and the means of enforcing it) which was characteristic of the Catholic Church and preserved family life wherever it operated. Lately, this charge has taken the form that birth-control is the result of disobedience to the Church, and that therefore fertility is highest where the Church is strongest.

These two sets of charges seem mutually contradictory, and that there is something of a dilemma here has been admitted by Catholic writers.[2]

The development of the argument naturally starts with the defence by Catholic writers against the charge that the Church is a depopulating influence. The implication of this defence is always that the true barrier to increase is found in the ethics of 'progressive' man. There is also a direct attack: that Protestantism at least has sexual ethics far more barren than Catholicism, since it carries the idea of asceticism into the marriage, where it does not belong, and thereby makes it infertile.

This argument is not necessarily the work of Catholic writers. Certainly its most famous exponent was Max Weber, whose *Protestant Ethic and the Spirit of Capitalism* gained wide acceptance as a guide to the connexion between religion and social behaviour:

> The sexual asceticism of Puritanism differs only in degree . . . from that of monasticism; . . . and on account of the Puritan conception of marriage, its practical influence is more far-reaching than that of the latter. For sexual intercourse is permitted, even within marriage, only as the means willed by

[1] For sources, see Spengler, *French Predecessors of Malthus*, esp. Colbert, Montesquieu.

[2] See J. A. O'Brien, ed., *The Vanishing Irish; the Enigma of the Modern World* (London, 1954). That the apparent contradiction between the ideals of chastity and of the family is not a real one, has been shown by a number of writers who have traced the origins of Catholic sexual ethics. A good exposition, and further material: G. Mackenroth, *Bevölkerungslehre* (Berlin, 1953), pp. 344 ff.

God for the increase of His glory according to the commandment, 'Be fruitful and multiply'.[1]

Weber cited, amongst others, the seventeenth-century Kidderminster divine, Richard Baxter, in support of this view. A number of other German writers have called this attitude 'Anglo-Saxon Puritanism' (e.g. Mackenroth) and similar names, but there is evidence that German Lutheranism did not always follow Luther's own emphasis on the content of marriage.[2]

Both Catholics and Protestants, each vying with the other in appearing pro-populationist,[3] proclaim that the road away from religion leads to the decline of the family and thus population. This is not surprising when one remembers that even though Malthus was a parson, the neo-Malthusians, in practice his most important disciples, were mostly secularists. From the beginning the advocacy of birth-control was connected with rationalism. The best-known exponent of birth-control in England was Charles Bradlaugh—but he himself gained most notoriety as the first atheist to take his seat in the House of Commons. Everywhere the neo-Malthusians were called blasphemers—the present condemnation by the Roman Catholic Church of contraceptive practices is no more vehement than opinion in the Church of England eighty years ago. It is recalled that the Swedish economist Knut Wicksell was sent to prison for blasphemy—i.e. advocacy of family limitation.[4]

Already in the eighteenth century Catholic writers began to point out that their Church withdrew only a handful of men and women from family life—their opponents always over-estimated the number

[1] M. Weber, *The Protestant Ethic and the Spirit of Capitalism* (T. Parsons, trans., London, 1930), p. 158.

[2] G. Mackenroth, loc. cit. One recalls an old cartoon from *Simplicissimus* (the famous satirical journal published in Munich), showing a Protestant parson and his wife sitting on a sofa. She asks him whether he considers their love a sin, to which he replies, 'Only pleasure is a sin'. For a good summary of beliefs on population matters at the time of the Reformation, see O. Jolles, 'Die Ansichten der deutschen nationalökonomischen Schriftsteller des sechzehnten und siebzehnten Jahrhunderts über Bevölkerungswesen', *Jahrbücher für Nationalökonomik und Statistik* (Neue Folge, 1886), xiii. 193 ff.

[3] See J. J. Spengler, *France Faces Depopulation* (Durham, North Carolina, 1938), p. 174, note 109.

[4] It is only fair to point out that, *par contraire*, the other side equally condemned all Christianity. 'Le Christianisme n'a pas proprement pour objet de peupler la terre; son vrai but est de peupler le ciel' wrote one of the *Encyclopédistes* (vol. xiii, p. 92), following this up with specific instances of how the Church obstructs marriage, &c. There is an error of logic here: only the baptized can go to heaven, so births must in fact be encouraged.

of people in monasteries and convents. Instead, the Church was an element of stability in national life; as Moheau pointed out, it kept morals pure, and proscribed 'every act of pleasure which does not tend to generation'.[1] He called strongly for an extension of the Church's influence to encourage population; his opponents demanded equally strongly the removal of this baneful obstacle to higher fertility. This is what we would expect. But in the post-Malthusian period a curious situation arises. The Catholics could continue to preach their dogma—they were never good Malthusians—and if Catholic Ireland was the first country to act on Malthus's advice it was not due to the priesthood. The Catholic Church has consistently condemned mechanical contraception and abortion. But its opponents needs had to stand on their heads. Having proved, in the eighteenth century, that Catholicism prevented marriage, were they now to call boldly for more Catholics to stem the tide? Not at all: a new school of thought arose which showed, quite clearly, that religion encourages children where reason rejects them! Thus Sismondi based his charge in this direction on the fact that the Church condemned foresight—it commanded trust in God and proscribed shabby calculations.[2] In this he was probably right—had not Luther preached that God would send food for all their mouths? In the Ireland of Sismondi's time the priesthood, financially dependent on marriage fees, it was later alleged, encouraged the marriages of very young people without capital, income, or prospects—and this was what both Malthus and his opponents, for different reasons, sought to prevent.

Here again we repeat the experience found in other fields; only this time it is something undesirable rather than desirable which, in one context, is held to produce depopulation, in the next, over-population. There were always those who did not like the Church, or religion, and the application of this prejudice varies according to circumstances, just as did the advocacy of education or equality.

The further investigation of the effect of religion has been carried out on a fairly large scale in recent times.[3] Some, like Julius Wolf, threw the responsibility for over-population on religion or irrational

[1] M. Moheau, *Recherches et considérations sur la population de la France* (Paris, 1778), part ii, quoted in J. J. Spengler, 'Moheau, prophet of depopulation', *Journal of Political Economy* (1939), xlvii. 665 ff.

[2] J. C. L. S. de Sismondi, *Les Nouveaux Principes d'économie politique ou de la richesse dans ses rapports avec la population* (2nd ed., Paris, 1827, 2 vols.), ii. 292 ff.

[3] For bibliography, see United Nations, *The Determinants and Consequences . . .*, p. 81. One of the works investigating this problem is R. v. Ungern-Sternberg, *Die Ursachen des*

thinking *tout court*. Religious culture, said Wolf, declines to face the facts either as to numbers or quality of population.[1] That means that adaptation to conditions as they are can only come with complete emancipation from religion and tradition. A number of writers saw in religion simply the institutionalized prejudices, superstitions, and obstacles to all progress in any society. For them, arrest of growth is a sign of health. To the writers who follow the teaching of the churches, by contrast, the same phenomenon is a sign of mortal sickness, or decadence.

Geburtenrückgangs im westeuropäischen Kulturkreis während des 19. und 20. Jahrhunderts (Archiv für Bevölkerungswissenschaft (Volkskunde) und Bevölkerungs-Politik, Paris, 1938). He was convinced that Catholicism arrested the decline in the birth-rate through its teaching, and that the Protestant churches had the opposite effect. He even said that the Anglican Church had expressed itself strongly in favour of birth-control. His evidence for this curious statement was a letter which appeared in *The Times* in 1919, signed by the Bishop of Birmingham. Anglicans here would hardly think that Bishop Wakefield was likely to speak for the whole Church. Ungern-Sternberg also said that Anglican clergymen's families are usually small. He should have known them in the days of Karl Marx and George Eliot.

[1] J. Wolf, *Nationalökonomie als exakte Wissenschaft* (Leipzig, 1908), pp. 189 ff. The French demographer Landry, writing twenty-five years later, also stressed the common influence of religion and tradition. He pointed out that fairy tales usually ended with the information that 'they married, had many children, and lived happily ever after' (*La Révolution démographique* (Paris, 1934), pp. 35–36).

VII

THE BEGINNING OF GENERALIZED SOCIAL THEORIES OF POPULATION: SOCIAL BIOLOGY AND STATISTICAL THEORIES

I. THE EMERGENCE OF THE INDIVIDUAL AND SOCIAL EQUILIBRIUM

WE have so far been concerned with a number of theories which related the decline of fertility in individuals either to just one aspect of their mode of living or environment, or a series of features associated with a particular phase of economic or political development. The range has been from such narrow attempts at pin-pointing as the eighteenth-century strictures on the habit of putting out infants to nurse, to fairly wide theories like Dumont's. But we must now turn to more ambitious attempts to relate the movement of population, and especially the decline in fertility, to the whole context of human life. This means, in many cases, that the ideas we must trace move along the borderlines of political, social, and biological thought.

This, in the nature of our subject, is not surprising. There can be no clear distinction between the consideration of human beings, their attempts to live together in society and to earn a living, and the interaction of their natural and their created environment. The difficulty lies in the fact that there always exists a temptation to extend the sort of theorizing which is normal in the natural sciences to the social sciences. As we have previously noted, the eighteenth century suffered from a compulsive urge to bring human behaviour in line with that of stars and crystals. Unfortunately, this tendency never died out, and we shall be able to show variants on the general theme that the movement of population is subject to laws of nature which tend to produce an equilibrium. That is to say, where population grows too fast, forces are brought into operation which retard this growth, and vice versa. Such 'laws' would not be worth quoting were it not for the fact that quite often their mechanism of operation includes phenomena which fit into our general theory.

For convenience, rather than on chronological or local grounds, we may begin with theories which relate to the supposed adjustment of the individual or the family to an increasingly dense environment, and go on to those views which stress the total social effects of density on population. In the latter case, naturally, the operation through the individual has also to be implied even if it is often not expressed.

First, however, there is a further distinction to be made. The amateur writers in population theory are notoriously careless with their language. In particular, they do not always tell us whether they are concerned with fecundity, the reproductive capacity of human beings, or with fertility, the actual number of children they produce. In the case of Spencer and his followers, it should be made quite clear that they are concerned with fecundity, and therefore concentrate on the effects of changes in environment on the individual human body, and especially on the nervous system. We might therefore call these physiological theories. Very few writers now accept this type of explanation.[1] It has been pointed out that reductions in the fecundity of a married couple, short of absolute sterility, are unlikely to have much effect on the number of children they produce. Were it not for voluntary family limitation, family sizes would probably be the same as a hundred years ago, even if one could prove, say, a 20 per cent. reduction in reproductive capacity.[2]

But this does not mean that we can dismiss the work of the social biologists. It is probably best to assume that they were merely guilty of offering a wrong explanation for a phenomenon they accurately observed. The explanation can be translated from biological into social terms. In this way we may take their hypotheses as contributions to modern theory. The point was clearly made by J. A. Field:

> The laws thus announced partly describe influences supplementary to the economic check, but in each case either the law itself, or the popular understanding of it, really involves the principle of prudential restraint from economic motives that were not perceived.[3]

The same analysis applies, whether the cause of the decline in fecundity is social (as with the theories relating to the emergence of the individual), or economic (as in Doubleday's food theory), or physical (the density theory of Sadler). In each case we must concentrate more on the basis of the hypothesis than on the hypothesis itself.

[1] See United Nations, *The Determinants and Consequences of Population Trends* (New York, 1953), pp. 74–75.

[2] Ibid., para. 28, references to the work of E. Lewis-Faning and others, and criticisms of these.

[3] J. A. Field, *Essays on Population and Other Papers* (H. F. Hohman, ed. and comp., Chicago, 1931), p. 67.

Field himself thought that M. Muret was Spencer's first predecessor. But it would probably be more correct to say that there are three distinct streams of theory in this direction: the one that stems from Muret relates to automatic compensation for increasing density, and leads through Sadler to Pearl; the second begins perhaps with Ortes and the idea of the evolution of higher forms of animal being, and was taken up by Jarrold and Hickson. The third begins with Spencer's synthesis of the other two: at least he took the fact of some compensatory mechanism for granted, and explained it by the necessity for a higher form of nervous development in order to ensure survival under conditions of greater density. This process he called individuation.[1]

The difference between the two earlier ideas lies in the emphasis which they place on psychological and physiological causes of declining fertility. On the whole those who favoured automatic compensation paid little attention to the development of the mind—indeed many of them thought that the 'density' rule applied to animals, or even plants, as well as to human beings. In that sense Malthus may be numbered amongst them. The other group, which paid attention to man's social behaviour, laid as much, if not more, stress on his mental reaction to new conditions.

It is not suggested that the differentiation between the behaviour of men and animals was new. But what distinguishes the writers starting from Muret and Ortes from earlier attempts to describe the regulations of numbers is that they attribute some powers of reasoning to man which prevent him from sinking to his lowest natural state. Where the generation of Süßmilch had still spoken of a 'divine order' and had only very indirectly questioned whether man could alter his destiny by his own efforts, the investigators of society in a more sceptical age were to discover principles of human organization which hardly depended on divine providence and yet, often, showed this to be the best of all possible worlds. Finally, Spencer and the biologists brought the matter back to laws of nature. But the operation of these laws looks suspiciously like something quite calmly and deliberately arranged by very calculating human beings.

[1] See the discussion of the effect of the emergence of the individual in ancient Greece by Ludwig Elster in 'Bevölkerungwesen', *Handwörterbuch der Staatswissenschaften* (4th ed., Jena, 1924), ii. 736. He quotes Pohlenz: 'In Sparta ist der Staatszweck nur durch das Ganze bestimmt, in Athen wertet man das Individuum für sich.' But did any classical writers realize the implications of this contrast? Further views on the same subject in G. Glotz, *The Greek City and its Institutions* (N. Mallinson, trans., London, 1929), pp. 295 ff.

Giammaria Ortes (1713–90) was an Italian economist and social theorist of wide interests. Though he seems to have had some practical experience, his books have a rather theoretical flavour. As far as population is concerned he is something of a forerunner of Malthus, and his economics place him amongst the precursors of Marx. He assumed the possibility of a geometrical increase, but having demonstrated that such a progression would in practice have led to an impossible position within a few hundred years of any given starting-point, he enunciated a law which would limit further increase. Animals had similar powers of generation, but their numbers were limited by force. He could see 'generazioni negli uomini limitate de ragione'. Celibacy would spread, and an equilibrium prevail.[1] Reason here limits marriages, not fertility. The matter was taken a step farther by Thomas Jarrold's *Dissertation on Man*. Jarrold's view may be thought to have been influenced by his practical knowledge of human beings in a rapidly industrializing society: 'As the faculties of the mind are unemployed, as the man sinks down towards the animal, he is prolific; as he ascends above them, his fruitfulness decreases.'[2] But what are the activities of the higher stages of life? Those who engage in pursuits which put them constantly on their mettle. Those who tax their nerves, who are over-burdened with anxiety and hate; honest men come to grief through bankruptcy—all these have few children. All those who exert their minds a great deal in civilized countries are subject to the same influence. Greece provided an example of high refinement of mind and body leading to depopulation.[3]

The theme was taken up by William Hickson, the proprietor and editor of the *Westminster Review*, who indicated, unlike Jarrold, was taken seriously by the liberal economists of his time. He, too, remarked on the great fecundity of the lower orders in the animal kingdom and amongst human beings.[4] He agreed with Doubleday on the question of diet. But above all he thought that the future development

[1] G. M. Ortes, *Riflessioni sulla popolazione delle nazioni per rapporto all'economia nazionale* (Venice, 1790), in *Scrittori classici italiani di economia politica*. Parte moderne (Milan, 1904), xxiv. 32–36, quoted in C. E. Stangeland, *Pre-Malthusian Doctrines of Population; a Study in the History of Economic Theory* (New York, 1904), p. 336.

[2] T. Jarrold, *Dissertations on Man, Philosophical, Physiological and Political; in Answer to Mr. Malthus' 'Essay on the Principle of Population'* (London, 1806), p. 250. K. Smith in *The Malthusian Controversy* (London, 1951), p. 62, also characterizes Jarrold as a forerunner of Spencer.

[3] Jarrold, ibid., pp. 256–7, 267–8, 283, 366.

[4] W. E. Hickson, *Malthus; an Essay on the Principle of Population, in Refutation of the Theory of the Rev. T. R. Malthus* (London, 1849), p. 73.

of society in which he expected the best possible arrangements for production and distribution would lead to such large physical as well as moral changes as to amount almost to the creation of a new race.

The presumption is, that under such circumstances, the strength of the merely animal propensities would diminish, and that in accordance with the law that the highest organizations should be the most slowly developed, the ratio of increase would be less than at present.[1]

Herbert Spencer

Thomas Doubleday's *True Law of Population* is a good case of one explanation of well-attested phenomena being rejected as spurious by a critic who promptly substitutes another. In this case, it was Herbert Spencer who wrote the notices which reviewed a number of books, including Doubleday's, in Hickson's *Westminster Review*. Spencer did not say that the food thesis was without foundation; but he felt it was no law of nature since it did not disclose a 'self-rectifying arrangement'.[2] Instead, he postulated that among vertebrates 'the degree of fertility varies inversely as the development of the nervous system'. It is not to the bulk of the body as a whole but to the bulk of the nervous system that fertility stands related among the higher animals.

In social terms this meant that individual life could only be maintained under the increasingly complicated circumstances created by an overcrowded and specialized society, by a highly developed nervous system, and then only at the expense of fertility.[3] There will be a continuing tendency in this direction: the ability to survive improves and fertility decreases, until at last some sort of equilibrium is reached. Eventually such a highly developed individual mind will be necessary to keep alive at all, that fertility will be seriously impaired—then no further pressure will be added and existing aptitudes will be sufficient.

So the antithesis of 'individuation and genesis' emerges—the more modern man behaves like a civilized and intelligent being (because he has to), the less he will reproduce himself. The subject was further developed by Spencer on a large scale in his *Principles of Biology*, published in 1867. We see clearly how an apparently biological principle

[1] Hickson, loc. cit. Similar suggestions of the results of social reforms are frequent. Compare above, remarks on Condorcet and Godwin, Ch. V. Most socialists assumed some diversion of sexual energy in a more perfect state. See J. J. Spengler on Fourier in 'French Population Theory since 1800', *Journal of Political Economy* (1936), xliv. 749–53.

[2] H. Spencer, *A Theory of Population, Deduced from the General Law of Animal Fertility* (New York, 1852, reprinted from *Westminster Review*, xvii), pp. 427 ff.

[3] Ibid., pp. 495, 499.

is related to social questions. Fertility is said to increase with idleness and to decrease with restless activity. Excessive mental labour is likely to produce barrenness. Further development will lead to the increased 'skill, intelligence and self-control' necessary to find subsistence. We might now be inclined to say that these three attributes would also be necessary to exercise effective birth-control. Spencer persisted in explaining the matter the other way round by saying that the need for these qualities drained the substance necessary for generation. He even mentions that the process involves more intense education for the children—but not that the expense arising from this is a deterrent![1] But there are also indications that Spencer did not believe that the biological changes would alone be sufficient to produce the natural balance to be envisaged. He was disturbed at the possible effects on the composition of society if there were the slightest interference with the processes of nature. The Poor Laws, for instance, tended to keep one section of the community in a state of idleness, and thus allowed them to multiply themselves. (This may be said to be acceptable under the Malthusian or the Spencerian systems.) The other part of the community, which had to pay poor-rates, would be forced to work harder to support themselves and the ever-growing idle pauper body, and would thus become more infertile. A new process of natural selection would be in operation—the survival of the least fit. (Spencer was sceptical of much of Darwin's work.) The only solution will be for man's emotional nature to evolve to a stage where a new sense of morality will prevent improvident marriages which cannot support children: '. . . with a higher moral nature will come a restriction on the multiplication of the inferior'.[2]

We find therefore that Spencer not only explained phenomena by biological means which most of his contemporaries thought psychological, but he did not even trust his own system to produce anything but a crude balance between population and subsistence—certainly not a desirable society. At least those who followed Malthus and Darwin to the bitter end and allowed the process of selection to take place without any aid to those who would perish produced a consistent system.

Spencer had a considerable following. There were those who believed, like him, in a harmonious whole—Providence has arranged

[1] H. Spencer, *The Principles of Biology* (London, 1899, 2 vols.), ii. 509 ff., paras. 366–76.

[2] Ibid. His attitude to Darwin is clarified in a footnote to para. 373. The concluding paragraph (376) again states the unmodified biological theory.

things well, and the more people there are, the less will they tend to add to their numbers. The American anti-Ricardian economist Henry Carey (1793–1879) believed that agriculture was subject to increasing returns—so that mankind had a long way to go before any real danger existed. But eventually even the best system of production and distribution might result in pressure on subsistence—and then he called the Spencerian system into action. The reproductive power is lessened when man's various capabilities and activities are multiplied. So as civilization increases, more food is produced, but the act of producing also strains the nervous system sufficiently to lessen reproduction, so that equilibrium is attained.[1]

In Germany the statistician Ernst Engel put forward similar views. Man being the highest product of creation, is also the least fertile. Not only will greater numbers provide more opportunities for greater division of labour, but advance means diminished powers of reproduction.[2]

Spencer's curious thesis provoked a number of statistical investigations. Some of these would not appear to have proved very much according to modern notions, but to contemporaries they bore out a large number of the theories put forward by the early sociologists. In Scotland J. Matthews Duncan's *Fecundity, Fertility, Sterility and Allied Topics*, published in 1866, presented some of the earliest tables of differential fertility. These prove a variety of correlations, but not the truth of the theory of nervous development. Nitti and Spengler both list a large number of French writers who followed Spencer either in theory or in their interpretation of their statistics. Among the converts there were such notable figures as the historian of theory, Charles Gide, co-author with Rist of the *Histoire des doctrines économiques* and a prominent left-wing politician, who in his *Principes d'économie politique*, first published in 1883, stated his belief that fecundity stood in an inverse relationship to the intellectual and moral improvement of the individual. This presented a sharp contrast to Dumont's idea of a relationship between deterioration and infertility.[3] But on examination

[1] H. C. Carey, *Principles of Social Science* (Philadelphia, 1858–60, 3 vols.), iii, chs. xlvi–xlix. He mentioned the wider distribution of property as one of the prerequisites both for greater production and the growth of rational preoccupation (see esp. iii. 263 ff.).

[2] E. Engel, 'Über die Bedeutung der Bevölkerungsstatistik mit besonderer Beziehung auf die diesjährige Volkszählung und Produktions- und Konsumtionsstatistik im Königreich Sachsen', *Z. des stat. Bureaus des k. sächs. Ministeriums des Innern* (1855); quoted in Elster, op. cit. ii. 785.

[3] J. J. Spengler, *France Faces Depopulation* (Durham, North Carolina, 1938), p. 140;

most of these authors prove to accept more readily the general conditions under which a decline of population, or decline in the birth-rate, sets in, than the master's physiological explanations of why this was so. One point which was specially attractive to the writers of the period was the idea of an eventual balance. Many had, in their lifetime, seen a period of pro-populationist policies, the rise of the Malthusian spectre of over-population, and yet another change-over to a renewed bogy of decline. How convenient if in fact there were a law of nature which made it unnecessary to worry! Once again they seem to return, on a scientific basis, to the once theological belief in a rightly-ordered universe. If one substitutes institutional and physiological changes for the scourges and favours of God, one can see echoes of men like Canon Derham of Windsor.[1]

The conditions of equilibrium

The notion of a general equilibrium proved attractive to many investigators. One of the earliest to formulate it exactly was that famous Pastor Muret whom Malthus cited extensively. In introducing his account of the population of Leyzin in Switzerland, he asked, answering his own question as to the underlying cause: 'Is it not that, in order to maintain in all places a proper equilibrium of population, God has wisely ordered things in such a manner as that the force of life in each country should be in the inverse ratio of its fecundity?'[2]

The physical implications of the conditions of equilibrium had long been known, and superficial likenesses between the physical world and human society were fashionable already in the eighteenth century—in fact there were earlier precedents.[3] But few of the writers who used the

F. S. Nitti, *Population and the Social System* (English ed., London, 1894), pp. 70–79, 156–8. See also there for references to P. Jacoby and G. Delaunay, 'La Fécondité', *Revue scientifique* (Oct. 1885). The passage by Gide is in *Principes d'économie politique* (3rd ed., Paris, 1891), pp. 348–51. Another Spencerian cited by Nitti was the Swiss-French botanist Alphonse de Candolle, the author of *Histoire des sciences et des savants depuis deux siècles, suivi d'autres études sur des sujets scientifiques, en particulier sur la sélection dans l'espèce humaine* (Geneva, 1873).

[1] W. Derham, *Physico-theology; or, A Demonstration of the Being and Attributes of God from His Works of Creation... etc.* (6th ed., London, 1723), contains a picture of a cruel but remarkably wise God sending plague and abundance in necessary sequence. Süßmilch was less naïve.

[2] M. Muret, *Mémoires, etc., par la Société Economique de Berne* (1766), pp. 48 ff., quoted by T. R. Malthus, *A Summary View of the Principle of Population*, reprinted in *Introduction to Malthus* (D. V. Glass, ed., London, 1953), p. 166.

[3] Equilibrium as an end of policy, rather than a law of nature, had already been Aristotle's theme. For an evaluation, see R. Gonnard, *Histoire des doctrines de la population* (Paris, 1923), pp. 35 ff.

concept were able to distinguish between a purely theoretical long-term equilibrium with the assumption of an impossibly static social background, and the real world where indeed forces might be at work propelling society towards the balanced state, but never accomplishing their work since the conditions of equilibrium were constantly changing. Malthus himself had rejected the idea of possible stability with his notion of a tendency for the human race to increase beyond the available means of subsistence. Admittedly, as most of his adversaries pointed out, at any one moment all living human beings were matched with the available nurture, otherwise they would not be alive. But this was not a stable equilibrium, in the sense of a position which could be maintained for long. The same could be said of the processes implied in Lassalle's Iron Law of Wages. By contrast, the Spencerians and later biological investigators of population looked for long-term stability, and their findings were mostly optimistic in the extreme. In part they even resemble Godwin's and Condorcet's sanguine expectations of a decline in reproductive activity when mankind was lifted on to a higher plane.

The biological theories concerning the role of the individual in society merge imperceptibly into wider cultural theories with which we shall have to concern ourselves at a later stage. When contraceptives came to be widely used the physiological changes supposed to result from social changes could be pushed into the background. It mattered very little that a decline in *fecundity* could not be proved —the decline in fertility was apparent, the means by which it was achieved were well known, and so only the ultimate motive had to be explained.

But in Spencer's day, in the absence of any strong faith in the efficacy of moral restraint, let alone restraint after marriage, the need for some assumption about the physical effect of the new pattern of society was obvious.[1]

2. SOME PARTICULAR TYPES OF EQUILIBRIUM THEORIES

The influences described by Spencer and others in retarding the rate of increase of population under certain conditions might be said to have two special characteristics: they assume that these changes will be brought about as mankind advances to a higher state of development,

[1] See reference to Spencer's follower, Walter Bagehot, above, p. 177. Bagehot also thought that government by discussion raised the general level of intellectual activity and thus adversely affected fertility (Bagehot, op. cit., p. 199).

and on the whole they are dependent on biological assimilation to the new environment. As Field pointed out, however, the latter point is weak, and in a sense insignificant, since it matters very little whether the adjustment is automatic or volitional.

From this group of social biologists we distinguish another, which included a good many statisticians. This latter group made no assumptions about the state of development—it relied purely on the increase in numbers to produce the counteracting principle. It constitutes a curious assortment of people, from those who believed that this effect was part of the divine order of the universe, to those who demonstrated it merely as a statistical fact without attaching theological significance to the circumstances.

Already Sir William Petty had written of his belief that as numbers grew so the rate of increase would fall off,[1] and Süßmilch followed the same line.[2] Sir James Steuart, in his *Principles of Political Economy*, first published in 1767, produced the typical mechanistic analogy:

> The generative faculty resembles a spring loaded with a weight, which always exerts itself in proportion to the diminution of resistance. When food has remained some time without augmentation or diminution, generation will carry numbers as high as possible; if, then, food comes to be diminished, the force of it becomes less than nothing, inhabitants will diminish. . . .[3]

This statement was quoted by Frédéric Bastiat in his *Harmonies of Political Economy* (first French edition 1850), a work written in the full flight of an almost mystical liberal enthusiasm, with the characteristic motto, *digitus Dei est hic*. It is indeed only as part of a general belief in the goodness of the deity that one may understand the 'reasoning' behind this type of statement. After 1800, despite Malthus's ample demonstration that the deity would not help man if man did not help himself, this apparent law of nature was still pronounced, with many variants.

The best-known exponent of this view is a notable English reformer, Michael Sadler, whose voluminous *The Law of Population* (the title, like Doubleday's, is significant) was published in 1830. He was a

[1] Sir W. Petty, 'Another Essay in Political Arithmetic, Concerning the Growth of the City of London . . . etc.' (London, 1682), pp. 24–25, in *Economic Writings* C. H. Hull, ed. (Cambridge, 1899, 2 vols.), ii. 468–9.

[2] Quoted in Stangeland, op. cit., p. 217.

[3] Quoted by E. T. Hiller, 'A Culture Theory of Population Trends', *Journal of Politica Economy* (1930), xxxviii. 525, and there cited from Frédéric Bastiat, *Harmonies of Political Economy* (Edinburgh, 1880 ed.), p. 402. The original Paris 1850 ed. does not have this reference. See also Hiller, op. cit., pp. 530–4, for further references to automatic compensation theories and criticisms of these.

man of parts, largely self-taught, a prolific writer and agitator in the turbulent atmosphere of Leeds in the time of Poor Law and Parliamentary and Factory Reform. Anti-Malthusianism was to him, as to so many others, a natural consequence of a reformer's life, and his book, the product of much enthusiasm rather than scientific training, was a fighting pamphlet that grew into an extended treatise on social science. In detail, the work incorporates much that is found elsewhere concerning the effects of progress on fertility—in its pages are found both old wisdom such as the effects of luxury, and rather newer ideas, such as those concerning the effect of over-eating. He knew of the differentials between town and country, rich and poor, nobility and peasant. Yet all these manifestations were to him, as it were, minor manifestations of a universal law: 'The prolificness of human beings, otherwise similarly circumstanced, varies inversely as their numbers.'[1] He was never clear in his own mind about the connexion between this 'law' and all the other characteristics of fertility changes. To us it seems reasonably clear that he derived his theory from a look at a number of 'advanced' societies, and this first glance showed that they had this one thing in common: that they lived at high densities. Nothing further was needed. It was, in any case, a most useful debating point against Malthus: if the one said that the danger-point was reached when the earth was full, the other maintained that precisely at this point all was well.

Obsessed, like many others who lived after Smith even if they were not his followers, with the endless possibilities of the Division of Labour, he could see nothing but advance coming from density; and the manifestations of that advance were changes in modes and standards of living which produced the desired result. His misunderstanding of the situation is already clear in the phrasing of his law, 'otherwise similarly circumstanced'. The point was, that if people of similar occupations, background, income in money terms, &c., could really live at various densities, they could never in any true sense be similarly circumstanced—the *cetera* would never be *pares*. If his Leeds woollen workers lived at densities to the square mile ten times higher than in the time of Defoe, it was because their productivity, thanks to machinery, was higher. Sadler claimed that they were less fertile than their ancestors. Of this he could not have evidence, because it was not true. But even if it had been so, he could not have claimed that they were

[1] M. T. Sadler, *The Law of Population: a Treatise in Six Books; in Disproof of the Superfecundity of Human Beings, and Developing the Real Principle of their Increase* (London, 1830, 2 vols.), ii. 352.

'similarly circumstanced'. Their incomes in real terms were probably higher at some times, and lower at others; they performed different sorts of labour, and different skills were in demand. But in any case Sadler should have known that people could even live at ever-increasing density, and become more miserable and fertile in the process—he was familiar with Irish conditions. He would then have said that it was poverty that made them breed—in other words, density is not really relevant. But he made his point, forcibly and often, and in its simplicity, like Doubleday's law, it had its following.[1]

Although no other 'law' of nature was stated with quite such precision after Sadler's time by enthusiastic laymen, the search for some universal statement concerning population, to counter Malthus's progressions, went on in the ranks of the mathematicians. Clearly, their attempts were not so naïve as to suppose that human society followed such well-defined courses as the stars, as men had thought in the eighteenth century, for purely physical reasons—i.e. in accordance with laws which could be deduced with certainty and experimentally confirmed. Instead, they knew that the forces whereby the supposed result was accomplished were largely psychologically conditioned adjustments to circumstances. Nevertheless, this group of writers believed that this adjustment was, on the average, so predictable as to warrant a 'law'.

One of the earliest such attempts was made in Sadler's own time by the Belgian mathematician Adolphe Quételet (1796–1874). His book, published in 1836, was subtitled, significantly, *An Essay in Social Physics*—a title reminiscent of Bagehot's later volume *Physics and Politics*. In the early chapters, he discussed various influences on births and deaths, and his important conclusion for our purposes is curiously enough the same as Malthus's: 'La population tend à croître selon un programme géométrique.' This statement is followed, however, by the description of the geometric function which he meant: 'La résistance, ou la somme des obstacles à son développement, est, toutes choses égales d'ailleurs, comme le carré de la vitesse avec laquelle la population tend à croître.'[2] The law of resistance growing as the square of velocity

[1] For a good account of Sadler's theories, see Smith, op. cit., pp. 190 ff. Also S. H. Coontz, *Population Theories and the Economic Interpretation* (London, 1957), pp. 22 ff. On Macaulay and his criticism of Sadler (in the *Edinburgh Review*), see H. A. Boner, *Hungry Generations; the Nineteenth-Century Case against Malthusianism* (New York, 1955), pp. 116–18.

[2] L. A. J. Quételet, *Sur l'homme et le développement de ses facultés, ou, Essai de physique sociale* (Brussels, 1836), bk. i, ch. vii, p. 288.

was, of course, taken from physical science—one of a number of similar analogies made by Quételet and his followers.

It was obviously a case of hoisting Malthus with his own petard. Everybody knew he was wrong—many suggested vaguely that there was a counteracting principle—now there was an answer using Malthus's own language. Quételet himself charged Malthus with having deliberately suppressed mention of the total effect of the obstacles of which he knew. This seems a meaningless charge since in fact Malthus had a simple enough formula: total potential population minus casualties due to positive checks minus children not born through preventive checks equals actual population. What Quételet meant to say was that the incidence of the checks followed as precise a pattern as the potential expansion curve of total population. The precision Quételet introduced was, of course, spurious. He himself seems to have had doubts, for he charged a former pupil, Pierre-François Verhulst, also a Belgian, to undertake a thorough examination of the statistical data available.[1] At first Verhulst seems to have been uncertain of the exact nature of the relationship between expansion and obstacles, but later he formulated the hypothesis that 'the obstacles increase in proportion to the ratio of the superabundant population to the total population'.[2] The result of applying this braking force to a growing population is to produce what Verhulst called 'the logistic curve'—an S-shaped curve bounded by upper and lower asymptotes. Although such a curve has scientific pretensions, it may be classed essentially, like all other 'final' anti-Malthusian arguments, like Sadler's, or Spencer's, or Doubleday's, as a rationalization of influences welcomed by most people, into a universal system.

The logistic curve in its extreme form may have had few followers until it was revived in this century by Pearl and Reed,[3] but the fascination of the possibility of some such law of nature affected the thinking of a good many writers who were not otherwise given to speculation. Even Wilhelm Roscher, as sober an historical economist as one could

[1] For a full account of Verhulst's work and his relations with Quételet, see J. R. Miner, 'Pierre-François Verhulst, the Discoverer of the Logistic Curve', *Human Biology* (Dec. 1933), v, no. 4, pp. 673–89. Also Hiller, op. cit., p. 525 (where he is called Verlust).

[2] P.-F. Verhulst, *Recherches mathématiques sur la loi d'accroissement de la population* (Nouveaux mémoires de l'Académie royale des sciences et belles-lettres de Bruxelles, xviii, 1845). For details, see Miner, op. cit.

[3] For a full account of the cyclical theories of Pearl and others, notably Warren Thompson, see United Nations, *Determinants and Consequences* . . ., p. 29, and D. G. Cowgill, 'The Theory of Population Growth Cycles', *American Journal of Sociology* (1949), lv. 163 ff.

find in Germany at the end of the nineteenth century, could write that

> A basin entirely filled with water can be made to contain more only in case it is either increased itself, or a means is found to compress its contents. Otherwise as much must flow out on one side as is poured in on the other. And so, everything else remaining stationary, the fruitfulness of marriages must, at least in the long run, be in the inverse ratio to their frequency.[1]

The relationship between the standard of living and the possible size of population already noted by Cantillon found more exact expressions in the writings of several French economists of the mid-nineteenth century. They contended, in general, that the 'size of a country's population varies inversely with the *per capita* consumption, which in turn varies directly with the degree of inequality of incomes'.[2] These formulations are as meaningless as the logistic curve, since they tell us nothing about the ways in which population is in fact held in check—naturally at any one time, as Malthus could have told them, the number of people in a country is determined by the minimum amount of subsistence required by its inhabitants. If the minimum rises there can be fewer of them; if their numbers increase the minimum will fall, or the additional people will die. For our purpose, these authors are only interesting in so far as they relate the influences at work in raising the requirements of individuals, and thereby turn their thoughts to voluntary restraint.

As statistics were developed by mathematicians and economists, the attempts to translate generalized observations into precise formulations increased in number. By and large, however, these statistical contributions did nothing to provide fresh arguments in the whole complex of theories we are here examining. Instead, they did indispensable work in proving or disproving hypotheses—mostly the latter, since the unitary explanations, of which the nineteenth century was so fond, were almost always wrong in detail. The whole trend was towards the modern complex theories of interacting forces.

3. CHANGES IN SURVIVAL-RATES, IN MEDICINE AND PUBLIC HEALTH

There remains one particular type of equilibrium or 'adjustment theory' which has the advantage that it is, to a large extent, based on accurate statistical observation and not like the propositions of the first two

[1] Quoted by Hiller, loc. cit., from W. Roscher, *Principles of Political Economy* (New York, 1878, 2 vols.), ii. 276–7.

[2] United Nations, *Determinants and Consequences . . .*, p. 29, para. 31.

sections of this chapter, grounded mainly on the unproven hypotheses, religious beliefs, or social philosophy of their authors. We have already remarked, in the section on children, that a change in the expectation of life, especially for new-born children, would tend to influence attitudes towards family size. When the attainment of adolescence was a cause for deep thankfulness for the parents, it is to be expected that they would not treat a new-born child as an individual—it would be unwise to attach too much importance to each newcomer. If one wished to ensure the continuation of the family name, it would be best not to plan for any limited number of children. A study of any family tree, or burial register, of the eighteenth and early nineteenth century shows gradually increasing, but still not over-high, chances of survival.[1] Such statistics do not take into account the high proportion of miscarriages which were so common in England (and still are in some countries and some sections of all populations) that they were not even recorded in the annals of families, let alone officially.[2] Even a prudent couple therefore might not have felt it necessary to practise abstinence, or contraception if they had any such knowledge, until improvements in health increased the chances of the ultimate survival of the foetus. It is impossible to determine exactly at what stage a sufficiently large decrease of infant mortality occurred to affect family decisions sensibly.

There is also another aspect of this question of the expectation of life. Every variant of the wage-fund theory advises labourers not to produce more children than are needed to replace wastage through death or retirement. Therefore equilibrium will only be preserved if couples do not marry until there is a place vacant for them, and if as a whole they do not produce more births than burials in their class. Every time therefore that the average age of death, or retirement, is raised the labouring classes will have to adjust the age of marriage, and the size of their family, accordingly. Lionel Robbins has pointed out that the presentation of this truth by Adam Smith constitutes a sort of standard-of-living theory—a high standard is desirable, and can only be preserved at the expense of a low birth-rate. Any change in mortality must be linked with changes in reproductive habits.[3]

[1] About 1772 Dr. Percival thought half the children born in London died before they reached the age of two, half those in Manchester before five. See G. T. Griffith, *Population Problems of the Age of Malthus* (Cambridge, 1925), p. 242.

[2] See statistics in D. V. Glass, *Population: Policies and Movements in Europe* (Oxford, 1940), for Germany. Nothing is known of the percentage of voluntary abortions.

[3] L. Robbins, 'On a Certain Ambiguity in the Conception of Stationary Equilibrium', *Economic Journal* (June 1930), vol. xl, no. 158, p. 196. The reference is to bk. i, ch. viii

Since neither the equilibrium system of classical economics nor the theory of wages concerns us here, we must be content to note what the acceptance of the idea just described implies. If any general economic or social movements raise the standard of nutrition, of housing, clothing, and popular education, mortality will undoubtedly be reduced. If, however, this change is not followed by a corresponding reduction of fertility, then the original gain will be nullified through the increased pressure of population on the available subsistence. This is a purely Malthusian argument, yet if we link it with the proposition with which we began this section, i.e. that reduced mortality will increase the individual value of children in the eyes of their parents, and thus lead to greater care for them, then we have in essence an anti-Malthusian proposition. In actual fact, it would be left to the observer to devise an interpretation for the observed phenomenon according to his lights: if diminished mortality led to fewer births, he could say that this was a providential arrangement, or he could claim that the labouring classes were exercising moral restraint as a result of having been taught political economy. (He could even, like Ariès, ascribe it to an increased interest in one's children's welfare.)

We have examples of both attitudes. The first is that of Pastor Muret. He believed God had 'wisely ordered things in such a manner as that the force of life in each country should be in the inverse ratio of its fecundity'.[1] Those, like Bastiat, who believed in some general God-given equilibrium in the world were to write much the same sort of thing, perhaps in less simple fashion, in the following century.

The second attitude may best be shown in Malthus's criticism of Muret. Are we to suppose, he asks, that providence renders women less fertile in healthy countries? 'Or to suppose, as experience warrants, that the smaller mortality of healthy and improved countries is balanced by the greater prevalence of the prudential restraint on marriage and population?'[2] He went on to explain why he thought that his surmise was right, committing himself to the view that in this case good health produced prudence, and not vice versa. But he thought a process of interaction was more usual. If there is no prudence, and limited subsistence, no amount of 'natural healthiness could prevent an excessive

of A. Smith, *An Inquiry into the Nature and Causes of the Wealth of Nations* (11th ed., London, 1805; E. Cannan, ed., New York, 1937, 2 vols.), i. 123–6. Note that Smith there assumes that only half of those born will survive to the age where they earn, so that the labourer must have four children to replace his wife and himself.

[1] As quoted by Malthus, *Summary View* . . ., p. 166. Muret's observations were made in 1766.

[2] Ibid., pp. 166–7.

mortality'. It is difficult to know what this is supposed to mean, but by implication we come to the conclusion that the greater the natural advantages, in health and situation, of a given population, the greater will be the effort required of them to keep their numbers within bounds.[1] Once again we are faced with an insoluble contradiction. Either it is true, as he said at the beginning of his account, that an increase in health and expectation of life changes people so as to keep births down to a reasonable figure, or else health is irrelevant and what matters is that people should keep within the limits set by the means of subsistence, with the help of prudential habits. Malthus could evidently quite well see that something beyond the teaching of political economy had a chance of influencing social behaviour—but whenever he saw it, he made a point of minimizing it, or explaining it away.

The habits of the Swiss continued to exercise the minds of those who sought universal principles of population for a considerable time. Laing the elder, as we have seen, re-examined D'Ivernois's figures, as did Quételet. Edwin Chadwick, in the report of 1842, also looked at the Geneva registers. The parallel course of the curves was noted, but not explained:

> . . . the progression of the population and the increased duration of life has been attended by a progression in happiness: as prosperity advanced marriages became fewer and later; the proportion of births were reduced, but greater numbers of the infants born were preserved and the proportion of the population in manhood became greater. . . .[2]

At first, he thought, barbarous conditions produced large families and early deaths. But as civilization advanced, so both fertility and mortality declined, until, in 1836, the expectation of life even in Geneva was forty-five years, and births barely balanced deaths. His inference followed: the labouring classes of England were still living under barbarous conditions, for they exhibited the high figures which he had found characteristic of rude societies. Clearly Chadwick is here treating reduced infant mortality as a sign of causes, rather than a direct cause, of the decline in fertility. There are many examples of these shades of attitudes; of course each writer had to fit the observed facts, as best he could, into his own preconceived scheme of ideas. Unless, that is to say, they were of a sufficiently scientific turn of mind to state the corre-

[1] Malthus, op. cit., p. 168.

[2] *Report from the Poor Law Commissioners on an Inquiry into the Sanitary Condition of the Labouring Population of Great Britain* (London, 1842), Edwin Chadwick, secretary, p. 175.

lation, and leave the matter at that. As more accurate vital statistics became available, writers in all countries noticed the effect stated.

Chadwick's reasoning found an immediate following amongst the more enlightened administrators and economists. The correlation was a strong incentive to sanitary reform, the provision of housing—in fact, every conceivable measure to raise the standard of living of the poor. Thus the anonymous translator of Sismondi's works, in his prefatory essay,[1] was at pains to point out that: 'sanatory improvements, and whatever tends to lengthen life, are the most effectual means of restraining a too great increase of population.' Richard Jones, who contributed so much to the understanding of voluntary restraint, arrived at the connexion between the expectation of life and fertility independently from Chadwick, and probably before him. But it was still, at that time, a matter of logic rather than accurate statistical assessment, and some time elapsed before less speculative material became available.[2]

The statistical inquiries were carried out in various countries in the middle of the nineteenth century. Amongst the earliest in Germany was J. E. Wappäus's, who was virtually the founder of modern German demography, and who pointed out that parents first begin to think about the limitation of children when the first, second, or third child fails to die within the first few years of life.[3] That this was no mere middle-class rationalization was shown by another German medical statistician, Arthur Geissler, starting from Wappäus's work, but drawing his material from observations amongst miners' families.[4] It is interesting to compare the approach of Wappäus, who still retains something of a belief in the kind intentions of nature, and general social harmonies, and therefore finds it most fitting that lower infant mortality should be matched by lower fertility, and, on the other hand, the more scientific analytical study of Geissler. He found that the most probable reason for this lower fertility was the longer interval

[1] J. C. L. S. de Sismondi, *Political Economy and the Philosophy of Government: a Series of Essays Selected from the Works of M. de Sismondi . . .* (anon. trans., London, 1847), preface, p. 81.

[2] R. Jones, *Literary Remains, Consisting of Lectures and Tracts on Political Economy* (W. Whewell and Cazenove, eds., London, 1859), pp. 170 ff.

[3] J. E. Wappäus, *Allgemeine Bevölkerungsstatistik* (1859, 2 vols.), ii. 322–3. In a later volume (1861) Wappäus found a more general relationship between low fertility and low mortality.

[4] A. Geissler, 'Über den Einfluss der Säuglingssterblichkeit auf die eheliche Fruchtbarkeit, mit besonderer Berücksichtigung der Ehen im Bergmannsstande', *Zeitschrift des statistischen Bureaus des Kngr. Sachsen* (Dresden, 1885), xxxi. 23.

which would naturally occur between pregnancies where the last child born was being reared to maturity. This interval might be a matter of physiological necessity (although by this time few subscribed to the theory of Charles Loudon that women were unable to conceive while they were still breast-feeding their babies),[1] but a number of writers stressed simply the inconvenience of having children in too quick succession.[2]

In France statistical inquiries were carried out at a time when Malthus was still fashionable, although the facts, had they been known, would have led already to very different conclusions. Evidently even in a country much less industrialized than England the urban influences were much the same as those observed by Chadwick. Thus, A. H. Moreton quotes some tables from M. Chabrol, relating to Paris, which clearly show that

> the immediate effect of the suppression of a cause of mortality is rather to diminish than to increase the number of births.

Moreton had no doubt that in England, as in France, there was going on a process by which

> the same change in the condition of society that occasions a reduction of mortality, occasioned at the same time a reduction in the number of births.[3]

One would expect high birth- and death-rates amongst the poor, and low ones amongst the wealthy. When statistics in England on this subject became available, with the annual reports of the Registrar-General, they confirmed the anticipation of the earlier observers.

[1] C. Loudon, *The Equilibrium of Population and Sustenance Demonstrated, Showing, on Physiological and Statistical Grounds, the Means of Obviating the Fears of the Late Mr. Malthus and His Followers* (Leamington Spa, 1836). This belief about the efficacy of breast-feeding as a method of contraception was widespread, and has not yet died out everywhere. It forms another instance of the close connexion between folk-lore and population theory.

[2] Geissler quoted the work of J. E. Horn, *Bevölkerungswissenschaftliche Studien aus Belgien* (Leipzig, 1854). Some later studies are cited in United Nations, *Determinants and Consequences . . .*, p. 81.

[3] A. H. Moreton, *Civilization, or, a Brief Analysis of the Natural Laws that Regulate the Numbers and Conditions of Mankind* (London, 1836), pp. 131–3. The quotation is from *Recherches statistiques sur la ville de Paris et le département de la Seine. Recueil de tableaux dressés et réunis d'après les ordres de M. le comte de Chabrol, Conseiller d'état, préfet du département* (Paris, 1823).

VIII

THE SYNTHESIS OF SPECIAL THEORIES: CIVILIZATION, CULTURE, AND INDUSTRIALIZATION

In this chapter the attempt will be made to draw together the threads presented in earlier sections. We have seen how acute observers in all ages and places recognized that the checks to population increase may be found at least as much in the conditions influencing the decision to marry and to have children, as in the positive checks of war, famine, and disease. A thorough examination of these conditions brings us back at once to Malthus's own preventive check—the first of the causes which, in England, as he saw them, kept the increase of population in bounds. But for some of his value judgements, we should count Malthus in amongst those who saw the picture in its entirety. One such reservation arises from his summary dismissal, in his first essay, of these conditions as 'vice'. Men who do not marry, from prudential motives, cannot remain single and chaste, so vice results. In this he is nearer the eighteenth century than the nineteenth—it was before his time that the failure to marry was most often put down to a vicious disposition, and after his time that this failure most often became a virtue.

If voluntary restraint, then, is not a permanent vice, an inherent sin committed by the human species, it must be seen as a response to certain stimuli. As we saw, the attempts to describe these causes in terms of narrow fronts were not very successful. The question then is: what are the total social and economic conditions under which these pressures against marriage and procreation are brought to bear? In what atmosphere are the preventive checks or voluntary restraint most likely to be effective? The short answer, as we now see it, is this: when societies advance to a higher stage of civilization, or culture, or when they become industrialized. The distinction may seem artificial, as to some extent it undoubtedly is. The usage here adopted is largely dictated by national approaches. Civilization, in the French and English sense, means essentially the adoption of ways of life which lift a nation out of the barbaric stage. It includes the introduction of forms of government, ways of speech and manners, even arrangements for domestic comfort, eating and drinking, which present, in the view of anyone using the word, an advance on a more primitive stage.[1] But the word implies no general or consistent body of theory concerning the composition of the society or the conduct of its citizens. (Except in such notoriously meaningless phrases as 'our Western Civilization'.) Culture has many different meanings. Modern anthropologists speak of 'primitive' or 'advanced' cultures in the sense of distinct patterns of social and economic organization and moral systems as they are found in particular societies. In the German sense, in which it is also sometimes used in English, it describes an aspect of life in a society which, if it possesses it, is thereby distinguished from a state of barbarism. In that sense it is not so far removed from the meaning of the more usual English word 'civilization' since it may be taken for granted that a state which is based on culture (*Kulturstaat*) is a civilized state. Again, we use the word 'cultural' to describe activities which are pursued chiefly for non-economic ends. These artistic or recreational pursuits may take place in an environment which is otherwise quite uncivilized. Confusion thus arises where 'culture' is pursued by barbaric means, as it was in Nazi Germany. Conversely, the process of 'civilization' as occasionally carried on in colonial territories has the effect of destroying a native culture.

Since there is not, then, a perfectly clear method of separating the two terms, either normatively as regards the historical use-patterns, or in any objective or scientific manner in their present context, we shall have to group writers according to the content which they ascribe to that state of society which they describe as being 'civilization' or culture. The difficulty is purely linguistic, for however loosely the word is used, it is always intended to describe an environmental effect on population growth.

These considerations apply *a fortiori* to industrialization. Certainly, civilization and culture can be carried to a very high level without any industrialization. On the other hand, it will be possible to industrialize a country with a minimum advance in culture or civilization—even a backward movement may be found, as in Lancashire in the early Industrial Revolution.

Nevertheless, the three rather vague concepts are in practice found to be closely allied. What their originators lacked in precision, they made up in acute recognition of the developments going on around them.

[1] See Edmund Burke: 'civilisation had two principles to distinguish it from the barbaric state: the spirit of a gentleman, and the spirit of religion' (*O.E.D.*, quoting from *French Revolution*; *Works*, v. 154).

There is, naturally, no particular starting-point to the insights here described. It seems that only in the second half of the eighteenth century was any attempt made to relate changing social behaviour to a changing social background. Few of the earlier writers would have claimed that the manners of their times constituted an advance of civilization on their beloved model—the Graeco-Roman civilization. The concept, in the earlier eighteenth century, even assumed something of a pejorative meaning, precisely because some of its manifestations were so shocking to the moralists. Was not the model of behaviour the simple unlettered rustic, and the arch-fiend the complicated dandy?[1]

What rehabilitated civilization was the more positive belief in human progress which informed the moral philosophers in England and Scotland, and the *philosophes* and *encyclopédistes* in France. Their essential stress was on the power of human will and reason to accomplish desired aims, to overcome obstacles, to control nature. This theme was to be the predominant one in many of the authors who refuted Malthus with theories of civilization.[2]

I. THE HIGHER WANTS

The change from condemnation to welcome is the more noteworthy because it actually took place before Malthus wrote. Wallace, in his *Dissertation on the Numbers of Mankind*, took the line that a certain amount of refinement was a necessary condition of moral advance. He

[1] The verb 'to civilize' was used—'civilization' only came into the English language rather late. One proof of the connotation the word had acquired is in a passage by W. Temple, the Trowbridge clothier, in the work cited previously, *A Vindication of Commerce and the Arts . . . etc.* (1768; reprinted in *A Select Collection of Scarce and Valuable Tracts on Commerce* (J. McCulloch, ed., London, 1859)), attacking Bell, who wished to cut out refinement because of its attendant evils. Temple says that 'civilisation is not a vice, nor poverty a virtue'. This volume was published in 1768. The *O.E.D.* gives the earliest instance of the use of the word to the seventies—Boswell is supposed to have persuaded Dr. Johnson to put the word into his Dictionary. This is certainly not its first use, but it is clear that the time is about the right one. The concept was old, but its use to connote a particular circumstance was new.

[2] Although some of these opponents are outside the scope of the present work they are worth mentioning by way of illustration. What they were stressing was a permanent attribute of man—his power to control his instincts, not a new development due to economic or social changes. Thus Coleridge, attacking Malthus's second edition: 'The whole question is this: Are Lust and Hunger both alike Passions of physical Necessity, and the one equally with the other independent of the Reason, and the Will? Shame upon our Race, that there lives the Individual who dares even ask the Question!' (Quoted in H. A. Boner, *Hungry Generations; the Nineteenth-Century Case Against Malthusianism* (New York, 1955), pp. 44–45.) Similar thoughts were expressed by Southey, Hazlitt, and others—no revolutionaries these, but believers in reason for all that.

expressly recommends the civilized state without being too precise as to its limits. He rejected the return to the uncultivated state; he was fond of a 'commodious' way of life, which gave rise:

> . . . to the invention of many true refinements, heightens the splendour and magnificence of society, tends to render mankind social and humane, begets mildness and moderation in the tempers and actions of men, and helps to banish ignorance and superstition out of the world; and thus far it contributes to the perfection of human society.

But there must be no overstepping the limit—we must not ever re-create the atmosphere of the fall of Greece and Rome, where luxury and vice prevailed, and duty was forgotten. This state, he says in a memorable peroration, 'must of course prevent marriage, give check to the increase of mankind, and hinder millions from ever seeing the light'.[1] Earlier in his work he had hinted that 'operose manufactures' of various goods made of metal, wood, or earth might not contribute anything to the increase of population; on the contrary the tastes they generate (or which create them) may well act as a hindrance to increase.[2] Wallace, then, may be said to be uncertain about the outcome.

On the other hand, a Frenchman, the Lutheran clergyman John Brueckner (of German origin), who was highly praised by Marx, saw that the inevitable concomitant of a higher state of life was a changed attitude to marriage. He did not think that the characteristic occupations and predilections of this stage of development created physical obstacles to fertility, but rather that psychological checks began to operate. One of the reasons he adduced for his belief that civilization reduced fertility was his observation of the rise of dangerous and painful occupations such as mining and navigation. The arts and sciences, in addition to their beneficial effects, also produce 'hidden poisons, which retard progress and which serve as correctives for the excess [multiplication they otherwise occasion]'.[3]

The hostile attitude to the wants of a more industrial state engendered by advancing civilization is to be found in the pages of that pamphlet by William Bell which gave rise to the refutation by William

[1] R. Wallace, *A Dissertation on the Numbers of Mankind, in Ancient and Modern Times* (Edinburgh, 1809), pp. 337–8.

[2] Ibid., pp. 23–24.

[3] For an account of Brueckner, see C. E. Stangeland, *Pre-Malthusian Doctrines of Population; a Study in the History of Economic Theory* (New York, 1904), pp. 233–7, and J. J. Spengler, *French Predecessors of Malthus* (Durham, North Carolina, 1942), pp. 234–5. Similar aspersions on the effects of industrialization elsewhere, e.g. C. J. Herbert, quoted in Spengler, ibid., p. 71.

Temple, cited previously. Bell's *Dissertation* had been published at Cambridge in 1756.[1] He was so certain of the depopulating effect of this advance that he recommended it as a specific for over-population—then such a remote contingency that his reasoning may be taken as an outright condemnation of any occupation save agriculture. In Temple's words (paraphrasing Bell):

> When you have brought this to pass [i.e. fullness of numbers] I would advise you to adopt Commerce and the arts, in order to lessen your numbers; which they will effectively do, and at last bring you to certain destruction.[2]

Bell's contemporary John Brown goes farther in actually distinguishing three stages of technical advance—the last of which: 'brings in Superfluity and vast Wealth; begets . . . effeminate Refinement among the higher Ranks, together with general Loss of Principle'.[3]

These attitudes, then, are common, and not unexpected as products of their age. On the one hand progress was visible to the naked eye, especially in the standard of physical comfort amongst the upper classes—on the other hand the accent was still on depopulation, and the enemies of the one were not slow to blame on it the incidence of the other.

But already the more far-sighted could discern the other side of the picture. Adam Ferguson, one of the first to understand the implication of a changed standard of living, went farther than Wallace even in welcoming the new criteria of judgement. His 'civilized man' who fails to marry because he cannot get what he considers necessary, had his full approval already in 1767.[4]

It should be pointed out that this sort of reasoning, derived from a sociological approach to the problems of contemporary society, is rather different from the kind of pamphleteering which we observe in, say, William Temple, when he defends manufactures and the higher standard of living they bring. He, of course, flatly denies Bell's charge that such advances bring depopulation, and blames infertility on excess which may occur at any level of individual or national living. But one has the feeling that even if he had observed adverse effects in this one direction he would have suppressed the evidence. Ferguson, on the

[1] W. Bell, *A Dissertation on the Following Subject: What Causes Principally Contribute to Render a Nation Populous? And What Effect Has the Populousness of a Nation on its Trade?* (Cambridge, 1756).

[2] Temple, op. cit., p. 488.

[3] J. Brown, *An Estimate of the Manners and Principles of the Times* (2nd ed., London, 1757), p. 153.

[4] A. Ferguson, *An Essay on the History of Civil Society* (4th ed., London, 1773), p. 286.

other hand, is mainly concerned with his insights into the harmonious working of social laws, without, however, being under a constant necessity to score points. In this respect he is in the Scottish tradition of observation and comment, of which Sir James Steuart and Adam Smith are other examples. Had this tradition continued all would have been well. But the controversies, first around the absolute size and movement of the population, then around Malthus's theme and the Poor Laws, did not permit such comparative objectivity, nor such a broad view. Nevertheless, the influence of the French philosophers' speculations about the necessary general conditions of human existence did occasionally, even in England, induce some thoughts on the probable effects of total environment on reproductive habits, even if they are generally by way of incidental glosses and afterthoughts rather than carefully reasoned statements of views on demography.

Civilization and human reason, then, were coming into their own. The highest expectations were those of the men who finally aroused Malthus's wrath—Condorcet and Godwin. For these visionaries, unlike Rousseau, did not preach a return to a simpler way of life. On the contrary (and this applies especially to Condorcet), they foresaw ever greater advances—and the ultimate control of the problem of population growth formed an integral part of this progress. Condorcet's glowing account of new thought over the centuries is, in effect, a history of civilization. In the tenth and last stage of his *Sketch for a Historical Picture of the Progress of the Human Mind* he visualizes the liberation of the human mind from the prison of barbaric ignorance. 'The time will therefore come when the sun will shine only on free men who know no other master but their reason. . . .'[1] His description of this happy future state leaves no doubt that what he means is an advance both in the physical attributes of civilization and the intellectual atmosphere which we now call culture. Equality in education and international equality would help to promote fresh progress in the sciences and the arts—progress in machines and looms as well as in the production of food. Larger physical possessions will match a more enlightened outlook. Finally, he gives the answer to those who think that one day population might become too great for the amount of subsistence available:

> . . . if we consider that . . . the progress of reason will have kept pace with that of the sciences, and that the absurd prejudices of superstition will have

[1] M.-J.-A.-N. de Caritat, Marquis de Condorcet, *Sketch for a Historical Picture of the Progress of the Human Mind* (1795; J. Barraclough, trans., London, 1955), p. 179.

ceased to corrupt and degrade the moral code by its harsh doctrines instead of purifying and elevating it, we can assume that by then men will know that, if they have a duty towards those who are not yet born, that duty is not to give them existence but to give them happiness; their aim should be to promote the general welfare of the human race or of the society in which they liveor of the family to which they belong, rather than foolishly to encumber the world with useless and wretched beings.[1]

It is usually assumed that what Condorcet meant to convey here was that any particular prejudices, such as those against contraception or even possibly abortion, would be set aside in order to achieve the greater moral purposes of society, namely the attainment of human happiness. At least this is the interpretation which Malthus himself put on the passage, and in its context it seems reasonable enough. This, then, was the atmosphere created by the visionaries—the zenith of the ambitions of all believers in scientific progress and human perfectibility. As we know, Malthus's first essay was the 'douche of cold water' that was poured on the prophecies of these great minds, and with Malthus's swift rise to fame, the hopes of many men of good will were dashed. Not surprisingly, therefore, some of the liveliest answers to the *Essay on Population* based themselves precisely on the notion suggested by Ferguson, and, in a different form, by Condorcet: that it is the very advance of human society that carries within itself the seeds of the limitation of population.

Malthus himself was not unaware of the effects of industrialization on population growth, and helped to furnish the answer to his own problem. Although for the most part he subscribed to the view that the demand for employment was the most powerful regulator of incomes, and therefore of marriage and fertility, he could also observe the possibility of a check arising from the different patterns of employment and consumption when a nation progressed from the agrarian state.[2] This realization dawned on him fully only by the time of the fifth edition of the *Essay* (1817). There he commented on the startling results on population size of the stimulus of the increased demand for labour combined with increasing productive power:

[1] Ibid., p. 189. James Mill, a quarter of a century later, also delicately referred to the 'superstitions of the nursery' when speaking of the opposition to birth control. (In the article 'Colony', *Encyclopaedia Britannica Supplement* (5th ed., 1818); see J. A. Field, *Essays on Population and Other Papers* (H. F. Hohman, ed. and comp., Chicago, 1931), p. 94.)

[2] For a full description of Malthus's views on industrialization, see J. J. Spengler, 'Malthus' Total Population Theory ... etc.', *Canadian Journal of Economics and Political Science* (1945), xi. 83 ff., 234 ff., esp. pp. 100 ff.

What has taken place is a striking illustration of the principle of population, and a proof that in spite of great towns, manufacturing occupations, and the gradually-acquired habits of an opulent and luxuriant people, if the resources of the country will admit of a rapid increase, . . . the population will not fail to keep pace with them.[1]

In this passage the tendency of urban occupations associated with industrialization to retard population growth is implied in so off-hand a manner that one would say that Malthus took this effect for granted. But one has the impression that this attitude is in reality a hangover from the eighteenth-century view that in general only agriculture can sustain a people, and that all manufacture of 'ornamental luxuries' adds little to total satisfaction. Gradually, Malthus came to discard this unfriendly or rather ostrich-like attitude towards industry which is still so evident in the first edition,[2] and from 1817 onwards described a little more carefully the beginnings of the international exchange economy which had begun to operate by then. Nevertheless, he could not and would not admit that in the long run the country could be saved from the effects of over-population merely by trading manufactures against food and raw material. The best that could be said for the change was that it might help people to cultivate prudential habits—by putting within their reach 'conveniences and luxuries' of a sort which engendered care and foresight. This point, as we have seen, Malthus elaborated many times. In the present context, it is particularly interesting to note the close connexion he established between industry, civil liberty, and habits of consumption. Especially in the third and fourth books of the later editions of the *Essay*, he contrasts the state of a poor country like Poland, where maldistribution of property and feudal customs prevent the growth of industry,[3] with the democratic arrangements in England where the whole structure is conducive to habits of foresight. When one reads a passage such as this, one really wonders how Malthus could have been such a spectre to his generation:

England possesses very great natural and political advantages, in which perhaps the countries that we should in this case compare with her would be found to be palpably deficient. The nature of her soil and climate is such, that those almost universal failures in the crops of grain, which are known in some countries, never occur in England. Her insular situation and extended commerce are peculiarly favourable for importation. Her numerous manu-

[1] Malthus, *Essay* . . . (5th ed., 1817), ii. 103–4; (Everyman ed.), i. 261.
[2] Ibid. (1st ed., 1798), chs. xvi–xvii.
[3] Ibid. (Everyman ed.), ii, bk. iii, ch. viii.

factures employ nearly all the hands that are not engaged in agriculture, and afford the means of a regular distribution of the annual produce of the land and labour to the whole of her inhabitants. But, above all, throughout a very large class of people, a decided taste for the conveniences and comforts of life, a strong desire of bettering their condition (that master-spring of public prosperity), and, in consequence, a most laudable spirit of industry and foresight, are observed to prevail. These dispositions, so contrary to the hopeless indolence remarked in despotic countries, are generated by the constitution of the English government and the excellence of its laws, which secure to every individual the product of his industry.[1]

We may take exception to this passage on several grounds (such as that many people were engaged in neither agriculture nor manufacture, but the provision of services, or that, as Ricardo had seen by that time, even the law did not secure to every man the 'product of his industry') but we are struck by the comparatively full environmental explanation given by Malthus to the phenomenon of a society exercising the prudential check.

There are in this part of his writings also a number of subsidiary and sometimes obscure reasons for the favourable effect of industrialization on population growth. One of these concerns the necessary social rearrangement of society: as the feudal system of agriculture is replaced by a trading and manufacturing system, so the proportion of the middle classes in society increases, and since they are, almost by definition, prudent, the tendency of the whole population to grow is thereby diminished, even if we cannot all expect to be middle-class.[2] The second additional reason for the supposed wholesome effect of industrial growth on population trends is hard to understand. While food is cheap, Malthus thought, the labourer will work only as many days of the week as he must to obtain necessaries, and idle away the rest rather than acquire 'conveniences and comforts'. But once food is comparatively scarce and dear, and the conveniences and comforts therefore relatively cheap, the labourer will exert himself not only to get all the food he needs, but, by comparatively small additional labour, also these other things for which the high price of food will give him a taste.[3] This relative position of prices can only occur, one would guess, in a manufacturing country depending on dear home-produced corn and marginal imports kept low by tariffs—in other words, the British position after 1815. But the argument sounds altogether improbable.

[1] Ibid. ii, bk. iv, ch. viii, pp. 206–7.

[2] Ibid. ii. 134.

[3] Ibid., p. 135.

2. AFTER MALTHUS

It should be noted that the first book to concern itself with 'civilization' as such, after Malthus's work, is not at all in the tradition we are here describing. Charles Hall's *The Effects of Civilisation on the People in European States*, published in 1805, is an early socialist work blaming many of the miseries, and consequently lack of foresight, of the poor on the refinements of civilization for the rich, bought at the expense of an impoverished multitude. So little faith had he, in fact, in the possibility of a real check to over-population merely by an increase of standards that he actually advocated, in an appendix, the eventual regulation of marriage, if required.[1] Nevertheless, the work is worth mentioning for the definition of civilization given at the start, which, from its tone, leads us to suppose that its author was not hostile to progress as such:

> We understand by civilisation that manner of living in societies of men, which is opposite to that of those who are called savages. . . . It consists in the study and knowledge of the sciences, and in the production and enjoyment of the conveniences, elegancies, and luxuries of life. . . .[2]

The tripartite definition of the last line echoes Malthus, foreshadows Nassau Senior, and, in itself, does not reproduce the anti-luxury arguments of the previous century. In a way, it is a pity that Hall, a vigorous and able writer, did not draw the proper conclusion from his own premisses—it stared him in the face.

But meanwhile others had eagerly seized both on Malthus's own hints as to the conduct of the English, and on their own observations. Thomas Jarrold's *Dissertations on Man, Philosophical, Physiological and Political*, published in 1806, were, as the title implies, an ambitious attempt to relate the whole of human society to its surroundings, and to explain the changes it was then undergoing. He used his wide practical experience as a doctor to refute Malthus's main arguments. The first part of the book was a detailed consideration of the Malthusian theory, but in the later chapters Jarrold developed his own ideas. These were clearly based on the understanding of Man rising from the beastly stage to the highest attainments of which he was capable—and when successive stages of civilization were reached, his fertility would be

[1] C. Hall, *The Effects of Civilisation on the People in European States* (London, 1805), with Appendix: 'Observations on the Principal Conclusion in Mr. Malthus' "Essay on Population".'

[2] Ibid., p. 1.

controlled to an ever-increasing degree. He has many assertions on differential fertility—rich and poor, urban and rural, educated and illiterate. He found, in fact, a large part of the population not subject to Malthus's checks of vice, misery, and moral restraint as such, and what was true of that part could one day be true of the whole.[1] The characteristic of a civilized society, he thought, was that men lived by exercising their minds—and that in itself, amongst other factors, affects their fertility. (Here, of course, he anticipates Spencer.) This, he felt, was only to be welcomed—if only as an answer to the fears that were abroad. A remark of his about the Greeks as an example of a nation brought to small numbers by a high development of their civilization would appear to lead to flights of high fancy, but he ended on a very prosaic note. His first reliance is on an increase in human intellect and a reduction of moral depravity: but, if it should happen that morals remain as bad as they were before, it is still quite possible that an increase in civilization alone will produce the desired result.[2] Here, obviously, civilization is taken to mean the outward trappings rather than the inner elevation of an advanced society.

Jarrold's theme is to be found in a number of other writers of the same period who did not always add fresh matter to the general environmental approach. Sometimes civilization appears as a short-hand term for the forces producing that automatic equilibrium which, as we saw, was so dear to our early writers. In this sense it was clearly used by Colonel Torrens, a liberal economist and opponent of the Corn Laws, who had no fears of the future since the prudential check on marriage was 'a function of those moral causes of instruction and civilization, which are ever gradual in their operation'.[3] This was a necessary belief in the face of the Malthusian 'tendencies'—for the efficacy of corn imports as a means of feeding the country's population would depend on some prospect of stabilization in the rate of increase of the people. Home production alone would soon lead to diminishing returns from cultivation, so the economists argued, hence we come to a declining standard of living, consequently high mortality and the familiar attitudes connected with this state of affairs, leading to high fertility.

[1] T. Jarrold, *Dissertations on Man, Philosophical, Physiological and Political; in Answer to Mr. Malthus' 'Essay on the Principle of Population'* (London, 1806), p. 267.

[2] Ibid., p. 366.

[3] R. Torrens, *An Essay on the Influence of the External Corn Trade upon the Production and Distribution of National Wealth . . . etc.* (2nd ed., London, 1820), p. 64. See also L. Robbins, 'On a Certain Ambiguity in the Conception of Stationary Equilibrium', *Economic Journal* (June 1930), xl, no. 158, p. 196.

Given the improvement in standards connected with cheap and plentiful food, there is then a chance for the general rise in standards here characterized as civilization. This, of course, is in direct opposition to one of Malthus's arguments.

John Weyland, in his *Principles of Population and Production*, was less concerned with imports than with the mechanism by which production in general responded to increases in population. This he had in common with many of Malthus's opponents. But, like the rest, he still had the residual point to explain away: suppose you have doubled, quadrupled, multiplied to the *n*th degree the food you produce—what then? Then, Weyland would say, we shall have reached such a high stage of development that a new principle will operate. He foresaw that ever-increasing numbers of people, in these advanced states, must devote themselves to urban employments, to the planning and directing of the huge effort involved. And so it comes about that:

> . . . as civilisation advances . . ., the number of those who spontaneously prefer the advantages of celibacy to those of the married state continually increases; and that the power of propagating their species in many of those who choose the other alternative is at the same time continually diminishing.[1]

Here we have a blend of physiological and psychological teaching—some will not, and some cannot. He does not seem to consider the possibility that some of those who do choose the alternative of marriage might also be amongst the 'will-nots'—like Malthus, he does not think of restraint after marriage. That was yet to come.

For the most part the investigators of the immediate post-Malthusian period had already abandoned the physiological approach altogether, but some helped to pave the way for Sadler and Spencer. Most prevalent was the notion of mankind passing through different stages of progress—not indeed usually in so utopian a manner as Condorcet's scheme had shown, but soberly enough reflecting on what had already been achieved. Simon Gray, whose essay on *The Happiness of States* had been written before Jarrold's, but was published only in 1815, foreshadows many later writers who became intoxicated with the notion of progress. Gray warned against superficial indices of material progress as guarantees of moral and intellectual advance. Yet all the circumstances of life in his age, it seemed to him, worked in the same direction. The greater density of the population and the consequent increased

[1] J. Weyland, jnr., *The Principles of Population and Production, as they are affected by the Progress of Society; with a View to Moral and Political Consequences* (London, 1816), p. 410.

struggle of the body and brain to keep alive, urban growth—all these were the concomitants of civilization.[1]

The most prevalent notion of the period, however, was once again the assertion that the human mind was capable of controlling its environment—not in any extreme or miraculous sense, but merely in the shape of the emergence of strong social pressures of standards which helped the individual to overcome his own weaknesses. This was intended to dispose of Malthus's sad observation that, in the individual, the mere desire to better his condition was not as strong as his sex instincts. Thus T. R. Edmonds calls civilization a stage of development where standards of conduct matter[2] and John Stuart Mill described it as the struggle against animal instincts, which had, so far, been least successful in the field of population, mainly because it had never been tried.[3]

Several authors even gave Malthus credit for having given pointers in the right direction. Amongst these was Robert Hamilton, Professor of Mathematics in Aberdeen, who, like Mill, was at least a conditional follower of Malthus. He also looked forward to an increased environmental influence:

> ... the rate of increase becomes slower with the progress of art and civilization. This arises from the difference of habits that accompany the change of the state of society, and is likely to operate still more powerfully as art and civilization are carried to a higher pitch, and without having recourse to harsh measures, may be expected to restrain the progress of population within the necessary limits.[4]

When Gray, Weyland, and Jarrold were writing, Malthus was still at the zenith of his power, and their theories bear the marks of their origins as rather desperate attempts to stand Malthusianism on its head. As time passed, and ever more distinguished names were added to the list of those who did not believe the dignified professor at Haileybury, there appeared rather better thought-out attempts to fuse the experience now available into consistent bodies of thought. Between Malthus's

[1] S. Gray, *The Happiness of States; or an Inquiry concerning Population, the Modes of Subsisting and Employing It, and the Effects of All on Human Happiness: in which is Developed the New or Productive System of Statistics* (2nd ed., London, 1819), p. 625; quoted in K. Smith, *The Malthusian Controversy* (London, 1951), p. 217. See also his fuller account of Gray, pp. 86–91, and *passim*.

[2] [T. R. Edmonds], *An Enquiry into the Principles of Population* ... (London, 1832), pp. 77, 87.

[3] J. S. Mill, *Principles of Political Economy... etc.* (6th ed., London, 1902), part 1, bk. 2, ch. 13.

[4] R. Hamilton, *The Progress of Society* (London, 1830), p. 352.

first *Essay* and the time of Senior's *Lectures*, the population of England had increased by something like 50 per cent.—and yet there were many more people than previously who were enjoying a high standard of living. The Poor Law, admittedly, had become a worse burden than ever—but on the credit side there were a new middle class and a new artisan class, created by the growth of industry and commerce, whose habits did not suggest that they were particularly subject to the positive checks. Their psychology repaid study. A high proportion of their numbers, at any rate, received some sort of education—indeed it was an indispensable condition of their livelihood. The general moral tone of society had distinctly improved as the influence of the Evangelical movement increased. It did not take Victoria's succession to produce a widespread condemnation of the morals of Regency England.[1]

3. THE CONSTANT ADVANCE

This new society of sober, industrious citizens, with their cherished standards of property and proprieties, engaged the analytical eye of Nassau Senior. In the chapter of his *Outline* in which he describes the operation of his treble standard of necessities, decencies, and luxuries, he comes to the conclusion that the only sure protection against over-population lies in: 'prudence in contracting marriage, and of considerable superfluous expenditure.'[2] But such expenditure cannot be achieved until there has been considerable progress:

> And as the former habits exist only in a civilized, and the latter only in an opulent society, it appears equally clear that, as a nation advances in civilization and opulence, the positive checks are likely to be superseded by the preventive.

If this be so, the positive checks fall victims to constant improvement. It is necessary for these standards to change, too—so as to ensure constant diffusion of notions of comfort to ever lower ranks of society, until finally the threat disappears. We note that there is now a clear distinction between 'civilization' and 'opulence'—the former word evidently denoting the refinement of manners, and the latter the physical means which went with them. It appears possible to have opulence without civilization, but hardly, in Senior's usage, the other way round. The age of the Impoverished Gentlewoman was yet to come.

[1] See M. Jaeger, *Before Victoria; Changing Standards and Behaviour, 1787–1837* (London, 1956).

[2] N. W. Senior, *An Outline of the Science of Political Economy* (London, 1938 ed.), p. 42.

Contemporary with Senior, but far less clear in his interpretation of the developments of the age, was A. H. Moreton, the Gloucestershire landowner and Member of Parliament, who was obviously torn between his readiness to accept Malthus's explanations of the misery of the poor, and his more optimistic observations of the habits of large numbers of people. His book, characteristically, was called *Civilization, or, a Brief Analysis of the Natural Laws that Regulate the Numbers and Conditions of Mankind.* He had read Sadler, and was impressed with the density argument.[1] But his reasoning was more subtle than that of others who thought that the retardation of increase was a mere consequence of numbers. As we have seen, he was aware of French researches showing the connexion between lower mortality and lower fertility, of the failure of the aristocratic families to maintain their line, and other aspects of differential fertility rates. These observations he grouped together into the idea that development meant diffusion of comforts, hence greater survival rates, and at the same time greater opportunities for the lower classes to improve their position. Hence, differential birth-rates are not 'exceptions to the benevolence of Providence'[2] but on the contrary, an important principle for the happiness of mankind. On this progress of civilization depends the effective answer to Malthus. (Though he does not expressly repudiate Malthusianism, he is far too optimistic to be classed amongst its adherents.) Moreton is thus one of the first to realize clearly that the different manifestations of the exercise of prudence are aspects of the same general process—where social pressures, individual advantage, and moral judgement all combine to alter fertility patterns. If one takes this view, then a society in which fertility was fixed, or equal amongst all sections of the community, could easily be branded as backward. This thought has survived to some extent in the modern notion of primitive as against advanced demographic régimes, with their fluctuating but consistently high birth- and death-rates—high, that is, compared with advanced societies.

Perhaps the fullest statement of the position came from George Rickards, in his work *Population and Capital.* Here the ideas of the conditions of progress were further analysed in the light of increasing experience. We are aware that first Senior, and then Rickards, both wrote in the full flood of the liberal triumph. Adam Smith is justified

[1] A. H. Moreton, *Civilization, or, a Brief Analysis of the Natural Laws that Regulate the Numbers and Conditions of Mankind* (London, 1836), p. 128.

[2] Ibid., p. 143.

beyond doubt. Malthus had cast a shadow over the empire of *laissez-faire*—was there not one point where Nature, left to itself within the free economic system, threatened to wreck the beautiful edifice? Would not Government have to take stern measures to inculcate into its citizens that sense of responsibility they so obviously lacked? No, indeed not: for lo! the system left to itself produces its own happy antidote. Man's genius has advanced subsistence, in its widest sense, faster than population could increase, and the resultant taste of comforts has automatically stopped, at least those who benefited from these developments, from too-rapid increase.

'The true interests of individuals and of the community coincide', Rickards was pleased to observe.[1] Competition leads not to fear of distress, but to the stimulus of social emulation. The middle ranks of society have benefited from this competition. Their outlook is good. But how to get the lower orders to share in this advance? Obviously by making sure that the whole of society advances in every way.

As Arts and Sciences improve, so:

> ... the cheapening of production by mechanical agency places within [their] reach, at a trifling cost, conveniences and luxuries, which in former times even the highborn and wealthy could not command.[2]

There is another way in which this advance operates, and that is through the very mode of industrialization, which ensures that the intellectual development keeps up with the material:

> The progress of industrial invention gradually devolves upon machinery the harder and ruder processes of labour. Of the work left for human hands to do, less is thrown upon mere brute strength, more and more upon intelligence and skill.[3]

And so it goes on. Steam-power creates refined and delicate operations, a higher standard is demanded, and wages rise. The proportion of skilled to unskilled labour must increase. There is a real hope that one day the lower classes will cease to behave like lower classes and conduct themselves like English gentlemen. This, of course, can only be ensured by complete freedom, and so there follows the familiar statement of liberal doctrine, in a form not very different from Malthus's.

The check to population which this kind of conduct implies, Rickards concludes, is part and parcel of human nature—it stands in

[1] Sir G. Rickards, *Population and Capital: Being a Course of Lectures Delivered before the University of Oxford in 1853–54* (London, 1854), p. 204.

[2] Ibid., p. 251.

[3] Ibid.

the same category as the principle of reproduction itself: '. . . moral restraint is a check which Nature herself spontaneously developes in the progress of civilisation'.[1]

It should be noted that there were also one or two voices at this time, amongst the chorus of self-satisfied optimism, asserting that the decline of fertility associated with industrialization was not necessarily a sign of growing comfort and skill. Marx, later on, was emphatic in denying any connexion with an elevated standard of living, and writers like the tory radical Samuel Laing in England and the early socialist F. Schmidt in Germany, may be seen as forerunners of Marx. Schmidt suggested that there would be a reduction in fertility when there was a change to capitalist enterprise in a fully settled country. This, he thought, was due to the fact that capital accumulation was only possible when there was reduction in the supplies required for consumption, and therefore a Malthusian effect is produced—population fails to rise as industry develops. He used this observation to express opinions in support of Sadler's density theories.[2]

Laing had a different view of industrialization. Realistically, he took a less rosy view of the ascent of the population under the factory system. Under a régime of production where individuals could really expect to rise to respectability and affluence (and he thought, perhaps wrongly, that the old domestic system fulfilled that condition), it would be quite true to say that a civilizing influence would be exercised. But under the conditions of contemporary Lancashire, he felt there was no hope. 'The capitalist and operative are separated by a wide gulf which is becoming every day more and more difficult to pass.'[3] The result was that even where money wages were comparatively high 'improvidence and dissipation' were the rule. Moreover, he felt, the instability of the whole modern commercial world is such that people are deprived of any useful sense of security—people are affected by a system 'fluctuating with every political rumour and monetary derangement, from New York to Canton'.[4] This was not a very surprising observation to make

[1] Ibid., pp. 254–5.

[2] F. Schmidt, *Untersuchungen über Bevölkerung, Arbeitslohn und Pauperismus, in ihrem gegenseitigen Zusammenhange* (Leipzig, 1836); quoted in R. v. Mohl, *Die Geschichte und Literatur der Staatswissenschaften, in Monographien dargestellt* (Erlangen, 1858, 3 vols.), iii. 512–13. Mohl himself was an exponent of Malthusian views in Germany and advocated the official regulation of marriage in his monumental *Die Polizeiwissenschaft nach den Grundsätzen des Rechtsstaates* (Tübingen, 1866, 3 vols.).

[3] S. Laing (the younger), *National Distress: its Causes and Remedies* (London, 1844), p. 77.

[4] Ibid., p. 78.

in the year 1844, when the controversies generated by the renewal of the Bank of England's charter had given much publicity to the extremely sensitive position of the English banking system in a world affected by rumours and speculations. This was to be a familiar theme, but whereas Laing seems to have thought of this influence as one leading to recklessness, most later writers thought this insecurity to be a chief cause of sterility, or rather failure to marry, at least amongst those who might be affected by it.[1]

4. FRANCE FACES DEPOPULATION

So far, the majority of the writers examined have been British. This is as we would expect when we remember that 'civilization' in one sense, the diffusion of comforts amongst a great part of the population and the alteration in habits and manners which accompanies it, was seen to its greatest advantage in England and Scotland: for here the increasing productive capacity of industry and the spread of education made these changes possible. When writers in other countries spoke of 'industrialization' it was generally in connexion with observations made in England. But naturally this does not mean that French or German writers conceded to the British a monopoly of civilization, let alone culture. It was in France, where it had originated, that the theory of civilization reached its fullest development, and in Germany that culture was elevated to the same status.

The younger Dr. Bertillon gave his father the credit for the invention of the civilization theory.[2] Although the passage he quotes contains some good points, it is clear enough that there is nothing new in it compared with Senior, Moreton, or Rickards.[3] The influence of the factors connected with 'civilization' was particularly strong, he thought, where 'la civilisation est le plus universalisée, démocratisée, alors que la masse de la collectivité considérée est gagnée à la contagion de goûts plus relevés'.[4] This leads to the desire for security by the accumulation of capital, and thus the need to save. The existence of savings, or the

[1] A similar view of the effects of industrialization had been expressed by W. F. Lloyd, *Two Lectures on the Checks to Population, Delivered before the University of Oxford in Michaelmas Term, 1832* (Oxford, 1833), p. 68: 'The industrial revolution has produced a great increase of the labouring classes who have no hopes and prospects, and weakened by women and child labour, and poor laws, the responsibilities of the *pater familias*.'

[2] J. Bertillon, *La Dépopulation de la France . . . etc.* (Paris, 1911), pp. 128–9.

[3] The original article was entitled 'Natalité' and published in the *Dictionnaire encyclopédique des sciences médicales* (Paris *c.* 1874), pp. 89 ff.

[4] Bertillon fils, op. cit., p. 129.

desire for them, have been separately investigated in relation to fertility. The attitude towards them undergoes the familiar cycle: virtue, vice, object of scientific investigation. In Malthus's day thrift was to be promoted, and he himself advocated the establishment of savings banks as a means of encouraging the poor to practise foresight.[1] The point was taken up by a number of his followers, such as Count Pellegrino Rossi, who prepared the most important French edition of the *Essay*.[2] The writers who figure later in this chapter, like Bertillon and Leroy-Beaulieu, were then responsible for turning the habit into a vice, and declared it to be miserly accumulation due to excessive anxiety about status and so on.[3] Scientific investigations were begun by Tallquist in Finland in the eighteen-eighties.[4] In England, where the promotion of savings banks had been the object both of private charitable initiative and of legislation (Gladstone's Post Office Savings Bank), the movement towards small savings assumed sufficient proportions to be noticed by social investigators like Sidney Webb as a factor in reducing fertility.[5] Members of the Hearts of Oak Friendly Society, Webb noted, were claiming ever smaller amounts of lying-in benefits, just as Malthus would have predicted. Scientifically, the correlation does not bear examination in isolation, but as a prejudice it has a definite place in the history of the environmental argument.

Where the French writers differed from the British predecessors was in their approach, which was, on the whole, more generalized, discursive, and dramatic. Moreover, their object was to present the benefits of civilization in a doubtful light, or even, as in the case of Dumont, to condemn most of its aspects altogether. To some extent, to lay the blame for France's problem at the door of her over-developed civilization was to boast in the midst of lamentation. What other nation could claim this disaster? There is nothing really apologetic, for instance, in Leroy-Beaulieu's statement:

C'est au moment où, intellectuellement, socialement, par le développement de l'aisance, des arts, par l'élévation du niveau général, les nations paraissent s'être le plus perfectionnées et avoir atteint la situation la plus brillante qu'elles

[1] T. R. Malthus, *An Essay on the Principle of Population* (Everyman ed., London 1914, 2 vols.), ii. 242–3.

[2] See J. J. Spengler, 'French Population Theory since 1800', *Journal of Political Economy* (1936), xliv. 586.

[3] J. J. Spengler, *France Faces Depopulation* (Durham, North Carolina, 1938), p. 168.

[4] *Recherches statistiques sur la tendance à une moindre fécondité des mariages*, (Helsingfors, 1886), quoted in Bertillon, op. cit., p. 152.

[5] S. Webb, *The Decline in the Birth-rate* (Fabian Tract No. 131, London, 1907), p. 6.

donnent des preuves d'arrêt dans leur croissance et même de recul par la réduction progressive de la natalité.[1]

He, like many other writers, recalled the glories and fall of the Greek and Roman societies at the height of their intellectual development. The picture presented by these writers, however, is such that one can well understand the extreme reactions of men like Dumont. High intellectual development there may be, but how are we to regard 'personal and familial ambition', 'luxurious tastes', even 'shamelessness',[2] if not in the same light as the eighteenth-century moralists did? In truth, the wheel had come full circle, and the 'civilizationists' were like the pre-Malthusian writers—only that they tried to subordinate their moral indignation to the 'scientific' analysis of causes and effects. Leroy-Beaulieu's 'moral causes of decline' are not simply historical categories—they represent the bitter disappointment of a nation defeated in war by a once inferior neighbour, looking inside itself for the causes of decline. Civilization brings in its train the development of new classes of people—the professions, the administration, the middle-men—and their life is one of bitter competition. The politicians who rule them seek popular favour and thus are corrupt. This passage could easily have been taken from some Roman orator of the second or third century:

> Les politiciens contemporains, à tous degrés, depuis les conseillers municipaux des villes jusqu'aux ministres, représentent, pris en masse et la part faite de quelques exceptions, une des classes les plus viles et les plus bornées de sycophantes et de courtisans qu'ait jamais connues l'humanité.[3]

Careerism, abortion, feminism—all these came in for attack. Most would not answer the question clearly: do you, then, wish to turn the clock back? Instead, they recommended ways of strengthening the national character, and urged pro-populationist policies. Some bold spirits, notably Dumont, clearly said that civilization and democracy had gone too far. If our democratic civilization meant that the individual could defy and harm the state and society by his selfishness, then the power to do so must be taken from him. 'La solidarité doit remplacer la fidélité—la solidarité peut être imposée par les lois.'[4]

[1] P. Leroy-Beaulieu, *La Question de la population* (3e éd., Paris, 1913), p. 180. Leroy-Beaulieu had already published his ideas in an article in the *Revue des deux mondes* (Oct. 1897), pp. 851–89: 'La Question de la population et la civilisation démocratique'.

[2] Leroy-Beaulieu, *La Question . . .*, pp. 220 ff.

[3] Ibid., p. 262.

[4] A. Dumont, *Dépopulation et civilisation. Etude démographique* (Paris, 1890), headings to chapter 20.

The next stage in the history of population theory once again turned its back on this type of generalization. More coolly, statisticians began to investigate the individual processes which made up the 'civilizing' phase. Modern methods of census-taking made it possible to correlate more nearly fertility and its determinants, from domestic plumbing to higher education. Nevertheless, there are still people who believe that advancing civilization as such must needs involve some change in fertility,[1] and others who base on this relation their chief hopes for an eventual decline of fertility in the underdeveloped countries.[2]

5. CULTURE THEORIES AND DECADENCE

The notion of progress was already inherent in every definition of civilization as a depopulating factor. From this it is only a short step to the wider idea that nations undergo a process of social development in distinct stages, each with its own laws of population trends. Usually this process is depicted in three of its principal stages—a rising society, a society at the peak of its development, and finally in its stage of decline. The explanations for the variations in behaviour are then environmental—the prevailing 'culture' is said to exert pressures on various aspects of human life, and to force the individual to modify his reproductive behaviour in particular.[3] In very many cases, therefore, this type of theory is found in conjunction with hypotheses about the decline of human societies, since the most marked changes in the fertility pattern occurred round about the time of the change from growth to decay, and became, by definition, notorious when a nation died out, usually through its military impotence. The advantage of this type of explanation was that it reconciled the apparent contradictions we found, for instance, in Leroy-Beaulieu: the appearance, simultaneously, of the greatest flowering of the national genius, and *mœurs* bearing in them the seeds of inevitable downfall. As the centuries of the rising phase laid the preparations for the period of national greatness, so this period in itself wrought changes which meant its end.

[1] F. H. Hankins, 'Does Advancing Civilisation Involve a Decline in National Fertility?' *Publications of the American Sociological Society* (May, 1930), xxiv. 115 ff.

[2] United Nations, *The Determinants and Consequences of Population Trends* (New York, 1953), p. 41, note 177.

[3] For a general survey of culture theories of population, see E. T. Hiller, 'A Culture Theory of Population Trends', in J. J. Spengler and O. D. Duncan, eds., *Population Theory and Policy, Selected Readings* (Glencoe, 1956). The article was intended to show the limitations of biological and economic interpretations, and to plead for the substitution of a cultural approach.

The notion of cultural stages was already clearly outlined in Condorcet's *Sketch for a Historical Picture of the Progress of the Human Mind*, and in Godwin's *An Enquiry concerning Political Justice*. . . . Each stage had its own laws, including those affecting population, and, as we saw, Condorcet strongly believed that the most perfect stage would also see the control of that problem. But for these and their friends, the last stage was the millennium—nothing lay beyond it except paradise. Later writers often classified their society according to the typical mode of life and its associated fertility.[1] Few still believed that ultimately man would lose his sex-instinct, but many thought that culture itself was a substitute for merely animal enjoyment, and therefore each successive stage was bound to bring some lowering of sexual activity.[2]

This idea of progressive stages of culture, in which new interests and enjoyments arise to compete with the most primitive gratification, was particularly developed in Germany in the second half of the nineteenth century. The theories which arose there have sometimes been called simply *Wohlstandstheorien* or standard-of-living theories, but they are more correctly *Wohlstands- und Kulturtheorien*—theories of standards of living and culture together. Their principal characteristic is their stress on the operation of abstract cultural influences in an environment of some physical comfort. They differ from the French theories of civilization in stressing much less the negative, amoral effects of increased comfort in a competitive society; instead, they point to the elevating effect of this comfort. Where their French contemporaries speak of selfishness and ostentation, the German writers more often refer to the powers of reason, self-control, prudence, and abstinence—a vocabulary reminiscent both of the Malthusians and the anti-Malthusians.[3] Since most of these writers were in fact Malthusians in a limited sense, but on the other hand had no reason to criticize the demographic behaviour of their German contemporaries, this contrast is not surprising. Johannes Conrad thought that Malthus had underestimated the power of culture in its twofold impact: first through the moral

[1] Jarrold, op. cit., p. 275—nomads, farmers, traders, &c.

[2] See W. E. Hickson, *Malthus; an Essay on the Principle of Population, in Refutation of the Theory of the Rev. T. R. Malthus* (London, 1849): 'The presumption is, that . . . the strength of the merely animal propensities would diminish, and that in accordance with the law that the highest organizations should be the most slowly developed, the ratio of increase would be less than at present' (Summary, p. 73).

[3] e.g. J. Conrad, *Grundriss zum Studium der politischen Ökonomie* (6th ed., Jena, 1909–13), 2nd part, p. 557, quoted by L. Elster, in 'Bevölkerungswesen', *Handwörterbuch der Staatswissenschaften* (4th ed., Jena, 1924), ii. 792.

fibre it provides, secondly through increased economic output, which in turn depends on faster intellectual development.[1] The particular apostle of this type of theory was the economist Lujo Brentano, a Munich professor who had made a close study of British conditions as well as the life of the German working classes. The essential point to him was the introduction into the life of successive nations and classes of 'competitive enjoyments' to which he applied a sort of law of diminishing returns—or better, a theory of diminishing marginal rates of substitution. These enjoyments were both of the physical-comfort variety, and new sentiments which entered into peoples' lives. People will stop producing children when this act would deprive them of whatever other gratifications in life are rated at that particular level by the society in which they live.[2] This kind of assertion naturally ignores the question of birth-control—when that is widely known, there is no need even to reduce the amount of sexual enjoyment.[3] But the point is immaterial. Children themselves, most of the writers urge, are part of the pattern of society; they have both a useful economic role at a lower stage of development, and they afford gratification at a higher stage, so that their omission denotes both a higher form of economic organization and the choice of gratifications already mentioned.[4] Brentano, as an economist, did not seek to explain why these higher cultural stages should witness this change in needs and desires—that was the task of the sociologist. For him, it was simply a question of fact; he did not seek to judge this choice. This, too, was the approach of Marshall, who, at the beginning of his chapter on population declared his belief in a general culture theory, though he came to stress economic considerations in its later sections to a greater extent: '... society exercises pressure on the individual by religious, moral and legal sanctions, sometimes with the object of quickening, and sometimes with that of retarding, the growth of population'.[5] After the generation of Brentano and Marshall the economists usually did not even refer to the possibility of this wider set of population determinants, but sought to find the

[1] Ibid.

[2] L. Brentano, 'Die Malthus'sche Lehre und die Bevölkerungsbewegung der letzten Dezennien', *Abhandlungen der Historischen Klasse der Königlich Bayerischen Akademie der Wissenschaften* (Munich, 1909), xxiv, sect. 2, p. 606.

[3] See comments by R. v. Ungern-Sternberg, *The Causes of the Decline of the Birth-rate within the European Sphere of Civilization* (New York, 1931), p. 33.

[4] Brentano speaks of a 'more refined love of children' (*verfeinerte Kindesliebe*); see P. Mombert, *Bevölkerungslehre* (Grundrisse zum Studium der Nationalökonomie, Bd. 15, Jena, 1929), p. 331.

[5] A. Marshall, *Principles of Economics* (8th ed., London, 1930), p. 173.

answer in an analysis of economic fluctuations or rates of expansion. It was left to sociologists to pursue the other line.

Amongst those who explored more deeply the social aspects of the matter was Julius Wolf, an original and forceful writer who is in essence fairly close to the other writers mentioned here, although he attacked most of them rather heavily. Wolf played down the socio-economic aspects of the standard-of-living theory, and concentrated on the cultural concept.[1] He spoke of the effects of education in creating a new sense of 'order' amongst the masses—a sense of the fitness of things which was the result of a good many individual beliefs produced in modern society. Wolf knew of statistical observations available by his time, investigating all the factors we have already mentioned—the behaviour of aristocracies, of literate and illiterate people, the effects of urbanization, and so on. To none of these influences could a pre-eminent position be assigned—it is how these things excite the reaction of the individual that matters. No absolute rules were possible, but one had to ask which of these various influences predominated in a certain society. For his own time Wolf could see how the processes of western European culture were facilitating the spread of contraception. This point did not escape other writers of this time, and twentieth-century works on the theme of birth-control and its sociological significance are too numerous to mention.[2]

With Wolf and Brentano we have reached the most complex modern population theories, which belong properly to the field of contemporary demography rather than historical analysis. But the last variant of the civilization and culture theories has still to be mentioned, that which sees the decline in fertility as a characteristic of the last stage of development—decline, decadence, and death of a nation. As we have seen, Greece and Rome provided an example to writers of all periods. Neither British nor German writers of the nineteenth century had cause to think that their own nation had as yet entered the stage of

[1] J. Wolf, *Der Geburtenrückgang. Die Rationalisierung des Sexuallebens in unserer Zeit* (Jena, 1912), p. 32. He quotes Kautsky's rejection of vague terms—*Vermehrung und Entwicklung in Natur und Gesellschaft* (Stuttgart, 1910), p. 193: 'Statt uns mit der allgemeinen belletristischen Phrase von "Wohlstand und Kultur" zu begnügen. . . .'

[2] For a full account of the *Wohlstandstheoretiker* and others see G. Mackenroth, *Bevölkerungslehre; Theorie, Soziologie und Statistik der Bevölkerung* (Enzyklopädie der Rechts- und Staatswissenschaft. Abteilung Staatswissenschaft, Berlin, 1953), pp. 317 ff. He includes in this section *Gesinnungstheoretiker* or 'attitude theorists' who seem to be mostly the fascist successors of the culture theorists, and in some sense, like Le Play, are prophets of decadence. There is a distinct connexion between the lines of action recommended by Le Play, Dumont, and Nazi racial biologists.

decadence; but in France, as we have seen, men like Dumont and Leroy-Beaulieu thought that the point of greatness might have been passed. Even before their time critics were not lacking who pointed to a progressive deterioration of national life through the new influence brought in by the Revolution. Of these, the best known is Le Play, who felt that social cohesion and stability had been broken through revolutionary principles and legislation. His particular stress was on the 'unstable family', the product, he believed, of the inheritance provisions of the Napoleonic Code, a rootless organism which undermined the whole fabric of society. He looked back to the ordered customs of an earlier period, when the 'root-family' (*famille-souche*) formed the basis of social organization, with its strong ties to the family holding and a sense of mutual responsibilities.[1] The purpose of Le Play's writings, naturally, was to advocate remedies for the prevailing state of affairs, and although the general tone of his argument is one of regret at the prevailing decline, there is still hope for a reversal of the trend.

The analysis of progressive decline was taken up by other writers, and finally applied to Western civilization as a whole. The idea that the countries of the West had passed through the day of greatness was popular in widely different circles. We find evidence for this in contemporary comment on the 'decadent' movements in art and literature, particularly in the nineties. One of the first detailed studies of differential fertility, that of David Heron, prepared under the auspices of Galton and Pearson's Eugenics Laboratory, was published in a series characteristically called *Studies in National Deterioration*, financed by the Drapers' Company. The country was going to the dogs, and things were not what they had been. Into this atmosphere contemporary population theories seemed to fit admirably. Fahlbeck, one of the earliest scientific students of the habits of the aristocracy, believed that all nations underwent a sort of life-cycle, with distinct characteristics of behaviour in each phase, of which population movements formed part.[2] In Germany a theory of decadence was first outlined in general terms (but not with reference to contemporary German conditions) by G. Hanssen. His work distinguished three levels of population development, corresponding to three types of social strata—the landed proprietors, the *bourgeoisie*, and the proletariat. The processes of movement he

[1] F. Le Play, *La Réforme sociale en France déduite de l'observation comparée des peuples européens* (Paris, 1866, 4 vols.). Summaries from Spengler, *France Faces Depopulation*, pp. 146 ff.

[2] P. E. Fahlbeck, 'La Décadence et la chute des peuples', *Bulletin de l'Institut international de statistique* (Rome, 1900), xv. 367 ff.

described were mainly evidence of the effect of cities—their deadly exhausting organization which eats men and destroys the community. But he was constantly aware that urbanization was a cultural stage and that it gave rise to a great flowering of genius—only it carried within itself the seeds of its own destruction. Effeminate ways and luxury, he thought, were not the cause but the symptom of this decline which was bound to set in. As long as population grows there is still competition, and only those with special talents can assert themselves; they will displace those who have grown soft. But when, in the final stage, population ceases to grow, even the fool can maintain himself and come to riches and honours. So the nation progressively declines, tastes deteriorate, the nation's heritage is ignored. Infertility and the death of the nation occur together.[1]

The most comprehensive, as well as the best known, of these pessimistic views of developments is Oswald Spengler's *Decline of the West*. In this work, population only figures incidentally—infertility is just one rather minor aspect of the general catastrophe described by the author. He attributes it to the reasoning of civilized man—or rather his faulty reasoning, since it hastens his own doom. Primitive peoples had no thought about the number of their progeny—children were a natural phenomenon. But already in Greece (here, like everyone else, he quotes Polybius) calculation began, and Rome was worse. The peasant chooses for a wife a woman who will be the mother of his children. The modern town-dweller chooses, instead, a 'life companion'. This sort of woman (whom he later calls the *Ibsenweib*) is unfit to be a mother—in her own proud boast, she belongs to herself, and naturally she is infertile.[2] And so the rot sets in:

At this level there begins in all civilizations the stage, which lasts several centuries, of dreadful depopulation. The whole pyramid of human society capable of developing culture disappears. The destruction begins at the top of the pyramid, first the great cities, then the provincial ones, and in the end

[1] G. Hanssen, *Die drei Bevölkerungsstufen. Ein Versuch, die Ursachen für das Blühen und Altern der Völker nachzuweisen* (Munich, 1889), esp. p. 323. For further works on urban decadence as part of national decline, see Mackenroth, op. cit., p. 263. One of R. R. Kuczynski's earliest works seems to have been a factual critique of the Hanssen thesis.

[2] O. Spengler, *Der Untergang des Abendlandes. Umrisse einer Morphologie der Weltgeschichte* (Munich, 1924, 2 vols.), ii. 124. The attack on German women and their declining fertility in the general national deterioration had already been started by a German woman doctor a few years earlier. See Agnes Bluhm, 'Zur Frage nach der generativen Tüchtigkeit der deutschen Frauen und der rassenhygienischen Bedeutung der ärztlichen Geburtshilfe', *Archiv für Rassen- und Gesellschaftsbiologie* (July–August 1912), ix. 454–74, quoted in Hiller, op. cit., p. 531.

the countryside, which, by ever-increasing flight of its people into the cities, delays for a time the emptying of the cities. Only the primitive stock finally remains, but it is deprived of its strong elements, who might have had a future. So there develops the type of the fellaheen.[1]

Spengler's picture was a plausible one, and many of his observations of contemporary society woke his readers to further thought. His aptest pupils finally (though he would have repudiated them), were the early Nazis, determined at all costs to save the Fatherland from the fate Spengler had predicted.

Since Spengler's time, theories of decadence have been less popular, perhaps because the word came to be used in such dangerous context. But the idea of a life-cycle of nations retains its appeal to the imagination of the general public. The mental image conjured up by the word 'decline' includes now, as it did in Gibbon's day as well as in Dumont's, the care-and-pleasure-worn townsman, the deterioration of morals and religion, and the absence of a new generation.

[1] O. Spengler, op. cit., p. 125.

IX

SOCIAL THEORIES OF POPULATION AND THE POSITION OF MALTHUS

I. THE HISTORY OF AN ARGUMENT

As Marshall rightly remarked, the study of the factors which control population growth is not a modern phenomenon, for

> in a more or less vague form it has occupied the attention of thoughtful men in all ages of the world. To its influence, often unavowed, sometimes not even clearly recognised, we can trace a great part of the rules, customs and ceremonies that have been enjoined in the Eastern and Western world by lawgivers, by moralists, and those nameless thinkers, whose far-seeing wisdom has left its impress on national habits.[1]

With very few exceptions, these thoughts were directed towards an increase in fertility. The investigation was therefore usually into the causes of barrenness, of the reasons why men failed to marry, and of the causes of premature mortality. The infrequent writers on relative over-population, such as those one finds in Germany in the sixteenth century, would certainly not advocate any deliberate fostering of the obstacles to fertility which were so universally condemned.[2] Colonization, conquest, or redistribution of land would accomplish all that was necessary.

Therefore the entire weight of legislation as well as moralizing was brought to bear in the direction of greater fertility. Moreover the justification for the demand was held to be self-evident. There was no need to prove that the world was under-populated, or that the Crown lacked subjects. Legislation to reform manners, like the *Lex Papia Poppaea* or the *Lex Julia*, could state its justification in terms of the axiomatic need for a greater population or the propagation of a valuable part of the community. Even if scientific methods of investigation had

[1] A. Marshall, *Principles of Economics* (8th ed., London, 1930), pp. 173–4.

[2] See O. Jolles, 'Die Ansichten der deutschen nationalökonomischen Schriftsteller des sechzehnten und siebzehnten Jahrhunderts über Bevölkerungswesen', *Jahrbücher für Nationalökonomik und Statistik* (Neue Folge, Jena, 1886), xiii. 196–7, quoting Sebastian Frank von Wörd, *Germania Chronicon* (1538), Ulrich von Hutten, *Ad principes Germanos ut Bellum Turcis inferant, exhortatoria* (1518), and others.

been normal, nobody would have asked for numerical proofs of such necessity. As it was, an age which read Pliny or Bacon for its natural history (and they held sway well beyond their own centuries) could not be expected to question the superstitions attached to the vagaries of human reproduction.

The second stage of population theorizing arises out of the attempts at scientific systematizing which we associate with the early days of the Royal Society and the age of Newton. As the motion of the stars and the circulation of the blood yielded to tenable interpretation, as plants and animals began to be classified, so all forms of human behaviour, both in the individual and in society, attracted the philosophers into attempts at universal explanations. This was not only due to man's vanity. To explain everything in terms of universal laws was to extol the virtues of a beneficent and all-wise Creator. To accuse the Deity of random behaviour was to deny its principal attributes.

That was the mountainous array of ignorant prejudices and superstitions which faced the generation of David Hume and Adam Ferguson. It was their task to record, to measure, and to apply inductive logic to their findings. Metaphysics, which had been the ally of physics, now became, very gradually, a discredited occupation for a would-be scientist. Whereas Newton or Leibnitz were outstanding in times which produced a majority of speculators, Malthus or Senior a hundred years later found themselves appealing to a large educated public which might criticize their findings but spoke essentially the same language.

In the preceding chapters we have quoted at length from a number of writers of these earlier periods in order to trace the origins of beliefs which had some relevance in the later stages of investigation. To write the history of the transition is to attempt an account of the development of Western thought as such. This is out of place here. But it is worth pointing out a few salient features of the earlier systems of thought in order to appreciate to its full extent the impact which Malthus made on the whole subject.

The first point to note again is that very few writers indeed held a theory of population at all. The vast majority produced *obiter dicta* when discussing life and death, the strength of the state, or the duty of man to God. Thus the literature is overwhelmingly philosophical, political, or theological, or all of these at the same time. The titles are good indications: typical specimens include the great reformer Ulrich von Hutten's *Exhortation to the German Princes that they should wage*

War on the Turks (1518), Botero's *Reason of State* (1589), J. P. Süßmilch's *Divine Order* (1751), to mention only a few abbreviated versions of the sonorous titles in all languages of the time from the Renaissance to the Enlightenment.

Secondly, we have noted throughout the reliance of the majority of authors on two principal authorities: the classical writers and the Bible. Very rarely do medieval writings figure in these works. Partly, of course, this is the typical effect of the Renaissance as such, partly it is no doubt due to ignorance of medieval manuscripts which often came to be resuscitated only in the nineteenth century, but it is also inherent in the character of medieval writings as such. Perhaps for our subject the most significant observation is that made, for instance, by James Bryce: that the Middle Ages lacked all idea of change or progress, that their authors lacked critical judgement to such an extent that they really could not see the difference between themselves and their Roman or Greek models.[1] This difficulty, which was only gradually overcome in modern times, led not only to a static, and therefore false view, of population questions, but it also engendered the notion that statements about any topic of this kind must be universally and perpetually true.

The third significant characteristic of this early stage is the absence of statistics. The notorious inability of the ancient world to use figures, so often commented on by the writers we quoted in earlier chapters, like Beloch, Pöhlmann, Seeck, and Kahrstedt, was not exposed until the nineteenth century and examples are not lacking of the population estimates of the ancient world finding their way into modern treatises. Cities like Carthage, less than a square mile in extent, were cheerfully credited with 700,000 inhabitants (a figure even quoted by Mommsen without comment), and Antioch and Syracuse equally elevated to the status of cities of half a million people. This feeling that accuracy did not matter not only infected the writing of the historians, but it also led to the totally false view of the direction of movement when, in the eighteenth century, movement as such was discovered and the contemporary situation, for the first time, analysed with some attempt at precision. Hence the belief of Wallace's generation that the world had declined in population since ancient times.

[1] J. Bryce, *The Holy Roman Empire* (4th ed., London, 1890), pp. 260–1. See also P. Mombert, 'Die Anschauungen des siebzehnten und achtzehnten Jahrhunderts über die Abnahme der Bevölkerung', *Jahrbücher für Nationalökonomik und Statistik* (1931), III. Folge, lxxx. 499, quoting E. Bernheim, *Lehrbuch der historischen Methode und der Geschichtsphilosophie* (3rd ed., Leipzig, 1903), pp. 30 ff.: 'Es fehlte "die Anschauung, dass eine kontinuierliche Veränderung in allen menschlichen Verhältnissen vor sich geht".'

Malthus's impact on the political and economic thinking of his time therefore coincides with the discoveries of clay feet on various idols. The authority of the Bible as such had diminished in the period of Enlightenment, of Deism, of the *philosophes*, at any rate amongst thinkers. Lyell's *Geology* and D. F. Strauss's *Life of Jesus* were both published in the 1830's. Attacks on ancient chronology did not diminish the importance of the classical authorities as such, but statistics of another kind had been introduced into population discussion in the seventeenth century and therefore ousted the Greeks and Romans as sources of wisdom on this particular subject. Even Süßmilch quoted enough contemporary vital statistics to make it worth Malthus's while to misquote them, despite the general theological and teleological approach of the *Göttliche Ordnung*. The investigators of the English bills of mortality, the authors of the early life-tables and other actuarial workers, and finally the census officials headed by Rickman and Farr, made it unnecessary to worry about the size of Xerxes' army or whether the word *insula* in Rome meant a block of flats or a block of houses, except within the field of classical scholarship.

At the same time, round about the end of the eighteenth century, the notion of static societies, already shaken philosophically, finally crumbled. Not only did political events, like the rise and triumph of the American colonies, the French Revolution, and the arrival of the Australasian world in the consciousness of the Old World, upset any notions of a permanent distribution of population or balance of power, but the idea of change as a basic principle of social organization emerged, only to be superseded in turn by the Victorian notion of continuous and inevitable progress. No change–change–progress—only change, that is the progress of attitudes, and it applies in our field as it does in others. This does not mean to say that moral judgements were entirely absent from the new attitudes towards investigation. But the emphasis changes. Whereas in the case of so many of the French pro-populationists quoted, the threat of declining fertility served as a convenient stick with which to beat the loose behaviour of their times, we are faced, in such groups of writers as the English Poor Law authors of the period 1770–1830, with a utilitarian attitude. That is to say, they did not desire a reform of manners for its own sake, but they considered, or claimed to consider, the ultimate well-being of the population, and their concern about urban living standards or nutrition springs neither from a mercantilist anxiety about the numbers of the Kingdom, nor from a prophetic desire to castigate Sodom and Gomorrah, but from admittedly often highly individualistic notions of the best means of achieving happiness for present and future generations.

It will be seen that such a preoccupation is in itself bound up with the optimistic assumption that change is not only possible as such, but that it can be brought about by human agency. According to the political conceits of the author, it is best achieved by sweeping away all old obstacles to progress, or creating fresh machinery to deal with old complaints. At any rate the economists from Smith to J. S. Mill, and the political writers from Godwin to Macaulay, share the vision of a rise, whether they claim that all happiness lies before us, or that their world was already the best of all possible worlds.

To all such discussions the impact of the Malthusian theory lent added importance. It became obligatory for every writer on political or economic subjects to explain the effects of the system or policies he described or advocated, on the movement of population. Whether this took the form of asserting that the problem did not exist, or of showing that the world as it is, or as it is to be, contains sufficient checks to deal with the question, each author had to take his stand. As we have shown, many of them turned this necessity into a virtue, and roundly asserted that their favourite theory or policy was expressly designed to master the situation. This is particularly striking in the case of those authors who attacked poverty as conducive to high fertility, and proceeded to tell how they would overcome this menace by the redistribution of property and incomes.

The outstanding common feature of these writings is the sense of immediate relevance to the historical changes of their times which we feel in reading them. The hopelessly poor who have no hope of rising in the world are to be found, according to the bias of the author, in stationary agrarian societies like Ireland, or in the new slums of urban England. On the other hand, the ascending people who restrict their fertility to achieve promotion to a new social class, are also characteristic inhabitants of the new expanding industrial society—only they are to be found amongst those who are at least one stage removed from the lowest rung of the social ladder. As they rise, so the checks become more powerful, and in some cases are shown to require ever more powerful monetary incentives for their removal in fruitful marriages.

Again, every writer who investigated these standards of living in the industrializing societies, from Colbert's France to Bismarck's Germany, noticed that the commodities which entered into the calculations of the potential fathers varied not only from class to class, but also within each class, as the standards of requirements changed ever more rapidly. As we have seen, the relative nature of such a word as 'luxury' was recognized at an early stage, and in time it was abandoned completely. Even Nassau Senior's distinction of necessities, decencies, and luxuries did not survive for long in the face of a constantly increasing supply of diversified consumer goods to a public whose purchasing power increased in the long run, even if there were notable intermediate periods of stagnation and even retrogression.

Relative standards and prospects of promotion were only two of the more common social observations of the industrializing phase. Where incomes rose, there savings rose too, and savings meant the acquisition of property, whether in houses, land, or movable goods. In the early days franchise, at least in England, went with property, and in time it went with male, and finally female adulthood, and these concessions were a recognition of a *de facto* achievement of equal status in the community, though the extent of equality varied from country to country. With the more important industrial role of the worker and his civil rights went the ever-increasing standards of education demanded of him. His literacy was both the prerequisite and the result of the changed social and economic structure, and the same interacting processes may be observed in connexion with the rising status of women and the changed attitude towards children.

In fact, the short history of the social theories in relation to population trends is that we can only distinguish two major epochs: that of the preindustrial or stationary world, where separate checks to fertility are observed, and the industrializing world where the checks are never isolated, but work in conjunction with each other through the total environment of the individual and the family. To confine one's attention to these two rough classifications is not to ignore the important distinctions between different approaches within each. Nor does the existence of these categories in any way reduce the importance of Malthus, who, as we have seen, stands at the beginning of the second epoch and foreshadows many, if not all, of the component parts of the modern social theories of population checks.

2. THE POSITION OF MALTHUS

The attempt must now be made to place Malthus correctly into this long-term development of the social theories of fertility. To do this is to evaluate Malthus's teaching, and that in turn means summarizing not only the theories on which no two authorities have ever agreed, but also at least the most recent of those writers who have attempted their own restatement of the central propositions of the successive *Essays* and Malthus's other writings. Apart from Kenneth Smith's[1] and Joseph Stassart's[2] extended expositions, important systematic demonstrations have been published by Kingsley Davis,[3] Antony Flew,[4] Joseph Spengler,[5] and others.[6] Amongst fresh attempts to restate economic, as opposed to socio-economic, theories of population, there is Sydney Coontz's *Population Theories and the Economic Interpretation.*[7]

Most of these restatements aim at a clear recapitulation of the classical theory of population, either as Malthus formulated it, or as it emerged in the course of nineteenth-century discussion. All are agreed that there is need for it, since Malthus has been misrepresented and misunderstood for 160 years, often, as Paul Lambert remarks in his analogy between Keynesianism and Malthusianism, by people who have never read him.[8] More particularly, Malthus is often quoted only in a limited context, much in the way in which isolated passages have been cited in the earlier chapters of this volume. But this is not the way in which he ought to be read. Rather one should look at what Spengler calls 'Malthus' total population theory'. This total theory is so hard to state because Malthus was unsystematic in the extreme, because even in the *Summary View* of 1830 he never stated all his assumptions clearly enough, and because he often undid in a footnote or an appendix what had taken him several chapters to build up. Anyone else who was guilty of such untidy writing would have run the risk of immediate consignment to obscurity. But everyone knows why this fate did not overtake Malthus. Firstly, the *Essay* of 1798, much the crudest of his books, created an indelible impression on his generation, which was not weakened by the second and subsequent editions or their footnotes and appendixes. But even this first edition, crude as it was, contained

1 K. Smith, *The Malthusian Controversy* (London, 1951).

2 J. Stassart, *Malthus et la population* (Liège, 1957).

3 K. Davis, 'Malthus and the Theory of Population', in P. F. Lazarsfeld and M. Rosenberg, eds., *The Language of Social Research* (Glencoe, 1955), pp. 540–53.

4 A. Flew, 'The Structure of Malthus' Population Theory', *Australasian Journal of Philosophy* (1957), xxxv, no. 1, pp. 1–20.

5 J. J. Spengler, 'Malthus' Total Population Theory . . . etc.', *Canadian Journal of Economics and Political Science* (1945), xi. 83 ff., 234 ff.

6 J. J. Spengler and O. D. Duncan, eds., *Population Theory and Policy, Selected Readings* (Glencoe, 1956).

7 S. H. Coontz, *Population Theories and the Economic Interpretation* (London, 1957).

8 P. Lambert, Preface, in Stassart, op. cit., p. 7.

the germs of many valuable ideas which were later developed by Malthus himself and others. In the second place, then, Malthus could not be ignored because he was a much more acute observer, and a much better economist and sociologist, than his arrangement of ideas led readers to believe. In other words: no one could then, or can now, afford to ignore 'the Malthusian problem' even in its simplest form, because he managed so to formulate it that it is an ever-present problem, and also because both the *Essay* and the *Principles* were found, on examination, to contain such important parts of modern social and economic theory. There is, fortunately, no 'ranking' of the fathers of economics (after due reverence at the shrine of Adam Smith), but Malthus is generally placed with Ricardo and Senior at the head of classical economics. In population theory only his position is so unique as almost to defy classification. But he has not been given his due place as a sociologist. This is mainly because population discussion has been for so long, as was pointed out in the introductory chapter, a part of economics, and has so recently become chiefly sociological that the reader tends to concentrate on Malthus's arguments relating to quantities of food and the demand for labour, and to overlook the extensive passages dealing with social structure and individual and social psychology.

Malthus, then, has stood at the centre of discussion for so long that, like the Bible or the writings of Marx, he has had to suffer the indignity of not being taken as a whole, but dissected and reconstituted mercilessly. Some concentrated on querying the facts (or at least spending much time in analysing them). Some concentrated on finding the original works from which his ideas were said to be derived. Some refuted some part of his system (like his 'ratios'). Very many attacked his conclusions, for instance on the Poor Laws, and concluded that the man must be heartless, perverted, and arguing from false premisses. Others again pointed, as does Flew, to the 'few simple ideas and obvious facts'[1] which made up his system, and wondered what all the commotion was about. But certainly no one tried to ignore him, and as we have seen, his population theory, or something supposed to be like it, was prayed in aid of a great many reform movements of the nineteenth century, or else cited as proof that the movement was mistaken in its intentions. Those who wished to repeal the Corn Laws as well as the protectionists, the Poor Law reformers and their enemies, the Darwinists and the Spencerians, the educators and the opponents

[1] Flew, op. cit., p. 16.

of the franchise, they all found their chapter and verse in the *Essay*. To make a bibliography of such *Malthusiana*, fascinating though it is, is not to define his theory adequately. The position is summed up by Kingsley Davis:

> ... there are good reasons for using Malthus as a point of departure in the discussion of population theory. These are the reasons that made his work influential in his day and make it influential now. But they have little to do with whether his views are right or wrong.... Malthus' theories are not now and never were empirically valid, but they nevertheless were theoretically significant....[1]

Therefore even in this limited discussion of one aspect of population theory, that of the social checks to fertility, the only method of evaluation is to relate them to their place in the Malthusian system.

Davis himself went on to construct a 'frame of reference' within which to set the Malthusian system of deductive reasoning, or to which one might relate empirical observations. A similar framework is provided by Flew.[2] Alternatively, one may classify all arguments, including Malthus's, by reference to a number of basic assumptions about population movements in general, and the desirable directions of population policy, which in their variations provide a common basis for all writers on this subject. By examining these various methods we shall be able to provide a tolerably logical classification for the Malthusian pronouncements in our field.

Davis's frame of reference is the following:[3]

Capacity for population growth	*Checks to population growth*			
	Preventive checks		*Positive checks*	
Instinct of reproduction	Voluntary or rational limitations on births		All causes of mortality	
	Moral restraint	Vice	Vice	Misery
	Means of subsistence in each category			
	Land—Arts—Social organization in each category			

The meaning of this scheme is clear. The first two types of division are purely descriptive. Preventive checks, or those that relate to the voluntary or rational limitation of marriage and therefore births, relate

[1] Davis, op. cit., p. 541.
[2] Flew, op. cit.
[3] Davis, op. cit., p. 544.

to decisions made by human beings. Positive checks, or causes of mortality, include all influences outside immediate volitional control. The next subdivision, into moral restraint, misery, and vice, is not descriptive at all, but refers to Malthus's own moral judgement of contemporary social events. As Davis says, 'what is moral and what is vice varies from one culture to another, since it depends not on the facts but on the values and attitudes that one has'.[1] But leaving this difficulty, often described, we now find that the 'means of subsistence' is added as an element in each category. In other words, they are what Davis calls a 'master check' behind all other divisions. Positively, the lack of these means cuts off life. Preventively, the fear of lacking them leads to restraint. Nothing else can provoke the one, or induce the other, check. In turn, the supply of means of subsistence is determined by the amount of land, by the state of industrial organization and trade, and social factors such as the distribution of incomes.

The instinct of reproduction, then, is continuously pushing the population in an upward direction, and a number of economically and socially conditioned forces restrains its indefinite growth. For the purposes of study, the inadequate and misleading divisions into moral restraint, vice, and misery might as well be omitted. Nevertheless, we shall have to see later what Malthus meant by moral restraint, in order to determine his own place in the debate. There remains only the study of the mechanisms by which the master factors, operating through the general supply of the means of subsistence, affect mortality and fertility rates. This study is modern demography almost in its entirety. The subject of this book is the mechanism of the left half of the table only, including both moral restraint and 'vice' since the latter includes birth-control, abortion, and so on.

We arrive at a similar structure by using Flew's analysis.[2] He begins with the geometrical and arithmetical progressions as his first two basic Malthusian propositions. This is followed by the usual comparison between these two, either in its crudest form, or in the mild form of the *Summary View*, where the contrast is merely between the actual increase of population and that which would obtain were it to continue unchecked. This leads to the inquiry into the checks, which are represented either in a 'value-neutral' division (i.e. merely according to a mechanical division of positive and preventive checks), or in the 'strongly evaluative and prescriptive' division into misery, vice, and moral restraint. Now, as Flew points out, there are a number of

[1] Ibid., p. 545.

[2] Flew, op. cit., p. 3.

weaknesses in this structure, but they do not destroy it.[1] Even if we dispense with the ratios altogether, we shall still be left with the observed difference between what population actually is, and what it might be, or a justified assumption that we can conceive of a rate of multiplication of the human species which would lead to an impossible situation, whatever rate of increase we can imagine for our means of subsistence. This may conveniently be represented by Arthur Lewis's picture of world population doubling itself every twenty-five years so that by the year A.D. 2330 there would literally be 'standing room only', or one person per square yard of the earth's land surface.[2] Given the indisputable existence of checks then, we can also dispense with the evaluative-prescriptive division and simply look for the answer to what Flew calls 'Malthus' master speculative question': what are the reasons for which population does *not* grow as fast as it could do in theory? All that is necessary for an initial classification of these reasons is to divide them into those which are within human control and those which are outside it.[3] Though Malthus did not use this division, it serves well enough to receive all the checks listed in detail.

In this way Flew makes Malthus's position stronger than any of the *Essays* could make it, and it brings us back to the same point as Davis's analysis: that what we must mostly study are the checks within human control, that is, human reactions against the background of their social environment and economic development. The question that arises now is this: given that Malthus's system revolves round the question of the available means of subsistence and their interaction with population size, is it fundamentally operating in a different frame of reference from those of earlier and later writers? The answer appears to be this: writers differ from each other mainly as to what they think are the *tendencies* in the long-term or contemporary situation, in the policies they think are required, and as to whether they are more preoccupied with economic matters or social matters. The economists are more concerned with the physical production of the means of subsistence, and with the demand for labour, whereas the sociologists take this economic environment as given and concentrate on the individual's reactions to the pressures set up by the system of production and distribution.

These divisions may be set out as follows:

1. According to opinions as to the natural tendencies of population —to increase, to decrease, or to remain stationary, to grow within limits, or to fluctuate according to conditions.

[1] Flew, op. cit., pp. 5 ff. [2] Ibid., p. 13. [3] Ibid., p. 16.

2. According to what is thought desirable—a larger, smaller, or stationary population.
3. Amongst those who think that population tends to grow and think it ought not to grow so fast—those who believe that natural forces, if left free play, will ensure the correct result, and those who think that intervention is necessary to secure it.
4. Amongst those who think that natural forces will secure the necessary checks, those who think that voluntary abstinence is possible, and those who think that contraception is part of the natural scheme.
5. Amongst those who think that intervention is necessary to secure a check to population growth, those who would achieve it by marriage legislation, and those who would do it by birth-control propaganda by governments.
6. Amongst those who think population tends to decrease and ought to be encouraged, those who would confine themselves to negative means (prohibition of birth-control), and those who would give positive encouragement (family allowances).

The categories are not exhaustive, or mutually exclusive, and we know a number of authors who held more than one of these views during their lifetime. The division may also be presented diagramatically (see below, p. 242). In the diagram, the 'Irelanders' are those who point to Ireland as an example of how education and experience may produce the working of moral restraint without recourse to intervention or birth-control.

The picture now emerges somewhat as follows: Malthus and his Malthusians (the term is held to include his precursors such as Townsend) occupy a unique but by no means dominant position. The eighteenth century had seen a gradual decline of the cruder pro-populationist views. Whether the new thinking postulated a stationary, growing, or fluctuating natural trend, the emphasis was on *laissez-faire.* Few felt that there was any danger from over-population or depopulation without energetic measures to redress the balance. Into this relatively calm atmosphere came Malthus's warning. There were three possible reactions to this disturbance: to deny that the danger exists at all, to accept the danger but point to the existence of natural correcting influences, or to advocate energetic action to deal with the danger. The uniqueness of Malthus and the true Malthusians lies in the fact that, having given warning of catastrophe, they decided to do nothing at all. In H. L. Beales's words: 'The main contribution of his school

Direction		*Policy*	*Period or school*			
Natural	*Desirable*		*Pre-Malthusian*	*Malthus or Malthusian*	*Neo-Malthusian*	*Anti- or non-Malthusian*
Downwards	Upwards	Positive interventionist	Mercantilists, pro-populationists			Alliance Nationale, Welfare State, Fascists, &c.
Stationary	No Change	Neutral	Equilibrists			
	Slower	Relying on natural forces		Moreton, &c.	Standard-of-living theorists: birth-control as natural means to an end	'Irelanders'
Upwards (tendency unlimited)	Slower	Negative or through education only	Wallace	MALTHUS		Catholics
	Slower	Positive interventionist	Greeks	German states early 19th century	Propagandists	
Upwards (tendency limited)	No change		Condorcet, Godwin, &c.			Logisticists, Spencer, Sadler
Fluctuating according to conditions	No change	Improve conditions	Cantillon			Culture theorists, optimum theorists, socialists

is that the essence of social policy is that there should be no social policy'.[1]

It is true that they advocated at least the removal of those institutions—like the Poor Law—which, in their view, positively encouraged growth of population, and the establishment of organizations like savings banks which might help individuals to order their lives more advantageously.

Instead, Malthus's reliance was on the cultivation of moral restraint. The growth of this attitude of mind was the only possible acceptable alternative to the continued operation of the positive checks. What separates him from his opponents is not the admission of the existence of famine and disease, or moral restraint, but rather the different emphasis he placed on various matters. First of all he took a gloomier view than most of them of the operation of positive checks at all times. Secondly, he had a slightly different conception of the most likely origins of moral restraint. Thirdly, his methods of promoting it varied from the others. But it is at least possible to argue that the total Malthusian theory is much closer to the rest of population theory than is commonly supposed. To say this is not to minimize the importance of his work. His inconsistencies, and his refusal, at times, to face the consequences of his own discoveries, are a weakness in the man himself. We cannot for this alone dismiss him, as Marx did, as a plagiarist, or as so many others did, as totally wrong-headed. Whatever the merits of Wallace and Townsend,[2] they created no stir. It was the *Essay* of 1798 which put the cat among the pigeons. Here the dangers of unlimited growth were, for the first time, presented forcibly in language which would be understood by everyone. Those who did not bother to read the book could get all they wanted from about four sentences. If it is argued that the subsequent editions of the work modified the first impact, it can only be answered that the essential points remained unaltered. The addition of 'moral restraint' as a separate category of checks scarcely weakened the original violence, since it seemed obvious that the author himself placed very little reliance on it.

Yet this appearance is deceptive. Malthus did know a great deal about the forces which made for moral restraint, and his fault lies in the way in which he hid his observations amongst a mass of irrelevant or inaccurate arguments about the positive checks.

It is a far more serious charge against him that he does not separate

[1] H. L. Beales, 'The Historical Context of the *Essay* on Population', in D. V. Glass, ed., *Introduction to Malthus* (London, 1953), p. 22.

[2] See Smith, op. cit., ch. i.

out clearly the social and economic aspects of the question. This may be difficult, since they are linked, yet the attempt should have been made to avoid the confusion. To use Kingsley Davis's scheme again: the available means of subsistence, as conditioned by technical and social organization, determine how many people may be kept alive at any one time, given a stationary standard of living. Thus the economic forces are those which determine population through production and the demand for labour. In this sphere there is no need for a 'moral-restraint' category, or indeed the preventive check at all. But once we start assuming that people are frightened of a premature end, or of a lower standard of living, and adjust their marriages (or fertility) accordingly, we are concerned with social issues. Now Malthus's teaching was at its vaguest on precisely this question: whether there was a fixed standard of living, whether this was at a subsistence minimum or not, and whether this standard or standards could move independently of the size of population. It is this side of his work that we must examine most closely. Is it really true that he saw clearly the whole of the modern explanation of why population does not inevitably press against the means of subsistence?

We shall divide our answer into three parts. First, we must see what Malthus meant by moral restraint, secondly, we subject the concept of a 'standard of living' to a similar examination, and thirdly, we must see how far Malthus's scattered remarks build up to anything like a tenable social theory of fertility. We shall leave to the last section the question of whether this social theory is at all tenable as distinct from economic theories.

What is moral restraint?

The orthodox view of Malthus's teaching is that he held up the concept of moral restraint as the only desirable check to population growth, and defined it so narrowly as to make the possibility of its efficient action a remote contingency. It will be argued here that Malthus did not really take quite such a narrow view of the subject, and that one may disregard even the obstinate reiteration of his original assertion in the light of the remainder of his writings. It is likely that he meant by moral restraint the exercise of much the same judgements as those which have formed the subject of this book. He spent very little time on explaining the narrower concept, and devoted large sections both of the *Essay* and the *Principles* to an exposition of the operation of voluntary restraint in general. He warmly advocated measures to increase the operation of this check, and optimistically looked forward to its further spreading in England and elsewhere, in such a way as to leave no doubt that he regarded less-than-perfect moral restraint as the one desirable and practicable alternative to vice and misery. We shall now present some of the passages which may be quoted in support of this interpretation.

The first of Malthus's own statements providing useful evidence is the explanatory footnote which he added to the very first statement of the checks of population as it appeared in the second edition:

It will be observed that I here use the term *moral* in its most confined sense. By moral restraint I would be understood to mean a restraint from marriage from prudential motives, with a conduct strictly moral during the period of this restraint; and I have never intentionally deviated from this sense. When I have wished to consider the restraint from marriage unconnected with its consequences, I have either called it prudential restraint, or a part of the preventive check, of which indeed it forms the principal branch.

In my review of the different stages of society, I have been accused of not allowing sufficient weight in the prevention of population to moral restraint; but when the confined sense of the term, which I have here explained, is adverted to, I am fearful that I shall not be found to have erred much in this respect. I should be very glad to believe myself mistaken.[1]

This passage presents difficulties. First of all, it admits of a certain overlap between the terms 'moral' and 'prudential', without, however, allowing a complete identity. Moral restraint is restraint from marriage with an eye to the consequences to one's own economic or social future, accompanied by strictly virtuous conduct. Exactly the same type of calculated restraint from marriage (not a particularly virtuous proceeding in itself), accompanied by loose sexual behaviour, is merely prudential restraint, the principal part of the preventive check 'of which indeed it forms the principal branch'. But, turning back, we find there are only two branches to the preventive check, moral restraint and vice, and since we have just been told that prudential restraint is not moral restraint, it must be vice! No wonder then that moral restraint is, to Malthus, so unimportant as a factor in the future trends of population, as the last paragraph suggests.

Yet in the Appendix to the fifth edition Malthus seems to have gone back a little on the narrowest interpretation of his categories. This

[1] T. R. Malthus, *An Essay on the Principle of Population* (Everyman ed., London, 1914, 2 vols.), i. 14.

probably was the result of the accusations against him that he was unduly pessimistic and he justifies himself in quite unambiguous terms:

> Mr. Young has asserted that I have made perfect chastity in the single state absolutely necessary to the success of my plan; but this surely is a misrepresentation. Perfect virtue is indeed necessary, to enable a man to avoid *all* the moral and physical evils which depend upon his own conduct; but whoever expected perfect virtue upon earth?
>
> I have said . . . that it is our duty to defer marriage till we can feed our children; and that it is also our duty not to indulge ourselves in vicious gratifications; but I have never said that I expected either, much less both, of these duties to be completely fulfilled.[1]

Prudential restraint was better than premature death.

Now the logical outcome of this recognition should have been a conversion to the point of view of his most respected adversaries, like Nassau Senior. But Malthus was unshakeable in clinging to his lofty aim, for in the last rewriting of his thesis, the *Summary View*, the old classification was brought out again almost unaltered:

> Moral restraint, in application to the present subject, may be defined to be, abstinence from marriage, either for a time or permanently, from prudential considerations, with a strictly moral conduct towards the sex in the interval. And this is the only mode of keeping population on a level with the means of subsistence, which is perfectly consistent with virtue and happiness. All other checks, whether of the preventive or positive kind, though they may vary greatly in degree, resolve themselves into some form of vice and misery.[2]

He did not say in this passage what 'prudential' had, finally, come to mean. But from the context it seems that it was a form of moral restraint and *part* of the preventive check; at least on the previous page he mentioned only those two, and in the very next line after that ending in 'vice and misery' he speaks of the *remaining checks* of the preventive kind, all of them the familiar vicious ones. Yet there is nowhere an open admission of defeat.

Was there then always a clear distinction in Malthus's mind between the moral and the prudential check as, for instance, Kenneth Smith believes?[3] This would mean that he would set up the one as a lofty ideal, and the other, at best, as an expedient to cope with a desperate

[1] Op. cit. (5th ed., 1817), Appendix iii, p. 363.

[2] T. R. Malthus, *A Summary View of the Principle of Population* in Glass, op. cit., p. 153.

[3] Smith, op. cit., pp. 250–1.

situation. Yet there are so many passages where he praises the prudential restraint, and so many details about its operation, that one cannot be quite certain how real the distinction was to him. In the fourth book Malthus clearly stated that the term 'moral' had a meaning only in relation to conduct during celibacy, and that this was a subject with which his work was not concerned. Instead, he wished to discuss the duty of extending the period of restraint, and in this context he only uses the term 'prudential':

> And it is by no means visionary to indulge a hope of some favourable change in this respect; because it is found by experience that the prevalence of this kind of prudential restraint is extremely different in different countries, and in the same countries at different periods [but it has lately increased in Europe, especially in northern parts].[1]

In other words, the greatest hopes lie in the extension of prudence in the manner which we have come to recognize in our own civilization. Does he not admit by this that this is a lofty aim, not inferior to the moral restraint of which he spoke earlier?

The term 'visionary' certainly seems to suggest desirability. It was possible just because of this impression which he himself felt he had created, that prudential restraint was an eminently respectable exercise, that he added the footnote in the first book which we quoted at the beginning of this section.

There is another point which needs clarification in connexion with Malthus's system of moral restraint. In the footnote mentioned we come across the words 'restraint from marriage unconnected with its consequences', and this is commonly interpreted as meaning the consequences for oneself of not marrying, i.e. possibly loose sexual behaviour, and thus the whole sequence is tacitly put into the 'vice' category. But it is possible to put another interpretation on these words. At the beginning of Book IV, Malthus repeatedly speaks of the 'consequences' which follow from disobeying laws of nature, of the sort well known already: over-eating, bad temper, and so on. Then he goes on to demonstrate that similar or worse consequences follow from reckless marriages, and makes it a moral demand that one should refrain from early wedlock out of regard both for oneself and for others:

> From the inattention of mankind hitherto to the consequences of increasing too fast, it must be presumed, that these consequences are not so immediately and powerfully connected with the conduct which leads to them, as

[1] Malthus, *Essay*... (Everyman ed.), ii. 256–7.

in the other instances; but the delayed knowledge of particular effects does not alter their nature, or our obligation to regulate our conduct accordingly, as soon as we are satisfied of what this conduct ought to be.[1]

What is meant is made clear from subsequent passages, where other forms of conduct (such as stealing) are shown to have evil social consequences which eventually injure even the person who first benefited from them.

The implication here seems to be that restraint may be either purely selfish (and incidentally possibly vicious), or it may have a higher moral purpose. Surely this is moral restraint! If it is not, why then the long introduction to Book IV of which this forms part, entitled 'Of moral restraint, and our obligation to practise this virtue'?[2] Throughout this section of the *Essay*, the most detailed attention is given to the prudential motives for postponing marriage, and the 'moral' slant is provided by the continuous reference to the effects on others of our own weaknesses. If this interpretation is correct, then Malthus is revealed as the arch-utopian of them all. Godwin expected the passion between the sexes to diminish because of the growth of other enjoyments and the increased sensitivity to communal needs. This was the system Malthus had condemned out of hand, since he did not believe that even under a system of perfect equality people could subordinate their sexual instincts to social advantage: 'I cannot conceive a form of society so favourable upon the whole to population'.[3] Yet the very effect he denied in Godwin's system now seems to be at the core of Malthus's own. For all the sections devoted to the circumstances most conducive to the exercise of moral restraint describe alterations in society to which Godwin might well have subscribed. They were all designed to foster not only the individual's appreciation of the advantages of prudence, but also his social consciousness.

The most logical way of dividing Malthus's checks to population, then, would be this: first, there are the positive checks which cut short life. Secondly, there are the preventive checks which reduce fertility. These again may be divided into good, bad, and indifferent checks. The good one is moral restraint, i.e. restraint from marriage with virtuous conduct, and out of regard for the well-being for society, as well as one's own advantage. The bad one is self-seeking prudential restraint from marriage with loose sexual conduct. The indifferent one is prudential restraint mostly for selfish reasons, with an occasional

[1] Malthus, op. cit. ii. 152.
[2] Ibid., pp. 151–9.
[3] Ibid., p. 14.

human lapse presumably permitted. Malthus the moralist seems to have concentrated on the good and the bad preventive check. But Malthus the sociologist devoted a large part of his work to the promotion of the indifferent check. Since it is this (afterwards termed by Richard Jones 'voluntary restraint') which has occupied the greater part of this book, it is worth seeing how far Malthus anticipated his later opponents.

The standard of living and prudential restraint

What did Malthus have to say about the standard of living? How was it measured, of what did it consist, was it changing in his time, and what were his future expectations regarding it? Unfortunately, as we have come to expect, the answer is not clear or consistent. In various places, both in the *Essay* and the *Principles*, we find hints. In total, they amount to the foundations of practically the whole of classical and neo-classical population theory, as well as foreshadowing modern social theories. Individually, they often contradict each other.

The passages quoted here are intended only as a selection, containing some of the more useful ideas, and are by no means a comprehensive account of the various shades of meaning obtainable. For full treatment, the reader is referred to J. J. Spengler's 'Malthus' Total Population Theory'.

First of all, there is fairly widespread agreement that Malthus basically knew two sorts of operation of the standard of living: the one applied where there was a minimum subsistence, or 'corn' standard; the other where the inhabitants included 'conveniences and comforts' in their requirements. In the first case, there would be usually an automatic direct response of population to the amount of food, in the second case there would need to be an increase in the supply of other commodities as well in order to produce an increase of population. Again, in the first case any diminution of the demand for labour would at once lead to the operation of the positive checks, whereas in the second case, there could be a retrenchment of expenditure on other wants, with no danger to existence, while the adjustment to the new conditions through the preventive check took place.

But even this picture is not allowed to stand in such simplicity. Malthus hedges it around with reservations. For instance, he says that in countries with warm climates and rich soils, labour may not always respond to the availability of plentiful subsistence by early marriage and high fertility, but, owing to the 'inveterate habits of indolence fostered by a vicious government', prefer to work only part of the time.[1] Where prudential habits prevail, people will work industriously, but in order not to forgo the ingredients of the higher standard, there will be a similar failure of population to grow *pari passu* with the demand for labour.[2]

How does this then square with his constant assertion that the 'passion between the sexes' is so much more powerful than prudence, and that therefore the unhappy effects of the principle of population are everywhere in evidence? The answer is that he himself apparently did not believe that the sexual instinct was stronger than the desire for a reasonable standard of living. In the introductory chapter on moral restraint at the beginning of Book IV, he clearly states:

> The most powerful and universal of all our desires is the desire of food, and of those things, such as clothing, houses, etc., which are immediately necessary to relieve us from the pains of hunger and cold. It is acknowledged by all, that these desires put in motion the greatest part of that activity, from which the multiplied improvements and advantages of civilised life are derived; and that the pursuit of these objects, and the gratification of these desires, form the principal happiness of the larger half of mankind, civilised or uncivilised, and are indispensably necessary to the more refined enjoyments of the other half.[3]

Sex comes lower down, a page later, clearly labelled as being the second most powerful desire. That is to say, Malthus acknowledges the superiority of the 'prospect of a good meal, a warm house, and a comfortable fireside in the evening'[4] over sexual enjoyments—in any society where such things are to be had. If, of course, one takes this picture of comfortable domesticity against the background of the 'wretched inhabitants of Tierra del Fuego' in the first book, we may assume that Malthus was putting forward a peculiarly British point of view. But as we have seen, he was convinced that this applied to the larger half of mankind.

How, then, did this state of affairs arise? Some time or other the inhabitants of the civilized part of the globe must have passed from the minimum standard to that in which prudence prevailed. Here Malthus confuses us thoroughly, for he tells us, in so many words, that the only way in which the labourer can attain a higher standard of living is by exercising prudence, but he cannot be expected to exercise prudence until he has a higher standard of living, as the result of advances in

[1] Malthus, op. cit. ii. 139. [2] Ibid., p. 140. [3] Ibid., p. 153. [4] Ibid., p. 154.

technique which make the comforts of life relatively cheaper than food, and therefore create an effective desire for them in his breast:[1]

... the condition of the lower classes of society certainly does not depend exclusively upon the increase of the funds for the maintenance of labour, or the means of supporting more labourers.... the comforts of the lower classes of society do not depend solely upon food, nor even upon strict necessaries; and they cannot be considered as in a good state unless they have the command of some conveniences and even luxuries. Secondly, the tendency in population fully to keep pace with the means of subsistence must in general prevent the increase of these means from having a great and permanent effect in improving the condition of the poor. And, thirdly, the cause which has the most lasting effect in improving the situation of the lower classes of society depends chiefly upon the conduct and prudence of the individuals themselves, and is, therefore, not immediately and necessarily connected with an increase in the means of subsistence.[2]

This passage, with its distinction of necessaries, conveniences, and luxuries, nicely foreshadows Nassau Senior's similar triple classification, but otherwise it is as obscure as any, for it tells us that anything may happen, and not how we may judge which way the movement will take place.

He makes an attempt to clarify the issue later in the same chapter. After introducing such matters as the unhealthiness of industrial occupations, the uncertainty and fluctuations of employment in the more advanced societies, and the vagaries of fashion, he goes on to tell us that the disadvantages resulting from industrialization are outweighed by certain quite definite advantages which help to keep the population problem under control. The first of these is the emergence of a larger and stronger middle class in society. The second, and more important for our argument, is the fact that there will be a relative fall in the price of manufactured commodities compared with corn:

... the production of an additional quantity of corn will require more labour, while, at the same time, from the accumulation and better distribution of capital, the continual improvements made in machinery, and the facilities opened to foreign commerce, manufactures and foreign commodities will be produced or purchased with less labour; and consequently a given quantity of corn will command a much greater quantity of manufactures and foreign commodities than while the country was poor. Although, therefore, the labourer may earn less corn than before, the superior value which every portion which he does not consume in kind will have in the purchase of conveniences, may more than counterbalance this diminution. He will not indeed

[1] Ibid., pp. 130, 134–5.

[2] Ibid., pp. 129–30.

have the same power of maintaining a large family; but with a small family he may be better lodged and clothed, and better able to command the decencies and comforts of life.[1]

The inference from this passage clearly relates the emergence of the preference for the higher standard of living to the time in which Malthus was living. Then, for the first time, there was some point in altering the habitual pattern of expenditure. Corn was relatively dearer than before, but other goods were cheaper. Therefore voluntary limitation of family size brought not just a greater sufficiency of diet, as it might have done in earlier ages, but the prospects of substantial additions to the standard of living. The emergence of the higher wants is thus clearly connected in Malthus's mind with the technological possibility of mass production, importation, and consumption of goods which had not previously figured in the English labourer's pattern of life.

But the technological aspect is not the only one. Malthus continuously stresses the need for civil liberty and education. Only if the people had the fruits of their labour ensured by good government, and if their attention was directed towards the advantages of the more refined mode of living, could they be expected to take advantage of the new opportunities. The point is made a number of times, but the following quotation from the *Principles* may serve for the rest:

From 1720 to 1750 the price of wheat had so fallen, while wages had risen, that instead of two thirds the labourer could purchase the whole of a peck of wheat with a day's labour.

This great increase of command over the first necessary of life did not, however, produce a proportionate increase of population. It found the people of this country living under a good government, and enjoying all the advantages of civil and political liberty in an unusual degree. The lower classes of people had been in the habit of being respected, both by the laws and the higher orders of their fellow citizens and had learned in consequence to respect themselves. The result was, that their increased corn wages, instead of occasioning an increase of population exclusively, were so expended as to occasion a decided elevation in the standard of their comforts and conveniences.[2]

Here, for a change, Malthus derives the change of the demand structure in favour of conveniences and luxuries in terms of a relative fall in the price of wheat, rather than a rise, and still produces the same effect.

[1] Malthus, op. cit. ii. 134.
[2] T. R. Malthus, *Principles of Political Economy* . . . (London, 1836), pp. 228–9.

But this is not the main point of this passage, rather it is the indispensable precondition for the change to a new standard of living implied in the second paragraph. Similar passages are to be found throughout the *Essay*.[1]

There is little doubt that Malthus observed the tendency in his own time for additional 'comforts and even luxuries' to creep into the schedule of minimum requirements, and that he expected this process to continue. Yet this expectation is nowhere explicitly stated, since it would in itself have weakened his case too much. When discussing the census of 1811, he implied that the process of industrialization, while favourable to population through the increased demand for labour, also generated greater checks:

> This is a rate of increase which in the nature of things cannot be permanent. It has been occasioned by the stimulus of a greatly-increased demand for labour, combined with a greatly-increased power of production, both in agriculture and manufactures. These are the two elements which form the most effective encouragement to a rapid increase of population. What has taken place is a striking illustration of the principle of population, and a proof that in spite of great towns, manufacturing occupations, and the gradually-acquired habits of an opulent and luxuriant people, if the resources of a country will admit of a rapid increase, and if these resources are so advantageously distributed as to occasion a constantly-increasing demand for labour, the population will not fail to keep pace with them.[2]

As for future expectations, he had his hopes. Speaking of the desire for bettering oneself, the great *vis medicatrix reipublicae*, he said:

> Owing to this powerful spring of health in every state, which is nothing more than an inference from the general course of the laws of nature, irresistibly forced on each man's attention, the prudential check to marriage has increased in Europe; and it cannot be unreasonable to conclude that it will still make further advances.[3]

Then he goes on to say that where this desire is strongest, it cannot be said that vice is rife, and that one cannot expect any adverse results from such progress. He once more advocates the spread of national education, and efforts to instil into the poor the truth about their poverty, and so he ends his great work on a note of optimism which seems to have escaped most of his contemporaries. The last word of the book is 'success'. For Europe at any rate, he thought that the 'evils resulting from the principle of population have rather diminished than

[1] Malthus, *Essay* . . . (Everyman ed.), ii. 139.
[2] Ibid. i. 261.
[3] Ibid. ii. 257.

increased. . . . it does not seem unreasonable to expect that they will be still further diminished'.[1] Naturally, he saw in his work an important contribution to the task of making sure that the problem was understood, and that therefore the chances of its solution were increased.

Malthus's theory of fertility

In other parts of the *Essay* Malthus drew attention to various aspects of the social background to increased prudence, some of which we have mentioned in the appropriate sections. We were able to show that he knew the connexion between industrialization, civil liberty, and prudence. He repeatedly referred to 'luxuries' and the necessity for spreading them throughout the nation, to increase the desire for restraint, and analysed at great length the evils resulting from the concentration on production of useless frivolities for a small class of proprietors.[2] We have also seen that he implicitly accepted the argument that towns were unfavourable to population, though more so through the prevalence of the positive check than through the operation of greater moral restraint. On property, his views are again somewhat confused, though he was sure, as were his predecessors in the eighteenth century, that excessive concentration and primogeniture were obstacles to greater population. This did not lead him, however, to advocate such concentration, since the total amount of subsistence thus produced would also be less. He knew that excessive subdivision of property could also be an encouragement to superfluous population, as Ireland was to prove before 1846.[3] He observed that the redistribution of property in France after the Revolution had had beneficial effects in making the labouring classes more self-reliant, and 'more saving, and more prudent in marriage than formerly';[4] thus showing the superiority of the French revolutionary system over the English scheme of parochial relief. In this observation, he foreshadowed the findings of Le Play and other French sociologists.

What then are we to make of the Malthusian system? He recognizes that there is no simple effect connecting food and population. A greater demand for labour, or an increase in the amount of available subsistence, may or may not lead to an increase of population, depend-

[1] Malthus, op. cit. ii. 261.

[2] See Spengler, 'Malthus' Total Population Theory', op. cit., pp. 234 ff., esp. references to *Principles of Political Economy* . . ., pp. 373 ff.

[3] For views on property, see Spengler, ibid., pp. 92 ff.

[4] Malthus, *Essay* . . ., op. cit. ii. 69.

ing on whether the gain is taken out in extra leisure (idleness), in other commodities, or in marriage and more children. A rise or fall in the price of food (i.e. the corn value of labour as he calls it) may have similarly diverse consequences. The exact mode of operation will depend on the form of government, on the state of technology, on the system of distribution, on the state of education, and a number of other social factors. This much at least can be derived from the scattered references in his works. In this form it is unexceptional, and it is unlikely that a modern sociologist would quarrel with it, although he would very likely say that Malthus should have been more precise about the exact sequence of events and reactions in each case.

If we take all these statements together with his constant reservations about the operation of the 'Law of Population' in its crudest form, with the footnotes and appendixes and the concession to Arthur Young, with the correspondence with Nassau Senior, and so on, we can scarcely believe that Malthus himself could attach much importance to the scheme in the simple form in which we presented it at the beginning of this section. Instead, he may well have believed in the 'tendencies' only in their most attenuated form, where they describe a movement akin to the physical law which says that bodies will continue to move in the direction of any initial impetus unless some other force arrests or changes this movement. In other words, these tendencies exist in a vacuum. Instead, there are numerous forces, increasingly of the preventive kind, which stop the growth of population, and it is these forces which form the proper study of population, and which must be encouraged by all possible means.

But he could never bring himself to say so. He had a good case, but obstinacy prevented him from stating it. Richard Jones, Malthus's successor at Haileybury, criticized the original classification into misery, vice, and moral restraint as defective, mainly because he thought the term should be 'voluntary restraint'. He also tried to add a category of 'neutral' checks which he believed originated from the 'growth and changes of societies of civilised men'.[1] The latter included non-economic considerations not of a vicious character. One of his chief objections to the original categories was his liberal view that a man should not be denied credit for his 'moral restraint' because he was guilty of a single indiscretion. But as we have seen, Malthus himself did not believe in such perfection either! Jones, though probably a

[1] R. Jones, *Literary Remains, Consisting of Lectures and Tracts on Political Economy* (W. Whewell and Cazenove, eds., London, 1859), pp. 96–97 and 154.

careful student of Malthus, was evidently misled, and it is not surprising that generations of readers have continued to misunderstand Malthus's position—much to the detriment of the great core of truth which undoubtedly exists in Malthus's teaching.

If we accept the characterization of Malthus as the arch-apologist of the ruling classes, his refusal to see the implications of his own observations can also be attributed to malice. His injunction to the working classes to improve their lot by partial self-extermination may be seen as a form of charity which would save the upper classes their poor rates without affecting their purses adversely in any other way, at least in the short run. The other remedy for over-population was based on genuine advancement, on the redistribution of property and income, on popular education and competitive examinations, on greater rights for women and universal suffrage. If Malthus truly understood the efficacy of these remedies, then his refusal to include them must have been based on his general distaste for change.

But it is at least possible that Malthus was not such a good observer as some have made out. Despite the confusion over the word 'prudential', Malthus was on the whole a rational thinker. His economics have stood up better to the test of time than his population theory, perhaps because they were based a little more firmly on deductive reasoning. Whereas the core of his population theory was also deductive, he thought it necessary to bolster up his simple law with masses of so-called evidence—much of it derived from hearsay, such as his tales of the Far East and South Seas, and most of the rest incapable of bearing the interpretation he put on it. As to observations of the contemporary British scene, Malthus's work bears almost no evidence. His chapters on England seem to contain factual material only from such sources as Short and Price. There is no sign that even at the end of his life he knew anything in detail about industrialization. His thesis was based on the life of an island agricultural nation, and so it remained long after the exports of manufactures had begun to pay for the imports of large quantities of raw materials. If not much corn came in, the increase in the volume of foreign trade in his own lifetime was at least so startling that it escaped no one else. Fond as he was of mathematical methods of forecasting population, he never allowed that even in his period the rate of increase of population was already slackening. The results of the 1831 Census were out before he died, yet he never came to interpret them. Statistics apart, the main charge against him must be that he was a bad observer of his fellow human beings. He may have known much of the habits of English country gentlemen and their sons—he knew little of the rest. The great advantage of men like T. R. Edmonds was their close acquaintance with the habits of the people, and even those who had no first-hand knowledge learned to draw on Chadwick.

Malthusian theories after Malthus

The main subjects of the preceding chapters have been those who, like Malthus, granted the possibility of a rising tide, but thought they knew what would stop it. Some of these might call themselves Malthusians—probably because they misread Malthus and thought that he himself had foretold and welcomed the spread of voluntary restraint in England. Most of them, however, were anti-Malthusians, including those who have been misnamed neo-Malthusians. The difference between these two sets of people lies mainly in the timing of restraint. The anti-Malthusians mostly thought of the postponement of marriage induced by cultural and economic influences, the neo-Malthusians thought that early marriage was at least harmless and possibly desirable (e.g. Place), and provided the techniques for achieving the result the others obtained by late marriage. In this sense the anti-Malthusians are followers of Malthus (since they work through a cautious approach to marriage, for whatever reason) and the neo-Malthusians directly defy the master, since they are not interested in postponed marriages. One further distinction may be drawn: the early advocates of birth-control also differ essentially from Malthus in their anxiety to use positive, energetic intervention to counteract the threat he had described, by the dissemination of propaganda. In this they show themselves as immediately aware of the dangers as the German princelings who forbade their subjects to marry. On the other hand, once birth-control was firmly established, the emphasis somewhat changed. The generation of Julius Wolf took birth-control for granted. Their theory of population was essentially a development of the earlier arguments. Where Moreton, Edmonds, Jones, or Rickards had shown how advances in civilization and industry acted as brakes on growth through postponement of marriage, the writers after 1900 equally naturally showed the same brake operating through birth-control. These last-named authors, then, are as far removed from Malthus's own views as is consistent with the original thesis: that preventive checks need to operate if positive checks are to be averted. If one goes beyond this, one must reject the idea of catastrophe altogether, accept growth as natural, and explain how mankind will adjust itself to the new conditions.[1]

If this view forms one end of the spectrum, there remains the revival of the opposite belief—that the natural tendency is towards a decrease in population, and that only intervention will reverse the trend. This is the view, not unnaturally, which found most supporters in France in the days of the founding of the *Alliance Nationale*, and then spread to most Western countries. It has found the most eloquent expression in the pro-populationist policies of France, the fascist régimes in Italy and Germany, and to a lesser extent in the family-allowance systems of socialist countries. As far as the explanations of the causes of this decline are concerned, they do not in any point of substance differ from those advanced by the anti-Malthusians to show that the threat of over-population was not real. Once again it is merely a matter of a changing vocabulary. Emulation becomes *arrivisme*, the emancipation of women no longer appears an act of progress to a generation confronted by the *Ibsenweib*. The virtues have again become vices.

There remains a last category of writers, who cannot be included either as successors of Malthus or of the pro-populationists. They are the ones who are not committed to any particular trend of movement, but believe that there is a correct population (and even perhaps a theory of population) for each stage of culture, or of economic development, and that in some way not always specified, the adjustment of people and subsistence takes place. Those who postulated 'optimum' theories of population, particularly, were often guilty of vagueness as to the means of adjustment. Sir Alexander Carr-Saunders put forward the idea that the evolution of culture would bring with it a universal tendency towards the maintenance of the optimum appropriate to the technical skills and resources of any particular period, by the evolution of institutions and techniques which ensured this maintenance. It is difficult to see how this adjustment is supposed to function except in the terms already used by Malthus's opponents. But the ideas and standards of behaviour which evolved in the nineteenth century were not necessarily movements towards an optimum, as the example of France shows. The main difficulty lies in the fact that the appropriate social responses to the economic conditions of today are not likely to change the pattern of population within one generation, and by the time they have effect the economic conditions may have changed again.

[1] Mr. Colin Clark is the best-known exponent of this view.

Much the same may be said of such socialist theories as Lassalle's 'Iron Law of Wages'. In general, population theories in terms of economic conditions and cultural response have often had a socialist flavour. Inspired by Marx, they refused to accept a general tendency or a general system of response. Echoing Godwin and Condorcet, they thought the world would support far more people under one system of production and government than another. Whereas the capitalist system encouraged the formation of a large proletariat with all the characteristics of a Malthusian rabble, prudence would come with socialism. In this context they have made important contributions to the standard-of-living theories. Culture and civilization theories outside the socialist orbit, dating back to such diverse origins as Cantillon and Paley, have also been independent of any prior assumption about the probable or desirable direction of population movements. It is this last group of views which forms the basis of modern population research. Once the investigator dissociates himself from the polemical turbulence, which has obscured the issue since the days of Hume and Wallace, Malthus and Godwin, and renounces the right to make judgements of a moral or political character, he is better able to make statistical investigations of what are, in fact, the 'determinants and consequences of population trends'.

Such investigations seem a far cry from Malthus. Yet, in a sense, they start with him, because he claimed to do just what they are trying to do. Animated by the same sort of general benevolence which presumably also animates the modern social scientist, he focused attention on a major social problem and claimed to investigate it scientifically, by collecting facts and statistics. That his methods were faulty is in this context irrelevant. But the true path of science was nevertheless effectively blocked by the result, because, although he did not—at any rate to any important extent—advocate social policies, his followers adopted them for reasons provided by the study of his works (even if they were quite negative), and in his name such damage was done, that for a hundred years any debate on Malthus was almost bound to be emotional, political, and unscientific.

The best way of fitting Malthus into the history of the most important modern theories, then, is to say that he thought of many of them, yet he delayed their formulation. Without him, the ideas of Ferguson and Paley might have been built into a reasonable general system by Senior, Jones, or Mill. Thus we deny his merits but not his importance, for it is in fighting Malthus throughout the nineteenth century that the most important discoveries were made. Yet had he been less obstinate he might himself have built much of the edifice.

3. POPULATION THEORY AND THE STANDARD-OF-LIVING ARGUMENT

It is now possible to assess the ideas which have been presented in this book in the larger context of population studies as a whole, and of the social sciences in general. What was the purpose of the authors quoted? What do their explanations achieve? Do their systems form a valid part of the total picture of human society, or are they merely giving explanations for rather isolated sections of complex processes?

In general, we are here concerned with theories concerning human behaviour, with voluntary or involuntary movements of population through alterations in the pattern of fertility, against a background of social and economic change. This classification creates difficulties. We cannot be certain what a 'theory' means in this context. There are no obvious or widely recognized tools of analysis. We know very little about the precise relationship between the fertility changes in the foreground (which can be measured statistically) and the social and economic changes in the background (which can often be described only in rather vague terms). One could ask, for instance: are we basically dealing with changes caused by non-economic factors, but leading to far-reaching economic effects, or are we mostly dealing with the effects of economic development on the composition of human society? Both kinds of questions have been asked, and the answers often treated quite separately from each other. Again, many works have appeared putting forward a theory (or hypothesis) concerning the connexion between movements in fertility and one aspect of the background pattern (e.g. education) without reference to the rest of the possible influences.

In this last section we attempt to investigate the matter under these headings: (1) What contribution to the subject is made by the specialized approach of economists and sociologists? Can fertility theory be simply a part of a general economic theory of development? (2) What, in essence, is this 'standard-of-living argument' now so widely accepted as the principal determinant of fertility changes by a great number of writers, and can it stand as part of a general theory in the light of recent developments? (3) What are the fundamental difficulties which appear to be inherent in the subject, and do these differentiate population studies from other social sciences?

What is theory in population studies?

A systematic investigation of these questions would have to begin with an attempt to define what is meant by 'theory' in the social sciences in general, and population studies in particular. But such an undertaking is beyond the scope of a final chapter summarizing only the history of theories in general. It is only necessary to refer the reader to a number of recent essays in this direction, both those which put forward a consistent system, like that of Kingsley Davis,[1] and those which mainly point out the difficulties.[2] Some of these point to the probability that the difficulties raised are not by any means confined to population studies.[3] The word 'theory' is used sometimes precisely, and sometimes rather loosely, to describe anything from a working hypothesis to a complete system of relationships.[4] One cannot easily dismiss any of these definitions as being meaningless in our context. It is only when one is faced with a demand such as that put forward by Sydney Coontz, that theory should be appraised for its 'correspondence with observed fact, coherence, and successful prediction',[5] that one must at once either repudiate the suggestion, or dismiss the greater part of social theories in general, and those relating to fertility in particular, as quite useless, since they do not lend themselves to successful prediction. True, it was precisely this search for prediction which motivated so much of the work in Malthus's time and even today. The world required a formula which would yield an optimistic prognosis. But it was found in time that the movement of population was not to be compared to the life-cycle of a plant, the path of a comet, or the flow of the tides. Only reluctantly did the investigators begin to abandon the search for the 'why' which would also, in the end, yield the 'how' and the 'when'. Economists have long ceased to put forward this requirement of immediate value for prediction when discussing, for instance, the trade cycle. One looks instead for intelligent and consistent explanations of observed phenomena, for internally consistent hypotheses, and for a statement of remaining gaps and uncertainties which so far prevent prediction. If population studies were

[1] e.g. Davis, op. cit., p. 542.

[2] e.g. R. B. Vance, 'Is Theory for Demographers?', Spengler and Duncan, op. cit., p. 88. See also Coontz, op. cit., p. 2.

[3] See F. Lorimer, 'The Differentiation of Logical Levels in Social Enquiry', Spengler and Duncan, op. cit., pp. 97 ff.

[4] For a comprehensive use in English analogous to the German practice, see E. T. Hiller, 'A Culture Theory of Population Trends', Spengler and Duncan, op. cit., p. 37.

[5] Coontz, op. cit., p. 1.

clearly part of economic science one might not be faced with the demand for forecasts. But the social pressures for prediction have been strong, and in some senses they are still strong today, as the continuous discussions on the future of Asian populations show.

In sum, there is no general agreement as to what one means by 'theory' and what a theory should do. In the United Nations volume which we have already cited repeatedly, the chapter headed 'History of Population Theories', and in many other recent writings on the subject,[1] the word is allowed to have many different partial and comprehensive meanings, and this may serve for an excuse not to attempt the impossible—namely to state unequivocally what one expects from a theory and then to test the one under discussion according to these criteria.

Economics—the position of Marshall

Since there is not room here for an extended discussion of the methodology of population studies, or even a review of the more important recent writings on the subject, the difficulties of the investigation of fertility-differentials will be illustrated with the aid of two examples. One will be taken from neo-classical, the other from modern Marxist economics. Alfred Marshall wrote at some length on population, and his views have been systematically collected by J. J. Spengler.[2] Since Marx himself did not put forward any great amount of thinking on population, and contented himself with incidental observations arising out of the concept of a surplus army of labour, the question whether the scientific approach characteristic of him and his school helps us to resolve the central problem is best answered by analysing a modern exponent's attempt to apply the economic interpretation rigorously.

The essence of the economic interpretation of population growth is, of course, that marriage and fertility are governed by the amount of available employment and means of subsistence in real terms, as we pointed out in the section on Malthus. Typical 'economic' statements

[1] See the following article headings in the volume edited by Spengler and Duncan: 'Is Theory for Demographers?'; 'Towards a General Theory of Growth'; 'The Theory of Optimum Population for a Closed Economy'; 'Theory of Population and Modern Economic Analysis'; 'A Culture Theory of Population Trends'; 'The Theory and Consequences of Mobility of Farm Population'.

[2] J. J. Spengler, 'Marshall on Population', *Population Studies* (1955), viii. 264, and x. 56.

on population determinants in Marshall show at once that there is nowhere a belief in simple economic determination:

> Given the climate, the average age of marriage depends chiefly on the ease with which young people can establish themselves, and support a family according to the standard of comfort that prevails among their friends and acquaintances: and therefore it is different in different stations in life.[1]

Only under conditions of practically unlimited expansion, as in the new territories in the United States of America, are additional children an unqualified aid to their parents.[2] In medieval England labourers married when there was a vacancy in the village, and not otherwise.[3] In the eighteenth century, Marshall thought, a fairly rapid growth of population was ensured by demands for labour in the growing industrial districts, where the birth-rate was very high.[4] In the nineteenth century, he found, the marriage-rate varied with the quality of the harvest.[5]

These statements do not mean that Marshall believed that prosperity and economic opportunity could be taken in isolation. They are constantly linked with observations on the checks to marriage and fertility, which are either, in fact, sociological observations, or imply such observations. In the passage quoted, it is the customary standard of living in the society in which the young people live which checks marriage. He thought that the slower growth of population in the first half of the eighteenth century was 'partly caused by, partly the cause of, a rise in the standard of living: a chief element of which was an increased use of wheat in the place of inferior grains as the common food of the people'.[6] If he meant these words as they stand, they make nonsense of the classical view, since what they really convey is this: a population of a given size, growing slowly, changes over to a type of food not so readily procurable as that to which they had been accustomed (cause not stated). This change is made possible by the fact that the increase in numbers is halted (cause not stated, but implied that the higher standard demands greater care before marrying or having children). In turn, the arrest in growth makes it possible for further sections of the population to adopt the new mode. The arrest is then made almost permanent by the fact that the harvest will occasionally fail, thus inculcating even more prudence than usual. (It is not stated

[1] Marshall, *Principles of Economics* (8th ed., London, 1930), p. 181.
[2] Ibid., p. 183. [3] Ibid., p. 186. [4] Ibid., p. 188.
[5] Ibid., p. 189.
[6] Ibid., p. 188.

why the English, unlike other nations, did not revert to a simpler standard when harvests failed.)

We can easily see that this description of the events in the eighteenth century is only to a very small extent economic history (even supposing it were a correct description). It is partly political history (concerned with the balance of forces in the country, the growth of a strong and independent peasant and labouring class); it is partly an allusion to a social revolution of the past when the accustomed standard changed for reasons no longer clear. If our forefathers ate pease and rye, why did they decide to press for wheaten bread? If we say that it is in some way 'natural' that people should adopt any more pleasant way of living which offers itself, and are prepared to apply prudential restraint in order to obtain it, we are enunciating a law of progress which owes nothing to economic science.

This belief in the possibility, and even likelihood, of improvements in the standard of living is in strong contrast to any wage-fund theory, particularly the 'Iron Law of Wages' as propounded by Ricardo and Lassalle.[1] Even Ricardo, as Marshall pointed out, did not really believe in an immutable minimum standard of living just high enough to ensure survival and efficiency. Instead, there were many different standards, based on conventions, and these were decidedly not the results of economic pressures. 'It is only temporarily and provisionally that we can with profit isolate for study the economic side of [man's] life . . .'.[2] And so the check to the increase in population follows naturally from the existence of these higher standards, or, as he called it, 'the standard of life' which serves as a description for the whole of the existing pattern of family life, as determined by employment, production, distribution, tastes, and the number of children.[3]

And so it comes about that the check to the increase in population does not only occur when the 'dividend' allotted to labour falls below what is required for health and efficiency, but much earlier,

> because the population at large would not be likely to limit its consumption to bare necessaries: some part of the family income would almost certainly be spent on gratifications which contributed but little to the maintenance of life and efficiency.[4]

Marshall evidently considered the influence of this spending pattern to

[1] Marshall, op. cit., pp. 508, 690.
[2] Ibid., p. 85.
[3] Spengler, 'Marshall on Population', loc. cit. ix. 61.
[4] Marshall, op. cit., p. 691.

be more important than that exerted by the demand for labour on its own:

Thus economic causes play a part in governing the growth of population as a whole as well as the supply of labour in any particular grade. But their influence on the numbers of the population as a whole is largely indirect; and is exerted by way of the ethical, social and domestic habits of life. For these habits are themselves influenced by economic causes deeply, though slowly, and in ways some of which are difficult to trace, and impossible to predict.[1]

The passage has, unfortunately, a typical Marshallian vagueness and provision for a line of retreat, should its argument be attacked, but, read in conjunction with others, one feels that on the whole he would claim no more than that the pattern of economic activity was one of several influences which shaped the social determinants of fertility, and in this he would not be out of line with the majority of modern writers.

How the checks to fertility operated in detail, Marshall did not investigate, though he quoted others, apparently with approval, to support a general fertility differential based on income.[2] He also put forward the idea, already mentioned, that those subject to mental strain were unprolific, and that those who do 'high mental work' married late and therefore had fewer children.[3] He knew of the French theories relating to the influence of property on marriage and fertility and quoted from Levasseur in this connexion.[4]

Similar evidence can be cited from other economists of the nineteenth century. In sum, it amounts to the fact that though they treated population as one of the most important topics within the field of economics, they did not think that there was any simple process by which economic activity governed the size of population through marriages and births. As writers began to investigate the phenomena of fertility decline in an age of expanding economic activity, the original connexion was almost forgotten, and for many years the sociological or psychological approach prevailed.

The Marxist position

To one school of thought, however, this approach was anathema. Marxists believed that the prevailing economic system gave rise to an

[1] Ibid., p. 218.

[2] Ibid., p. 184, quoting Smith, Doubleday, Sadler, Charles Booth, and the Registrar-General.

[3] Ibid., p. 184.

[4] Ibid., p. 185.

associated law of population, and that all general theories, like Malthus's own, were as misguided as any attempt to derive population movements from such non-economic factors as changes in prevailing levels of ambition unconnected with opportunity. Socialists had traditionally attacked Malthus as an apologist for the ruling classes and an oppressor of the poor. Marx himself, therefore, dismissed the whole topic with rather few words, partly perhaps because it was not necessary for him to convince his readers of the futility of Malthusian theories of population. Following Marx, the methodical socialist discussions of the problem are few and far between. Some socialists were only emotionally anti-Malthusian, and in practice neo-Malthusian. As the standard-of-living theories gained ground at the end of the nineteenth century, socialists participated less and less in the general discussion, since their case would obviously be weakened by any admission, or implied admission, that the standard of living of the masses might have risen. To attribute the decline in fertility to a decline in economic activity, i.e. the demand for labour, would have been to invite ridicule from an age which prided itself on the almost continuous expansion of production, even during the so-called Great Depression.[1]

Yet it is curious that the subject was so neglected by Marxist writers, since other topics, perhaps hardly less difficult to handle from their point of view, like art or music, were the subject of numerous monographs. Even in the Soviet Union, judging by the works cited in the United Nations bibliography, population studies received little attention. Perhaps in part this was due also to a general conviction, shared for instance by Schumpeter, that the subject was not very interesting, 'an intermediate cause, incapable of bearing much weight'.[2] In his *History of Economic Analysis* he called it a 'semi-independent science',

[1] There appear to be no adequate recent accounts of socialist attitudes to population. Amongst earlier works are: H. Soetbeer, *Die Stellung der Sozialisten zur Malthusischen Bevölkerungslehre* (Berlin, 1886); L. Dumas, *Le Socialisme et le principe de population* (Paris, 1908); E. Lowenthal, 'The Ricardian Socialists', *Studies in History, Economics, and Public Law*, Faculty of Political Science of Columbia University (New York, 1911), xlvi, no. 1, pp. 5–105; L. Sonolet, *Principe de population et socialisme* (Paris, 1907); R. L. Meek's edition of the writings of Marx and Engels on Malthus (*Marx and Engels on Malthus* (London, 1953)) has some further references. See also S. Levin, 'Marx versus Malthus', *Papers of the Michigan Academy of Sciences, Arts and Letters* (1936), xxii. 234–48. For Soviet views, see United Nations bibliography, and A. Sauvy, 'Doctrine soviétique en matière de population', *Rivista italiana di demografia e statistica* (Dec. 1948), ii, no. 4, pp. 474–88.

[2] J. Schumpeter, 'Gustav Schmoller und die Probleme von heute', *Schmoller's Jahrbuch* (50. Jahrgang, 1926), pt. 1, p. 386.

with which he would deal to get it out of the way, since it was in any case on the way out.[1]

One major attempt has recently been made to bring Marxian methods to bear heavily against the prevailing point of view, the growth of which has been traced in this book. Sydney Coontz's *Population Theory and the Economic Interpretation* represents a consistent effort to 'return population theory to its natural habitat, the field of economics'.[2] The work echoes the dissatisfaction widely felt with the failure of generations of investigators in the field to produce anything like a workable theory—that is, one which is capable of producing accurate predictions. The recent failure of the birth-rate to fall further in connexion with the rising prosperity experienced in many countries is the most obvious case in point. Coontz rightly castigates a large number of the writers who have already been quoted for their failure to evolve satisfactory techniques, which made the failure of their predictions inevitable. The only method, the author asserts, of fitting population into its proper place, is to make it again a 'dependent variable, a function of civilization'.[3] This might at first sight appear to indicate a familiar position, until we remember that in this context civilization is necessarily explained as arising out of almost wholly economic determinants.

For Marx, the characteristic situation under capitalism had been the ever-present threat of over-population, to provide the reserve army of labour. However much labour tries to restrict its fertility (if it can do so at all), it can never improve its position owing to the continuous substitution of constant for variable capital. Ignoring the question of who is to produce the constant capital (today the origin of the earnings of a substantial part of the labour force), the Marxist argument centres on the fact that the relative reduction of variable capital must mean the purchase of less labour power. This then leads to the familiar proposition that a decline in surplus value arising out of the exploitation of labour follows from this process of substitution, and that a fresh cycle of frustrated attempts to make labour scarce will start. Here we have 'theory' at a high level. We have a frame of reference and a system of interactions accurately described under the heading of 'capitalism', and a number of propositions are logically deduced. The trouble with this

[1] J. Schumpeter, *History of Economic Analysis* (Oxford, 1954), pp. 578. But his editor records a marginal note in his manuscript to the effect that population studies came back again before the end of his life.

[2] Coontz, op. cit., p. 8.

[3] Ibid.

Marxist scheme was that observed phenomena did not usually fit the scheme. Employment has almost continuously increased, the proportion of constant to variable capital at any rate in Western countries is still increasing, despite intermittent crises causing set-backs. We can only sum up the development by pointing out that adjustments have continued all the time, and that in the end there was a vastly greater population in Europe and America with a greatly improved standard of life.

But despite all this evidence, the Marxist–Leninist belief that the demand for labour regulates population continues in an unchanged tradition, as the references in Coontz's work to the writings of Soviet demographers like Urlanis clearly show.[1] From this belief also follows the conclusion that under socialism there cannot be such a thing as over-population, nor under-population. Heedlessness cannot create supply problems, and excessive caution a labour problem. In practice, this pure approach appears already to have been abandoned in China, but at any rate for the purposes of the economic theory of population, problems of this kind cannot exist, since individual attitudes cannot be divorced from material pressures.

The failure which the Marxist school shares with many of the neo-classical economists lies in their omission of any explanation of the mechanism which translates this theoretical demand for labour into marriages and children, or, alternatively, turns an excessive labour force into a smaller one. In the latter case, in theory, Malthusian positive checks would do the work most quickly, but while this may have been observed in the past, it could hardly be demonstrated to the same extent today, even in underdeveloped countries. It is not until one begins to examine the wants of the population, as opposed to the requirements of the productive system, that one can understand the relationship at all, and it is precisely this reverse process which Marxists neglect. Population also exerts an effect on the economy, through its demand for goods and services. If it grows, then the only way in which the economy can remain stationary is by the operation of the crudest of wage-fund theories. If there is the slightest lack of elasticity in a downward direction in their standard of living, the people will require activity. There is thus a 'feed-back' effect which produces an oscillation about the long-term trend. It may well lead to an equili-

[1] Coontz, op. cit., pp. 128 ff. B. Ts. Urlanis, *Rost naseleniya v Evrope* (Moscow, 1941), according to Mr. R. E. F. Smith, who has consulted it on my behalf, appears to contain no concession to the possibility of an inverse relationship of prosperity and fertility.

brium at a lower level of activity, relatively, but certainly it is not a one-way operation. If, of course, one assumes that there is a high degree of inelasticity in the standard of living, the fall in the demand for labour may be very slow. This is a difficulty complementary to one which already Marshall failed to face. Marx thought that standards could be changed too easily: Marshall thought them, in some ways, immovable. In both cases, one feels that one must turn to sociology and perhaps political science to answer the question: What are the steps by which your level of activity is translated into the 'resultant' population?

It is precisely to answer such questions that Coontz attempts his reconstruction of population theory in the second part of his treatise. Much of this part of the book is occupied by a description of changes in the composition of the demand for labour in the later stages of capitalism. One important section deals with the position of the family, and here once again we move at least on the borderline between economics and sociology. There can be no doubt that the functions of the family have changed for all classes, but the reasons are not all economic. If a society decides to treat its children with a measure of humanity, and withdraws them from the labour market, and if it objects to its women doing work in mines, or if it accumulates property and transmits it to legal heirs, then undoubtedly there will be effects on fertility. The reasons for these changes are proper objects of sociological studies. Sometimes there are economic factors involved, as in the Lancashire spinners' demand for ten-hour days for their women and children, which was meant to shorten their own working day. But one cannot sweep aside the whole codex of nineteenth-century social legislation as being prompted by economic motives.

Again, it is a matter of opinion, when there is a complex process, which of the factors is to be designated as the master force. Coontz would argue that if a woman makes a great contribution to the family earnings, her status would be high and her fertility low. If she ceases to work, her status declines, presumably, and her fertility goes up. But it is equally arguable that if a wife ceases to go out to work because her husband's earnings have improved, she gains status, both because she does not work and because they now both belong to a higher class, and so she will be more careful about pregnancies than before because she does not wish to lose her new-found standard of living. Or alternatively, one could say that now she no longer works she has time to have children—or she ceases to work because a child is expected.

Coontz shows[1] why the neo-classical economists finally abandoned the demand-for-labour theory, and joined the opposition to Malthus by taking up the volitional approach: it was because they could not reconcile the classical approach with the observed facts. He therefore attempts to help them out by showing that there is a true economic explanation of the decline of Western fertility after all, and it lies in the shift in demand from that for unskilled manual labour to that for skilled or non-manual labour. The fall in the demand for the lower-paid types has led to a worsening of their situation, he thinks, but at the same time so many have transferred to the non-manual occupations that their ranks are overcrowded too. Thus, the differential has not been maintained, and everyone is worse off. Now this is obviously not so, as marginal analysis would demonstrate. It would be far more true to say that there has been such an expansion of demand for manual and unskilled workers in recent years that the differential has narrowed from below—their bargaining power has improved because their marginal product has increased vastly. At the same time, there is a continuous shortage of skilled men, precisely because the easy money earned by the unskilled makes it uneconomic to train for higher skills.

Similarly, Coontz attempts to show that the general slowing down of the rate of economic progress has led to a decline in fertility. But this is not proven. Indeed, it would be as true to say that in the later stages of advance in the economy such high degrees of skill are required from so many workers that their individual standard of living will rise, and this in turn will lead them to restrict their families. That the rate of progress will slow down is almost inevitable. The greater the achievement in production in the past—especially in a densely populated country like Great Britain—the harder it is to have a constant annual percentage increase in production. This does not mean that anyone is worse off than before, unless there is an abrupt cessation of demand for capital goods, and experience suggests that this may happen at least temporarily. Population may indeed grow more slowly under these circumstances, but this need not be due to misery, i.e. a dramatic failure of demand for labour.

In general, then, we must hold that the evidence is inconclusive. There can be no doubt that the rise in the American birth-rate since the depression of the thirties gave a jolt to the narrowest of orthodox Western 'prosperity theorists'. There is an undoubted increase in prosperity, although the rate of expansion is probably less than at the

[1] Coontz, op. cit., ch. 8.

peak periods of the nineteenth century. Whether fertility is proportional to these rates is hard to establish. But it is quite clear that this increase in prosperity is accompanied by still faster replacement of manual labour by machines tended by highly skilled technicians. The American educational system ensures what Coontz would call a relatively over-large supply of non-manual workers, since these are becoming extremely productive working with machinery that displaces some of them, and thus surplus value should fall still further. But in fact we hear no more about the Marxian concept at this stage, and this is as well, since it would defy application to the present American scene.

Coontz, in his summary,[1] chides both neo-classical and Soviet demographers for neglecting the qualitative changes in the composition of the labour force which change its supply price. But Marshall at any rate did not neglect it, and in his usual half-hearted manner agreed with earlier writers like Rickards, who thought that it was precisely in the need for more skilled labour that we had one of the best possible answers to Malthusian fears. If, as Coontz claims, the essence of the increasing population phase of the early industrial revolution was that the new processes demanded ever more unskilled labour, and therefore cheaper labour, because machinery spread 'the value of man's labour power over the whole family', and because less training was required, then the decline in fertility could indeed set in with the concentration on adult male skilled labour. But the fact is, as we know, that the increase in population took place long before there was a demand for women and children in factories, which did not occur until after 1820, and the increase also took place in areas where there were no factories. It affected rural Ireland, and it takes place today in areas which have not seen machines. Moreover, the decline in fertility occurred in countries where there was no great increase in the demand for skilled labour, and no change in the economic function of the family. To those acquainted with these facts, it sounds extremely theoretical when Coontz calls further population increases in Far Eastern countries 'inconceivable' unless there are changes in the demand for labour. In practice such an increase is not merely conceivable, but highly probable.

At the end, Coontz qualifies his thesis when he says that if the productivity of labour continues to increase with skill, and if there is no institutional check to progress, then the demand for labour might continue to expand.[2] Fertility might then rise, and on the other hand

[1] Ibid., p. 188. [2] Ibid., pp. 193–4.

it might not. It would, he says, depend on social institutions. This seems to bring us back exactly where we started from, to reintroduce a method of looking at population which was previously rejected. In his introduction, he demanded that good population theory should be capable of allowing predictions. But if higher skills may or may not lead to increased fertility, depending on social organization factors, it cannot after all be that a study of economic factors will enable us to predict movements. In his final sentence Coontz allows that it may not even be in the majority of cases, at all times, that the demand for labour regulates its supply, and that if man is ever emancipated from 'exigencies arising from scarcities',[1] a new law of population might come into existence. When this happens, economics itself will cease to have much meaning, at least in the Robbinsian sense, but it is not necessary to wait until then to decide that the economic determinant is not all-powerful.

It seems therefore right to conclude that, whatever the undoubted shortcomings of some sociological population theories, it is not really possible to put the whole subject into the category of a study of effects of economic changes on social composition. On their own showing, Marshall and the Marxist revert constantly to forces which are not only, or even mainly, determined by systems of production and distribution.

Sociology and psychology

The discussion of the economist's relation to population questions also serves, by implication, to answer the question whether the techniques of sociological and psychological investigation are likely to be more appropriate in providing criteria by which to judge the sort of ideas we have listed in this book. If we say that economic changes are never in themselves enough to explain population changes, we are also saying that they can at least help. This does not mean, theoretically, that sociological explanations, by analogy, are also incapable of providing an answer unaided. In terms of our particular problem: given a certain society which is undergoing a change in its fertility pattern, can we provide a framework on a sociological basis into which we fit all the variants proper to this discipline, and can we then use this as a starting-point for empirical observations? Thus formulated, the answer is obviously affirmative. First of all, we do not now require prediction, since sociology does not claim to be scientific in this narrow sense, and secondly, since this is a comparatively new social science,

[1] Ibid., p. 195.

it has not had to operate in a vacuum where other disciplines do not exist. Therefore economic influences, just as questions of climate, or religion, are taken for granted as part of the pattern of determinants. Sociology does not have to be exclusive. It is in itself a sociological question to ask: given the difference in the fertility patterns of an English country gentleman in Malthus's time and that of a Ukrainian peasant in Lenin's, what are the influences likely to have brought about this difference? It is assumed that the answer will include evidence ranging from the biological to the theological, and from the political to the climatic, since these are the fields which make up the pattern of society as a whole. In a way then, the answer seems perfectly simple: when studying population phenomena, use exactly the same criteria as those you would use for any other sociological investigation. Ascertain the facts as far as possible according to the theoretical framework you have constructed, amend your hypothesis as you fit them into the pattern, reinvestigate where there were gaps, and continue the process until a consistent scheme emerges. Yet such an answer is evasive. We know that it is precisely the glaring imperfections of the 'ground-plan' (the Schmollerian *Grundriss*) which is at the bottom of the many partial and unbalanced views we have already presented. Whether it is Spencer's 'Social Biology' or Spengler's *Decline of the West*, in all too many cases have plausible unitary theories been put forward on scanty evidence and made to serve as explanations for all past and future variations. The modern sociologist will reply to this by saying that since then techniques have developed a great deal, and no such attempts could be made today. Yet even a quick glance at the United Nations bibliography shows how large is still the annual output of apparently serious works of the same kind. It would be invidious to single out individuals. The best compromise is probably to say that if we define sociology widely enough (and include psychology), and if we make rather few demands on the sort of theory we expect it to produce in this field, then the methods of this discipline are appropriate enough. We may even go farther and say that if sociology develops in the way ballistics and meteorology have done, with the help of electronic equipment, it may even be possible one day for sociology to be scientific in the predictive sense. That is to say, given an investigation of the factors operating in society at any given time (and that means *all* the factors), and a theory of their interaction, we may even foretell the fertility pattern of the future. One remembers that, as the students of elections have found out, that in such cases the existence of a prediction in itself becomes a factor and affects the first prediction, though this in itself does not mean that the correct prediction is theoretically impossible. Whether it will be practicable is another matter.

The study of population

In these last chapters, it was shown that the construction of a theory involves a number of distinct operations, and that the majority of investigations failed in one respect or another. Quite often the omission was on the mechanical side. Having discovered some 'correlation' between two variables, and having given this correlation a place in their general theoretical framework, authors then failed to say what was the mechanism, in terms of human decisions, which ensured the existence of the parallel or opposite movement. In economics, this study of decision-making has now been recognized for its importance in providing the link, but in population studies this side is still in confusion, partly because of the constant possibility of the existence of both voluntary decisions and biological changes. The latter loom large in anti-Malthusian literature, but usually in the shape of hypotheses only. It is when we come to such large collective efforts as the evidence placed before the Royal Commission on Population in Great Britain that we find a combination of general theory and detailed investigation into mechanisms.[1] The complexity of such work shows the difficulty of providing the forecasts which, as we have seen, are demanded from the theorizers. There is, unconsciously or consciously, still the search for *The True Law of Population.* Yet clearly such a thing is an impossibility in the present state of techniques of investigations. Since the influences on population behaviour are, *tout court,* all possible future events affecting mankind, a forecast of numbers would involve a prediction of the future course of history. If less were asked, the task might be less comprehensive, but not, for that, any easier. One needs to pause to consider the enormous variety of matters which would directly influence behaviour. We know nothing as yet, with precision, about the effect of family allowances. We know even less about the future of the Welfare State. Will Great Britain be Catholic by 1970? Will atomic radiation affect fertility? Will the world begin to eat bread deficient in Vitamin E? The survey made here, though it covers only a fraction of

[1] See E. Lewis-Faning, 'Report on an enquiry into family limitation and its influence on human fertility during the past fifty years', Royal Commission on Population, 1948–9, *Papers,* vol. 1 [Cmd. 7695].

population theories, has shown how large a range of influences was known to operate even in Malthus's time.

Yet one premature comprehensive theory after another was attempted. They have ranged from universal laws such as Sadler's or Quételet's, to those underlying some of the forecasts of population made in the 1930's. These were usually of the type where a structure 'Z' is predicted for half a century ahead, assuming factor 'A' to remain as it is, the influence of 'B' to increase at the rate of the previous ten years, and the importance of 'C' to diminish at a similar rate. The advantage of this type of theory is that it need not concern itself with the probability of the factors mentioned behaving as in the forecast, let alone of new factors appearing on the scene.

Not only have such prophecies satisfied a popular need, but they have also provided politicians with a ready-made basis for action. As we have seen, the majority of writings on population have been calls for some active policy or other (with the exception of the equilibrists, from the eighteenth-century deists to the Spencerians, who saw no need for action; and the *fainéants* Malthusians).

The task of telling us what the probabilities are—that tuberculosis bacilli will lose their potency, that there will be unemployment, or that state education will reduce parental anxieties about the welfare of their children—falls on the bacteriologist, the economist, and the sociologist. The population theorist must make use of their services if he wishes to build a comprehensive edifice. But, though the task of fitting all these data into the mosaic is the substance of demographic research, it does not amount to the work of constructing a 'single' theory of population. A flood of light may be thrown on a multitude of problems in this way, but very little can usefully be said as a result on the question of general population movements.[1]

These limitations still apply even if all we attempt is an explanation of past phenomena. To explain is to reduce to a class of events, to fit into a scheme of evolution, or refer to a general law of behaviour. We can 'explain' the growth of English population in the eighteenth century in terms of the age of enlightenment, or we can say that society passed from the preindustrial into the industrial stage, or we can formulate laws like Spencer's and fit our observations into that. The result of this process of explanation is almost always the same: if the 'law', as stated, is unquestionably 'true', it is not useful for forecasting (i.e. by a pragmatic test, good enough in practice), or if it appears to be useful

[1] See F. Lorimer, *Culture and Human Fertility* (Paris, 1954), p. 20.

(that is, so precise that it can be applied to an existing situation), it can be statistically shown to be untrue. The Malthusian progressions are an example of the first type of historical explanations, and Sadler's law, of the second, in relation to the making of a general theory.

Theory can have another meaning, however, and one that is much more appropriate to the work of population investigation. It can mean 'working hypothesis': something to start with, whether an observation taken from another field (e.g. that the higher the order of animals, the fewer their offspring) or a mere speculation. Without such theories, no investigation could hope to start. The history of ideas in our field is unfortunately rich in examples of such hypotheses elevated into general laws with the very minimum of supporting evidence. Thomas Doubleday's *True Law of Population* and its successors are cases in point.

Lastly, 'theory' may mean an analytical tool. In economics the theories of price or value are such aids to the understanding of processes. In demography occasional attempts have been made to devise similar methods, e.g. the optimum theory. These, while again valuable as starting-points, do not furnish explanations of behaviour, nor are they useful for prediction. Their employment may be justified, however, on the grounds that they provide a framework into which to fit various expositions of individual processes.

The survey of theory-making, in this section, shows the extreme difficulties with which we are faced. All the brilliant short-cuts which have illuminated other social sciences, insights leading straight to the heart of the matter, seem to have been doomed from the beginning. No Marx, no Einstein, no Keynes. Instead, a mass of polemics, and amidst the polemics, some useful pieces of information which helped to build up the present body of opinion. Some of these contributions were in the nature of inspired guesses, others were based on painstaking factual investigations from census reports, or even the bills of mortality of the seventeenth and eighteenth century.

Historical theory

The work of detailed investigation helps to establish what we usually call historical theory. It can be as ambitious as the most sweeping generalization from general premisses, but it never progresses beyond the solid achievements of the past. It has no limits, and may never be completely finished. Each age brings new variables, and it may even have, as Marx said, its own particular theory. The making of historical theory in population enlists the aid of all the other sciences we have already mentioned as contributing to the understanding of relevant processes. What results is a whole system of knowledge, but not a law. An example may show the sequence. Many observers agree that the rate of population growth tends to vary with successive stages of industrialization. There is usually first a sharp rise in the rate of increase, and then a gradual slackening off. These movements are the result of the interaction of birth-, death-, and marriage-rates. The influences which have a bearing on the situation include the general standard of living of the population, in itself the result of changes in productivity and distribution, the degree of social mobility, the spread of contraceptive practices, and so on—in fact all the influences which have formed the subject of this book. The accumulation of data on this process is not made with a view to predicting events in another country, about to undergo the process of industrialization. This would involve the construction of a time-scale, of fixing such definite values to the variables as to achieve a formula applicable under any situation. The impossibility of doing this does not detract from the value of the investigation. Its results are useful, but in the sense climatology serves a purpose: the more we know about it, the better we understand the working of the entire social and economic system.

The defence of this method of building up knowledge would now seem unnecessary in other fields of the social sciences. But in the field of population theory, the tradition of the inspired guess and the search for the universal law dies hard.[1] Since experiments are ruled out, and historical statistics suspect, the more painful method of piecemeal investigation still seems to many writers to be as unnecessary as to Malthus's earliest opponents.

For these necessary inquiries there was, for a long time, not even a clear ground-plan. Schmoller, the chief exponent of the historical method in the last century, laid great stress on this *Grundriss* on which he would fit the data, survey the gaps, and arrange for new investigations to fill them. Nobody asked questions covering the whole field. Sectional interest, political necessity, and lack of scientific training produced a situation where not even the vocabulary of population studies achieved any sort of unity. Various meanings were attached to

[1] See L. Hogben, ed., *Political Arithmetic* (London, 1938), Preface, pp. 18 ff., where he attacks the sort of attitude typified by a sentence he quotes from Lionel Robbins, 'that the truth of a particular theory is a matter of logical derivation from the general assumptions of the subject'. Economic theory, Robbins had said, did not rest on appeals to history, or the results of controlled experiments.

such words as voluntary, moral, and prudential restraint. Fecundity and fertility, baptism and birth-rates, were used imprecisely. Order came late into the chaos. Even today the student reading his population theory successively in works on sociology, statistics, economics, genetics, social medicine and administration, geography and history is apt to think he is not dealing with one subject. Only fairly recently have demographers with wide training in the social sciences produced works of extensive analysis without appearing to labour under a compulsion to produce a comprehensive theory. The facts of the behaviour of human beings are even now only partially known. But the ethics behind that behaviour (to use Mackenroth's distinction) are still an uncharted field. Facts can be discovered from census reports and vital statistics—ethics require a questionnaire. Since the processes which lead to marriage and reproduction were not, until a generation or so ago, subjects of polite conversation, most writers were forced either to write from their own experience, or, more often, to make guesses as to other people's motives.

Yet it is precisely here, in the field of the ethics of human reproduction, that we may hope to find the true nature of the checks to population. Malthus could only say that sexual urges were strong, and all other influences feeble in comparison (though he would admit that reason had some modifying effect). Godwin was sure that in a different society there would be less interest in sex. Both men were guessing. So were most of the others who wrote about the factors affecting voluntary restraint. But inquiries into differential fertility, beginning round about 1900, gradually established 'the facts about the ethics'.

The inherent vice

It remains to ask, after presenting the history of these theories and the difficulties which have been faced, why the field of population should be bedevilled, to such a high degree, by aberrations of the kind enumerated. The physicist or mathematician may well consider it superfluous to go into these matters—the flat-earthers are a lunatic fringe and hardly worth a footnote. The economist may devote part of an appendix to Social Credit, and the historian knows of peculiar sects and strange messiahs. It is obviously otherwise in population. The camps of warring factions are more equally divided, both as to numbers and academic respectability. Some apparently absurd views found a ready following amongst respectable people, and eventually were found, by great scholars, to contain more than a grain of truth. Why should this be so?

The most charitable explanation is that it is necessarily so because population studies stand at the very centre of the social and moral sciences, in the sense that the numbers of mankind are the result of, and influence, all other movements in society, and are affected by considerations which form the subject of all other disciples. Although economics, for instance, has close relations with sociology and law, its connexion with biology, medicine, and religion is probably tenuous. The movements of population, on the other hand, cannot be separated from the totality of human institutions and beliefs, or physical manifestations affecting human beings.[1]

It means, amongst other things, that it is difficult to say much of substance about population without touching on emotional and political questions. How can one discuss the population of Ireland without reference to the English landlords or the influence of the Catholic Church? It may well be said that the historian of political questions, such as Home Rule or Free Trade, also faces subjects once the topics of emotional controversy. But it is infinitely easier to give an account of them at a short distance from the time at which they were topical, without necessarily taking sides or stirring up deep-rooted prejudices. The essence of the problem in our field is that it continues, and that it personally concerns everyone.

Another way of putting this difficulty is to say that population studies are basically concerned with primitive instincts—so primitive, so remote and fierce, and yet so near to consciousness, that the objectivity of any human (and therefore by definition directly involved) observer must always be in doubt unless he is content to describe facts. But, as we have seen, the challenge has lain in the ethics. The concern with human reproduction, as anthropologists have explained, is at the core of organization in human societies—openly in primitive tribes, suppressed but none the less real in modern states. One need not be a wholehearted follower of Briffault, or a Freudian, to know this to be true.

For this reason, Stangeland and other systematic historians of population theories have usually listed the first stage of opinion as being 'theological'. The priests were the first in the field, and have never quite left it, from the days of phallic worship to strictures on Family Planning

[1] This view is strongly urged by, amongst others, A. Messedaglia and F. S. Nitti; see C. E. Stangeland, *Pre-Malthusian Doctrines of Population; a Study in the History of Economic Theory* (New York, 1904), Introduction, pp. 13–14.

Clinics or even a Health Service. Starting with the biblical injunction 'Be fruitful and multiply', and the explanations which have been given for the phrase, there have been numerous parsons in the subject. Most of them, as Marx noted, were Protestants. (He took them to task for contributing to the increase of population to an unbecoming extent.) This, as we have shown, was the natural result of preoccupation with the *natural* order. The feeling that human beings, like the stars, should conform to an orderly pattern of movement was responsible for some of the early equilibrist theories. Even Malthus, inspired by Süßmilch, may have been attracted by the need to explain the system behind the chaos. Here, then, is one deep-rooted reason for the difficulties in ridding population studies of their inherent vices.

A similar difficulty exists in the next stages of the development of theories, dominated by politics and metaphysics. Beliefs about what population does have always been mixed up with what population must do in order to achieve other ends. This connexion may have had its origins in the Platonists' ideal of a *polis* with a fixed number of inhabitants—a sort of primitive optimum theory based more on political than on economic considerations. This inevitably involves control—encouragement if population falls short of the ideal, and, as Aristotle showed, rather extreme measures to keep it down if it exceeds the maximum. On suppositions of this sort were based the laws of Macedonia and Imperial Rome. We find strong political action in the Mercantilist era, in Nazi Germany, and in modern France. To say this is not to deny that those who fashioned policy would also seek to explain why population did not conform to the desired standard. But there must be an inherent bias. The explanation would need to justify the predetermined policy.[1]

The opinions of the Mercantilists and the policies they urged on governments to counteract the supposed decline in population are particularly interesting in this respect. What contribution was made by their theories regarding luxuries, towns, and religion we have already seen. Some measures they advocated were of the nature of mild encouragement, others rather sterner attempts to suppress undesirable practices. Naturally they aroused the fiercest controversies amongst the interested parties. The measures advocated by the Malthusians, if not by Malthus himself, culminating in the call to infanticide by the possibly

[1] This was the special skill of the Nazi apologists. See T. Valentiner, 'Die seelischen Ursachen des Geburtenrückganges', *Politische Biologie, Schriften für naturgesetzliche Politik und Wissenschaft* (München–Berlin, 1937), Heft 2.

spurious Marcus, caused even more violent battles.[1] Both sides claimed to be humanitarians, and both were inclined to call the other murderous. Later, the clamour subsided somewhat, but the twentieth-century reader familiar with the attacks of the popular press on those who utter warnings of coming over-population, or of the modern Marxists and Catholics on the Malthusians,[2] will know that passions can yet be inflamed by the fundamental issues of the debate.

There remains one further deep-seated reason why the history of population theories can show so much more prejudice than science. Many of the earliest views on the factors affecting fertility show signs of having originated from folk-lore. High living causes sterility: aristocracies die out, towns are graveyards, the countryside teemeth with men. Intellectual pursuits and gallantry diminish powers of procreation, whores cannot conceive. Idiots breed like rabbits. Such ideas were learned, we may surmise, by writers in their youth, and they found it hard to rid themselves of such beliefs. Scientific investigations partially confirmed these views, and this helped to keep them alive in their cruder forms. Some of the notions involved must be as old as mankind itself. One has only to read the younger Pliny on the subject of fertility to realize that superstition was a powerful regulator of marriage and the marriage-bed. Juvenal's golden couch and Paley's rice-eaters, Hippocrates' soft airs and the boots that help to beget a male child—all these form part of a powerful web of superstition. Students of medical history will recognize the prevalence of similar influences in their field until comparatively recent times—with this one important difference, that there the study of anatomy and physiology, as well as the possibility of experiments, presented an opportunity to damn the most outrageous views one by one. No such chance arose on the subject of population. While country doctors may still have practised something akin to witchcraft, the metropolitan faculties were already well on the way to the understanding of the therapeutical properties of organic and inorganic substances. Though inoculation and vaccination and anaesthetics were the topics of violent public disputes, they did at least find fairly united support from medical experts in time, and had to be defended mainly against theological and lay opinion. Amongst population experts, there was no such majority view. In other fields, Darwinists and Mendelians had to undergo their

[1] On Marcus, see H. A. Boner, *Hungry Generations; the Nineteenth-Century Case Against Malthusianism* (New York, 1955), p. 138, and notes, p. 213.

[2] See, for instance, Meek, op. cit., on Voigt, pp. 40–42.

period of public hostility and trial. Though they offended, at first, against deeply held religious or ethical beliefs, they did not strike at the roots of ordinary men's experiences and views as effectively as did Malthus or the neo-Malthusians.

To sum up the difficulties, of their own making and provided by others, which faced the writers on population who have formed the subject of this book, it is useful to quote Gustav Schmoller again:

> By cloaking propositions as 'laws', one gives them an appearance of necessity which they do not possess, or one gives too high an importance to comparatively insignificant truths, thereby misleading those who apply them. . . . One may attempt to set out some general formula of economic progress, or even of human progress in general. But one is then in the realm of the philosophy of history, of teleology, prophecy, hopes and forebodings. The broader the basis of knowledge on which such attempts are based, the greater value they will have. Bold syntheses of this kind will always be necessary for the purposes of practical action, and it need not be held against the genuine prophets of the day when they believe they have found a 'law of development'. Herbert Spencer and the theorists of social development, Mill and Comte, have attempted such formulae, as have the socialists and the 'Manchester' liberals. This sort of thing will, however, always remain far removed from what the natural scientist calls laws. . . .[1]

In our field, the excuse for studying the views of these precursors of modern theory is not only that they have a right to exist, a place in the scheme of things. It is rather that their ideas are so closely based on the events and preconceptions of their own times, that they form a valuable aid to the study of the social and economic development. The writings of Ferguson or Alison in Scotland, of Richard Jones or T. R. Edmonds in England, enable us to form some opinion of the impact of political and industrial changes in these countries. Moreover, they made a contribution to something that forms an integral part of the modern body of theory. Godwin and Condorcet interest the historians of the revolutionary and romantic periods, but their connexion with modern political theory is remote. Those who began to discern the powerful preventive checks to population were the founders of the modern sociological approach to the determination of population size.

To appraise the contribution of some is to understand the history of their time. To trace the origins of the aberration of others is to help us to rid our own thinking of prejudice. The debate on Malthus is not ended.

[1] Quoted in T. H. Hutchison, *A Review of Economic Doctrines, 1870–1929* (Oxford, 1953), p. 182.

Conclusion: the standard-of-living theory

We started this book by stating a consensus of modern opinion that the decline of fertility in Western countries in the last century has been caused by developments which we can summarize under the headings of material conditions, political institutions, and social organization, or, more traditionally, the standard of living, democracy, and civilization. This is the 'standard-of-living theory' for short. Having stated what is meant by theory, and having shown the inadequacies of many past attempts to work consistently in this field, we must now ask ourselves: does this widely held opinion amount to anything at all? In other words, is this only a convenient first approximation to an explanation of past behaviour, or is this the core of a population theory as such? For Coontz, the answer is obviously that it is less than either of these things. But even a more charitable observer feels bound to ask whether, for instance, the rising fertility of the United States since the depression is not so incapable of reconciliation with the whole or the part of the 'theory' as to invalidate it completely. The failure of the Marxist system to account for the rise in real wages (not even salvaged by the concept of relative proletarianization) is hardly greater than the failure of the culture and prosperity theories to account for the larger families of modern North American experience (not even salvaged by such ingenious ideas as that children may constitute part of a higher standard of living in the way that refrigerators and motor-cars were formerly regarded).

Reluctantly, the historian must at this stage decide that he is not competent to judge these present issues. It seems clear enough from the evidence cited in this book, that the connexion, *in the past*, at any rate in Western countries, between changing patterns of social and economic organization and changing patterns of fertility, was real enough. As living standards have improved, so fertility has gone down, and the two sets of observations are so linked as to warrant the assumption of continuous interaction. But more cannot easily be claimed. The description of the theories and their relation to historical events has, one hopes, illuminated both to some extent. But it remains, in perspective, a very partial description. At best, it must be regarded as a contribution towards the formulation of a theory. If one criticizes those who can only see one set of connexions, like Doubleday or Le Play, one must also concede that the whole apparatus of standard-of-living theories here described is in turn no more than a part of a vast whole. Quite obviously, if there is ever to be 'theory of population', it will have to take into account not only all the observations that formed part of the more scholarly of these particular theories, but also all the observations that could not have fitted into this framework, and the evidence of the economists, and other specialists.

No general rule can therefore be derived. We cannot feel convinced by our authors that there is a natural law of the standard of living, either in the simple sense that each society has a threshold of well-being beyond which people exercise foresight, or in a more complex system whereby the fact of progress in society as a whole makes its members wish to control their fertility. But we can be quite certain that during the great upheavals of the last 150 years, the consciousness of a connexion between the circumstances of human life and the levels of fertility arose in the minds not only of theorizers and cranks, but also, indirectly, out of the subconscious levels of popular belief. These social theories should be taken, therefore, not as important constituent parts of modern demography (although they are obviously treated as such by some scholars), but as additional evidence for the nature of the changes themselves. The Malthusian problem stood at the very centre of these changes, and the debate which started from his work contains within it not only the nature of the response to the break-up of the old society, but also the seeds of the reforms which eventually overcame the evils of the transition.

BIBLIOGRAPHY

Section I. *Books and articles published before 1900.*
Population theory and other works containing observations on population matters.

(*Note.* Greek and Latin authors, the Bible, and works of fiction omitted, since reference may normally be made to these authorities without the help of full publication details.)

Section II. *Books and articles published after 1900.*
Population theory and sociology.

(Fiction omitted.)

Section III. *Books on the history of population theories, and historical treatises containing references to theories.*

Section IV. *Articles in periodicals on the history of population theories.*

Note on editions: Except where more than one edition had to be used owing to important differences in text, only the edition actually quoted has been given here. In the case of Malthus's *Essay*, the dates of the second and subsequent editions have not been given here. The date of the first edition is also given where the one used has been a recent reissue.

SECTION I

BOOKS AND ARTICLES PUBLISHED BEFORE 1900

POPULATION THEORY AND OTHER WORKS CONTAINING OBSERVATIONS ON POPULATION MATTERS

Sir A. Alison, *The Principles of Population and Their Connection with Human Happiness* (Edinburgh, 1840, 2 vols.).

C. F. J. Auxiron, *Principes de tout gouvernment, ou Examen des causes de la splendeur ou de la foiblesse de tout état considéré en lui-même, et indépendamment des moeurs* (Paris, 1766, 2 vols.).

F. Bacon, *Works* (B. Montagu, ed., London, 1834, 15 vols.).

W. Bagehot, *Economic Studies* (R. H. Hutton, ed., London, 1888).

—— *Physics and Politics, or Thoughts on the Application of the Principles of 'Natural Selection' and 'Inheritance' to Political Society* (new ed., London, 1885).

A. H. Bailey and A. Day, 'On the Rate of Mortality Prevailing amongst the Families of the Peerage during the Nineteenth Century', *Journal of the Royal Statistical Society* (1863), xxvi. 49–71.

F. Bastiat, *Harmonies économiques* (2nd ed., Paris, 1851).

—— *Harmonies of Political Economy* (Edinburgh, 1880 ed.).

A. Bebel, *Die Frau und der Sozialismus* (1883; Stuttgart, 1911 ed.).

C. Beccaria, Marchese de Bonesana, 'Della popolazione', *Elementi di economia pubblica* (1769).

W. Bell, *A Dissertation on the Following Subject: What Causes Principally Contribute to Render a Nation Populous? And What Effect Has the Populousness of a Nation on its Trade?* (Cambridge, 1756).

K. J. Beloch, *Die Bevölkerung der griechisch-römischen Welt* (Leipzig, 1886).

A. Bertillon, 'Natalité', in *Dictionnaire encyclopédique des sciences médicales* (Paris, *c.* 1874).

G. Botero, *The Reason of State* (with a subsection, *A Treatise concerning Causes of the Magnificency and Greatness of Cities* (Robert Peterson, trans., 1606), P. J. and D. P. Waley, trans. and eds. (London, 1956).)

J. Brown, *An Estimate of the Manners and Principles of the Times* (2nd ed., London, 1757).

L. G. du Buat-Nançay, *Eléments de la politique; ou recherche des vrais principes de l'économie sociale* (London, 1773, 6 vols.).

Dr. W. Buchan, *Domestic Medicine; or, a Treatise on the Prevention and Cure of Diseases, by Regimen and Simple Medicines . . .* (1763; new ed., London, 1880).

J. G. Büsch, *Vermischte Abhandlungen, 2. Teil: Von dem Schaden für die Bevölkerung durch die Menge der Säugeammen* (Hamburg, 1777).

A. de Candolle, *Histoire des sciences et des savants depuis deux siècles, suivi d'autres études sur des sujets scientifiques en particulier sur la sélection dans l'espèce humaine* (Geneva, 1873).

R. Cantillon, *Essai sur la nature du commerce–général* (Paris, 1755; edited with an English translation . . . by H. Higgs (London, 1931)).

H. C. Carey, *Principles of Social Science* (Philadelphia, 1858–60, 3 vols.).

T. Chalmers, *On Political Economy, in Connexion with the Moral State and Moral Prospects of Society* (2nd ed., Glasgow, 1832).

B. de Chateauneuf, 'De la durée des familles nobles en France', *Académie des Sciences morales et politiques* (Paris, 1845).

M.-J.-A.-N. de Caritat, Marquis de Condorcet, *Sketch for a Historical Picture of the Progress of the Human Mind* (1795; J. Barraclough, trans., London, 1955).

N. Plumard de Danguel, *Remarques sur les avantages et les désavantages de la France et de la Grande Bretagne . . . etc.* (Leyden, 1754).

C. D'Avenant, *An Essay upon the Probable Methods of Making a People Gainers in the Ballance of Trade* (London, 1699).

W. Derham, *Physico-theology; or, A Demonstration of the Being and Attributes of God from His Works of Creation . . . etc.* (6th ed., London, 1723).

T. DOUBLEDAY, *The True Law of Population, Shewn to Be Connected with the Food of the People* (3rd ed., London, 1853).

J. K. L. [J. DOYLE], Bishop of Kildare and Leitrim, *Letters on the State of Ireland, Addressed by J. K. L. to a Friend in England* (Dublin, 1825).

A. DUMONT, *Dépopulation et civilisation. Etude démographique* (Paris, 1890).

[T. R. EDMONDS], *An Enquiry into the Principles of Population, Exhibiting a System of Regulations for the Poor; Designed Immediately to Lessen, and Finally To Remove, the Evils Which Have Hitherto Pressed upon the Labouring Classes of Society* (London, 1832).

—— *Practical, Moral and Political Economy . . . etc.* (London, 1828).

E. ENGEL, 'Über die Bedeutung der Bevölkerungsstatistik mit besonderer Beziehung auf die diesjährige Volkszählung und Produktions- und Konsumtionsstatistik im Königreich Sachsen', *Zeitschrift des Statistischen Bureaus des Königlich Sächsischen Ministeriums des Innern* (1. Jahrg., 1855).

G. ENSOR, *An Inquiry concerning the Population of Nations: Containing a Refutation of Mr. Malthus' 'Essay on Population'* (London, 1818).

A. FERGUSON, *An Essay on the History of Civil Society* (4th ed., London, 1773).

F. V. DE FORBONNAIS, *Elémens du commerce* (2nd ed., Leyden, 1754).

F. M. C. FOURIER, *Le Nouveau Monde industriel et sociétaire* (Brussels, 1840 ed.).

B. FRANKLIN, *The Complete Works, in Philosophy, Politics, and Morals, . . . with Memoirs of His Early Life, Written by Himself* (London, 1806, 3 vols.).

F. GALTON, 'The Relative Supplies from Town and Country Families to the Population of Future Generations', *Journal of the Royal Statistical Society* (1873), xxxvi. 19–26.

A. GEISSLER, 'Über den Einfluss der Säuglingssterblichkeit auf die eheliche Fruchtbarkeit, mit besonderer Berücksichtigung der Ehen im Bergmannsstande', *Zeitschrift des Statistischen Bureaus des Königreichs Sachsen* (Dresden, 1885), xxxi. 23.

C. GIDE, *Principes d'économie politique* (3rd ed., Paris, 1891).

W. GODWIN, *Thoughts occasioned by the Perusal of Dr. Parr's Spital Sermon, preached at Christ Church, April 15, 1800* (London, 1801).

A. DE GOUDAR, *Les Intérêts de la France mal entendus* (Amsterdam, 1757, 3 vols.).

J. GRAHAME, *An Inquiry into the Principle of Population: Including an Exposition of the Causes and the Advantages of a Tendency to Exuberance of Numbers in Society, a Defence of the Poor-Laws, and a Critical and Historical View of the Doctrines and Projects of the Most Celebrated Legislators and Writers, Relative to Population, the Poor, and Charitable Establishments* (Edinburgh and London, 1816).

J. GRAUNT, *Natural and Political Observations made upon the Bills of Mortality* (London, 1662; Baltimore, 1939, reprint).

S. GRAY, *The Happiness of States: or an Inquiry concerning Population, the Modes of Subsisting and Employing it, and the Effects of All on Happiness: in which is Developed the New or Productive System of Statistics* (2nd ed., London, 1819).

C. HALL, *The Effects of Civilisation on the People in European States* (with Appendix: 'Observations on the Principal Conclusion in Mr. Malthus' "Essay on Population" ') (London, 1805).

R. HAMILTON, *The Progress of Society* (London, 1830).

G. HANSSEN, *Die drei Bevölkerungsstufen. Ein Versuch, die Ursachen für das Blühen und Altern der Völker nachzuweisen* (Munich, 1889).

C. J. HERBERT, *Essai sur la police générale des grains, sur leurs prix, et sur les effets d'agriculture* (Berlin, 1755 ed.).

W. E. HICKSON, *Malthus; an Essay on the Principle of Population, in Refutation of the Theory of the Rev. T. R. Malthus* (London, 1849).

J. E. HORN, *Bevölkerungswissenschaftliche Studien aus Belgien* (Leipzig, 1854).

D. HUME, 'Of the Populousness of Ancient Nations', *Essays and Treatises on Several Subjects* (1742; new ed., Edinburgh, 1825, 2 vols.), Essay XI, pp. 373–443.

SIR F. D'IVERNOIS, *Matériaux pour aider à la recherche des effets ... du morcellement de la propriété foncière en France* (Geneva and Paris, 1826).

—— *Sur la mortalité proportionnelle de quelques populations, considérée comme mesure de leur aisance et de leur civilisation* (Geneva, 1832).

—— *Enquête sur les causes patentes ou occultes de la faible proportion des naissances à Montreux* (Geneva, 1837).

P. JACOBY and G. DELAUNAY, 'La Fécondité', *Revue Scientifique* (Oct. 1885).

T. JARROLD, *Dissertations on Man, Philosophical, Physiological, and Political; in Answer to Mr. Malthus' 'Essay on the Principle of Population'* (London, 1806).

R. JONES, *Literary Remains, Consisting of Lectures and Tracts on Political Economy* (W. Whewell and Cazenove, eds., London, 1859).

P. JÖRS, 'Die Ehegesetze des Augustus', *Festschrift, Theodor Mommsen zum 50-jährigen Doctorjubiläum überreicht von Paul Jörs* (Marburg, 1893).

ANAXAGORAS VON OCCIDENT [i.e. J. H. G. VON JUSTI], *Physicalische und politische Betrachtungen über die Erzeugung des Menschen und Bevölkerung der Länder* (Smirna, i.e. Karlsruhe, 1769).

K. KAUTSKY, *Der Einfluss der Volksvermehrung auf den Fortschritt der Gesellschaft* (Vienna, 1880).

S. LAING (the elder), *Notes of a Traveller on the Social and Political State of France, Prussia, Switzerland, Italy, and other Parts of Europe, during the Present Century* (2nd ed., London, 1842).

—— *Observations on the Social and Political State of the European People in 1848 and 1849, in 'Notes of a Traveller'* (Series 2, London, 1850).

S. LAING (the younger), *National Distress: its Causes and Remedies* (London, 1844).

BARON E. DE LAVELEYE, *Luxury* (2nd ed., London, 1891).

F. Le Play, *La Réforme sociale en France déduite de l'observation comparée des peuples européens* (Paris, 1866, 4 vols.).

E. Levasseur, *La Population française . . . etc.* (Paris, 1889–92, 3 vols.).

W. F. Lloyd, *Two Lectures on the Checks to Population, Delivered before the University of Oxford in Michaelmas Term, 1832* (Oxford, 1833).

A. Loria, *La Legge di popolazione ed il sistema sociale* (Siena, 1882).

C. Loudon, *The Equilibrium of Population and Sustenance Demonstrated, Showing, on Physiological and Statistical Grounds, the Means of Obviating the Fears of the Late Mr. Malthus and His Followers* (Leamington Spa, 1836).

J. Lowe, *The Present State of England in regard to Agriculture, Trade, and Finance . . . etc.* (2nd ed., London, 1823).

J. R. McCulloch, *The Principles of Political Economy* (new ed., Edinburgh, 1843).

[T. R. Malthus], *An Essay on the Principle of Population* (London, 1798).

—— *An Essay on the Principle of Population* (1803 ff., Everyman ed., London, 1914, 2 vols.).

—— *Principles of Political Economy considered with a view to their practical application* (1820; 2nd ed., London, 1836).

—— *A Summary View of the Principle of Population* (London, 1830; reprinted in *Introduction to Malthus* (D. V. Glass, ed., London, 1953)).

J. F. Melon, *Essai politique sur le commerce* (Paris, 1736).

J. Mill, 'Colony', *Encyclopaedia Britannica Supplement* (5th ed., 1818).

J. S. Mill, *Principles of Political Economy . . . etc.* (1848; 6th ed., London, 1902).

—— *The Subjection of Women* (2nd ed., London, 1869).

V. Riquetti, Marquis de Mirabeau, *L'Ami des hommes, ou traité de la population* (Avignon, 1758, 3 parts).

M. Moheau [i.e. A. de Montyon], *Recherches et considérations sur la population de la France* (Paris, 1778).

R. v. Mohl, *Die Polizeiwissenschaft nach den Grundsätzen des Rechtsstaates* (Tübingen, 1866, 3 vols.).

C. de Secondat, Baron de Montesquieu, *Lettres persanes* (Paris, 1721; J. Davidson, ed. and trans., London, 1922)).

—— *De L'Esprit des lois* (*Œuvres complètes de Montesquieu*, E. Laboulaye, ed., Paris, 1877, tome v).

A. H. Moreton, *Civilization, or a Brief Analysis of the Natural Laws that Regulate the Numbers and Conditions of Mankind* (London, 1836).

F. Müller-Lyer, *The Evolution of Modern Marriage . . . etc.* (Isabella C. Wigglesworth, trans., London, 1930).

M. Muret, *Mémoires, etc., par la Société Economique de Berne* (1766).

B. G. Niebuhr, *Römische Geschichte* (Berlin, 1828–32).

F. S. Nitti, *Population and the Social System* (English ed., London, 1894).

A. von Öttingen, *Die Moralstatistik in ihrer Bedeutung für eine Socialethik* (3rd ed., Erlangen, 1882).

G. M. Ortes, *Riflessioni sulla popolazione delle nazioni per rapporto all' economia nazionale* (Venice, 1790).

W. Paley, *The Principles of Moral and Political Philosophy* (9th ed., London, 1793, 2 vols.).

The Pamphleteer (anon.) (A. J. Valpy, ed., London, 1813–28, 29 vols.).

British Parliamentary Papers: Report of House of Commons Committee on the state of the Circulation in Promissory Notes under £5 in Scotland and Ireland (1826) [421].

British Parliamentary Papers: Three Reports of the Commissioners on the Condition of the Poorer Classes in Ireland, the various Institutions established by Law for their Relief, and the further Remedial Measures for ameliorating the Condition of the Irish Poor (1835–36), [5818].

British Parliamentary Papers: Report from the Poor Law Commissioners on an Inquiry into the Sanitary Condition of the Labouring Population of Great Britain (HL., 1842; Edwin Chadwick, Secretary), [6682].

H. Passy, 'De la division des héritages et de l'influence qu'elle exerce sur la distribution des richesses', *L'Académie des Sciences morales et politiques* (2e série, 1839), tome ii.

Sir W. Petty, *Another Essay in Political Arithmetick, Concerning the Growth of the City of London . . . etc.* (London, 1682, in *Economic Writings*, C. H. Hull, ed. (Cambridge, 1899, 2 vols.), ii).

F. Place, *Illustrations and Proofs of the Principle of Population, Including an Examination of the Proposed Remedies of Mr. Malthus and a Reply to the Objections of Mr. Godwin and others* (1822; N. Himes, ed., London, 1930).

R. von Pöhlmann, *Die Übervölkerung der antiken Großstädte in Zusammenhange mit der Gesammtentwicklung städtischer Civilisation dargestellt* (Leipzig, 1884).

P. J. Proudhon, *De la Justice dans la révolution et dans l'église* (Paris, 1858).

G. Purves [Simon Gray], *Gray versus Malthus. The Principles of Population and Production Investigated, and the Questions: Does Population Regulate Subsistence, or Subsistence Population . . . etc. Discussed* (London and Edinburgh, 1818).

L. A. J. Quételet, *Sur l'Homme et le développement de ses facultés, ou, Essai de physique sociale* (Brussels, 1836).

D. Ricardo, *Principles of Political Economy and Taxation* (London, 1821; 1895 ed.).

Sir G. Rickards, *Population and Capital: Being a Course of Lectures Delivered before the University of Oxford in 1853–54* (London, 1854).

W. Roscher, *Principles of Political Economy* (New York, 1878, 2 vols.).

Count P. Rossi, *Cours d'économie politique* (Brussels, 1840–2).

J. J. ROUSSEAU, *Political Writings* (C. E. Vaughan, ed., Cambridge, 1915, 2 vols.).

M. T. SADLER, *The Law of Population: a Treatise in Six Books; in Disproof of the Super-fecundity of Human Beings, and Developing the Real Principle of their Increase* (London, 1830, 2 vols.).

H. M. MARSHAL DE SAXE, *Reveries, or, Memoirs concerning the Art of War . . .* (Edinburgh, 1776 ed.).

M. SCHIPPEL, *Das moderne Elend und die moderne Übervölkerung* (Leipzig, 1883).

F. SCHMIDT, *Untersuchungen über Bevölkerung, Arbeitslohn und Pauperismus, in ihrem gegenseitigen Zusammenhange* (Leipzig, 1836).

L. A. G. SCHRADER, *Grundgesetze der Natur in der Geburt, dem Leben und Tode der Menschen, als ein freyer Auszug, aus Süßmilchs Göttlicher Ordnung in den Veränderungen des menschlichen Geschlechtes . . . in veränderter Ordnung entworfen* (Glückstadt, 1777).

N. W. SENIOR, *Two Lectures on Population, Delivered before the University of Oxford in Easter Term, 1828, to which is added a Correspondence between the Author and the Rev. T. R. Malthus* (London, 1831).

—— *An Outline of the Science of Political Economy* (London, 1938 ed.).

T. SHORT, *New Observations, Natural, Moral, Civil, Political, and Medical on City, Town, and Country Bills of Mortality . . . etc.* (London, 1750).

—— *A Comparative History of the Increase and Decrease of Mankind in England and Several Countries abroad . . . etc.* (London, 1767).

J. C. L. S. DE SISMONDI, *Les Nouveaux Principes d'économie politique ou de la richesse dans ses rapports avec la population* (2nd ed., Paris, 1827).

A. SMITH, *An Inquiry into the Nature and Causes of the Wealth of Nations* (1776; E. Cannan, ed., New York, 1937).

H. SÖTBEER, *Die Stellung der Sozialisten zur Malthusischen Bevölkerungslehre* (Göttingen, 1886).

H. SPENCER, *A New Theory of Population, Deduced from the General Law of Animal Fertility* (reprinted from *Westminster Review*, vol. xvii, New York, 1852).

—— *The Principles of Biology. A System of Philosophy* (London, 1899, 2 vols.; vol. 3 of *A System of Synthetic Philosophy*, 11 vols.).

SIR J. STEUART, *An Inquiry into the Principles of Political Economy: Being an Essay on the Science of Domestic Policy in Free Nations, in Which Are Particularly Considered Population, Agriculture, Trade, Industry, Money, Corn, Interest, Circulation, Banks, Exchange, Public Credit and Taxes* (London, 1767, 2 vols.).

J. P. SÜßMILCH, *Die göttliche Ordnung in den Veränderungen des menschlichen Geschlechts aus der Geburt, dem Tode und der Fortpflanzung desselben erwiesen* (Berlin, 1775, 3 vols.).

J. V. TALLQVIST, *Recherches statistiques sur la tendance à une moindre fécondité des mariages* (Helsingfors, 1886).

SIR W. TEMPLE, *The Works of Sir William Temple*, 'Of Popular Discontents' (new ed., London, 1757, 4 vols.).

I . . . B . . . (M.D.) [i.e. W. TEMPLE], *A Vindication of Commerce and the Arts, proving that they are the Source of the Greatness, Power, Riches and Populousness of a State, Being an Examination of Mr. Bell's Dissertation upon Populousness, read in the schools and honoured with the Lord Viscount Townshend's Prize, by the University of Cambridge, wherein Mr. Bell's calumnies on trade are answered, his arguments refuted, his system exploded, and the principal causes of populosity assigned* (London, 1768; reprinted in *A Select Collection of Scarce and Valuable Tracts on Commerce* (J. McCulloch, ed., London, 1859)).

W. THOMPSON, *An Inquiry into the Principles of the Distribution of Wealth Most Conducive to Human Happiness; Applied to the Newly Proposed System of Voluntary Equality of Wealth* (London, 1824).

W. T. THORNTON, *Over-population and its Remedy; or, An Inquiry into the Extent and Causes of the Distress Prevailing among the Labouring Classes of the British Islands, and into the Means of Remedying it* (London, 1846).

—— *A Plea for Peasant Proprietors, with the Outlines of a Plan for Their Establishment in Ireland* (London, 1848).

R. TORRENS, *An Essay on the Influence of the External Corn Trade upon the Production and Distribution of National Wealth . . . etc.* (2nd ed., London, 1820).

J. TOWNSEND, *Dissertation on the Poor Laws* (London, 1817 ed.).

A. URE, *The Philosophy of Manufactures: Or, an Exposition of the Scientific, Moral, and Commercial Economy of the Factory System of Great Britain* (3rd ed., London, 1861).

G. S. DEL VECCHIO, *Gli Analfabeti e le nascite nelle varie parti d'Italia* (1894).

P. F. VERHULST, 'Recherches mathématiques sur la loi d'accroissement de la population', *Nouveaux mémoires de l'Académie royale des sciences et belles-lettres de Bruxelles* (Brussels, 1845), xviii. 1–38.

F. VILLANO, *L'ozio autunnale, ovvero discorsi economici politici* (Naples, 1768).

R. WALLACE, *A Dissertation on the Numbers of Mankind in Ancient and Modern Times* (2nd ed., Edinburgh, 1809).

J. E. WAPPÄUS, *Allgemeine Bevölkerungsstatistik* (1859, 2 vols.).

J. WEYLAND, jnr., *The Principles of Population and Production as they are affected by the Progress of Society, with a View to Moral and Political Consequences* (London, 1816).

SECTION II

BOOKS AND ARTICLES PUBLISHED AFTER 1900

POPULATION THEORY AND SOCIOLOGY

J. BERTILLON, *La Dépopulation de la France . . . etc.* (Paris, 1911).

A. BLUHM, 'Zur Frage nach der generativen Tüchtigkeit der deutschen Frauen und der rassenhygienischen Bedeutung der ärztlichen Geburtshilfe', *Archiv für Rassen- und Gesellschaftsbiologie* (July–Aug. 1912), ix. 454–74.

S. Budge, *Das Malthus'sche Bevölkerungsgesetz und die theoretische Nationalökonomie der letzten Jahrzehnte* (Karlsruhe, 1912).

J. de Castro, *Geography of Hunger* (London, 1952).

G. Cauderlier, *Les Lois de la population en France* (Paris, 1902).

J. Conrad, *Grundriss zum Studium der politischen Ökonomie* (6th ed., Jena, 1909–13).

S. H. Coontz *Population Theories and the Economic Interpretation* (London, 1957).

L. Dumas, *Le Socialisme et le principe de population* (Paris, 1908).

L. Elster, in: 'Bevölkerungswesen', *Handwörterbuch der Staatswissenschaften* (4th ed., Jena, 1924), ii. 687 ff.

P. E. Fahlbeck, 'La Décadence et la chute des peuples', *Bulletin de l'Institut international de statistique* (Rome, 1900), xv. 367 ff.

—— *Der Adel Schwedens (und Finlands). Eine demographische Studie* (Jena, 1903).

J. A. Field, *Essays on Population and other Papers* (H. F. Hohman, ed. and comp., Chicago, 1931).

D. V. Glass, *Population: Policies and Movements in Europe* (Oxford, 1940).

J. Goldstein, *Bevölkerungsprobleme und Berufsgliederung in Frankreich* (Berlin, 1900).

F. H. Hankins, 'Does Advancing Civilisation Involve a Decline in Natural Fertility?', *Publications of the American Sociology Society* (May 1930), xxiv, no. 2, pp. 115–22.

—— 'Has the Reproductive Power of Western Peoples Declined?', *Problems of Population . . . etc.* (G. H. L. F. Pitt-Rivers, ed., London, 1932), pp. 181–8.

E. T. Hiller, 'A Culture Theory of Population Trends', in: J. J. Spengler and O. D. Duncan, eds., *Population Theory and Policy, Selected Readings* (Glencoe, 1956).

L. T. Hogben, ed., *Political Arithmetic; a Symposium of Population Studies* (London, 1938).

U. Kahrstedt, 'Die Bevölkerung des Altertums', *Handwörterbuch der Staatswissenschaften* (4th ed., Jena, 1924), ii. 655 ff.

K. Kautsky, *Vermehrung und Entwicklung in Natur und Gesellschaft* (Stuttgart, 1910).

M. A. A. Landry, 'Trois théories de la population', *La Révolution démographique* (Paris, 1934).

P. P. Leroy-Beaulieu, *La Question de la population* (3rd ed., Paris, 1913).

E. Lewis-Faning, 'Report on an enquiry into family limitation and its influence on human fertility during the past fifty years', United Kingdom, *Royal Commission on Population*, 1948–49, *Papers*, vol. 1 [Cmd. 7695].

G. F. List, *The National System of Political Economy* (S. S. Lloyd, trans., new ed., London, 1904).

F. LORIMER, *Culture and Human Fertility* (U.N.E.S.C.O., Paris, 1954).

—— 'The Differentiation of Logical Levels in Social Enquiry', in: J. J. Spengler and O. D. Duncan, eds., *Population Theory and Policy, Selected Readings* (Glencoe, 1956).

R. LYND, *Home Life in Ireland* (3rd ed., London, 1910).

M. MACDONAGH, *Irish Life and Character* (London, 1905).

G. MACKENROTH, *Bevölkerungslehre; Theorie, Soziologie und Statistik der Bevölkerung* (Berlin, 1953).

A. MARSHALL, *Principles of Economics* (8th ed., London, 1930).

P. MOMBERT, *Studien zur Bevölkerungsbewegung in Deutschland ... etc.* (Karlsruhe, 1907).

—— *Bevölkerungslehre* (Jena, 1929).

J. A. O'BRIEN, ed., *The Vanishing Irish; the Enigma of the Modern World* (London, 1954).

K. OLDENBERG, 'Über den Rückgang der Geburten- und Sterbeziffer', *Archiv für Sozialwissenschaft und Sozialpolitik* (March 1911), xxxii. 319–77 (Sept. 1911), xxxiii. 401–99.

F. SAVORGNAN, *La Fecondità dell'aristocrazia* (Pisa, 1942).

MAX SCHELER, 'Bevölkerungsprobleme als Weltanschauungsfragen', in vol. 3, *Moralia*, of *Schriften zur Soziologie und Weltanschauungslehre* (Leipzig, 1929, 3 vols.).

G. VON SCHULZE-GÄVERNITZ, *Britischer Imperialismus und englischer Freihandel zu Beginn des zwanzigsten Jahrhunderts* (Leipzig, 1906).

L. SONOLET, *Principe de population et socialisme* (Paris, 1907).

P. A. SOROKIN, *Social Mobility* (New York, 1927).

J. J. SPENGLER, *France Faces Depopulation* (Durham, North Carolina, 1938).

—— and O. D. DUNCAN, eds., *Population Theory and Policy, Selected Readings* (Glencoe, 1956).

O. SPENGLER, *Der Untergang des Abendlandes. Umrisse einer Morphologie der Weltgeschichte* (Munich, 1924, 2 vols.).

R. VON UNGERN-STERNBERG, *The Causes of the Decline in Birth-rate within the European Sphere of Civilization* (Cold Spring Harbor, 1931).

UNITED NATIONS, DEPARTMENT OF SOCIAL AFFAIRS, POPULATION DIVISION, *The Determinants and Consequences of Population Trends* (New York, 1953).

T. VALENTINER, 'Die seelischen Ursachen des Geburtenrückganges', *Politische Biologie, Schriften für naturgesetzliche Politik und Wissenschaft* (München–Berlin, 1937), Heft 2.

R. B. VANCE, 'Is Theory for Demographers?', in: J. J. Spengler and O. D. Duncan, eds., *Population Theory and Policy, Selected Readings* (Glencoe, 1956).

S. WEBB, *The Decline in the Birth-rate* (Fabian Tract No. 131, London, 1907).

M. WEBER, *The Protestant Ethic and the Spirit of Capitalism* (T. Parsons, trans., London, 1930).

K. A. Wieth-Knudsen, 'Formerelse og Fremskridt, økonomisk-demografisk-biologisk Syntese . . .', from *Politisch-anthropologische Revue* (Hildburghausen, 8. Jahrgang, 1909–10), pp. 150–1.

J. Wolf, *Nationalökonomie als exakte Wissenschaft* (Leipzig, 1908).

—— *Der Geburtenrückgang. Die Rationalisierung des Sexuallebens in unserer Zeit* (Jena, 1912).

—— *Die neue Sexualmoral und das Geburtenproblem unserer Tage* (Jena, 1928).

SECTION III

BOOKS ON THE HISTORY OF POPULATION THEORIES, AND HISTORICAL TREATISES CONTAINING REFERENCES TO THEORIES

P. Ariès, *Histoire des populations françaises et de leurs attitudes devant la vie depuis le XVIIIe siècle* (Paris, 1948).

T. S. Ashton, *An Economic History of England: the Eighteenth Century* (London, 1955).

J. A. Banks, *Prosperity and Parenthood; A Study of Family Planning among the Victorian Middle Classes* (International Library of Sociology and Social Reconstruction, London, 1954).

H. L. Beales, 'The Historical Context of the *Essay on Population*', in D. V. Glass, ed., *Introduction to Malthus* (London, 1953), pp. 1–24.

K. J. Beloch, 'Die Griechen bis auf Alexander den Grossen', *Weltgeschichte*: I, *Geschichte des Altertums* (J. von Pflugk-Harttung, ed., Berlin, 1910), pp. 301 ff.

E. Bernheim, *Lehrbuch der historischen Methode und der Geschichtsphilosophie* (3rd ed., Leipzig, 1903).

H. A. Boner, *Hungry Generations: the Nineteenth-Century Case against Malthusianism* (New York, 1955).

J. Boswell, *Life of Johnson* (G. B. Hill, ed., revised ed. by L. F. Powell, Oxford, 1934–50, 6 vols.).

W. Boyd, *The Educational Theory of Jean-Jacques Rousseau* (London, 1911).

C. Brinkmann, ed., *William Godwin—Robert Malthus* (Stuttgart, 1948).

J. Bryce, *The Holy Roman Empire* (4th ed., London, 1890).

Sir J. H. Clapham, *An Economic History of Modern Britain* (Cambridge, 1926–38, 3 vols.).

K. H. Connell, *The Population of Ireland, 1750–1845* (Oxford, 1950).

G. G. Coulton, *The Medieval Village* (Cambridge, 1925).

K. Davis, 'Malthus and the Theory of Population', in P. F. Lazarsfeld and M. Rosenberg, eds., *The Language of Social Research* (Glencoe, 1955), pp. 540–53.

L. Friedländer, *Roman Life and Manners under the Early Empire* (L. A. Magnus, J. H. Freese, and A. B. Gough, trans., London, 1908–13, 4 vols.).

D. V. Glass, ed., *Introduction to Malthus* (London, 1953).

G. Glotz, *The Greek City and its Institutions* (N. Mallinson, trans., London, 1929).

R. Gonnard, *Histoire des doctrines de la population* (Paris, 1923).

G. T. Griffith, *Population Problems of the Age of Malthus* (Cambridge, 1926).

D. Heron, *On the Relation of Fertility in Man to Social Status, and on the Changes in this Relation that Have Taken Place during the Last Fifty Years* (Drapers' Company Research Memoirs. Studies in National Deterioration, I, London, 1906).

N. E. Himes, *Medical History of Contraception* (Baltimore, 1936).

T. W. Hutchison, *A Review of Economic Doctrines, 1870–1929* (Oxford, 1953).

M. Jaeger, *Before Victoria; Changing Standards and Behaviour, 1787–1837* (London, 1956).

R. R. Kuczynski, 'British Demographers' Opinions on Fertility, 1660 to 1760', *Political Arithmetic; a Symposium of Population Studies* (L. T. Hogben, ed., London, 1938), pp. 283–327.

E. Lowenthal, 'The Ricardian Socialists', *Studies in History, Economics, and Public Law, Faculty of Political Science of Columbia University* (New York, 1911), xlvi, no. 1, pp. 5–105.

R. L. Meek, ed., *Marx and Engels on Malthus* (London, 1953).

H. Michell, *The Economics of Ancient Greece* (Cambridge, 1940).

R. von Mohl, *Die Geschichte und Literatur der Staatswissenschaften, in Monographien dargestellt* (Erlangen, 1858, 3 vols.).

R. K. P. Pankhurst, *William Thompson, 1775–1833: Britain's Pioneer Socialist, Feminist, and Co-operator* (London, 1954).

R. von Pöhlmann, 'Römische Kaiserzeit und Untergang der antiken Welt', *Weltgeschichte*: I, *Geschichte des Altertums* (J. von Pflugk-Harttung, ed., Berlin, 1910), pp. 507 ff.

P. Reynaud, *La Théorie de la population en Italie du XVIe au XVIIIe siècle: Les précurseurs de Malthus* (Lyon, 1904).

M. I. Rostovtzeff, *The Social and Economic History of the Roman Empire* (Oxford, 1926).

—— *The Social and Economic History of the Hellenistic World* (Oxford, 1941, 3 vols.).

R. N. Salaman, *The History and Social Influence of the Potato* (Cambridge, 1949).

J. Saville, *Rural Depopulation in England and Wales, 1851–1951* (London, 1957).

J. A. Schumpeter, *History of Economic Analysis* (Oxford, 1955).

O. Seeck, *Geschichte des Untergangs der antiken Welt* (Stuttgart, 1920–2, 6 vols.).

K. Smith, *The Malthusian Controversy* (London, 1951).

J. J. Spengler, 'The Political Economy of Jefferson, Adams, and Madison', *American Studies in Honor of W. K. Boyd* (D. K. Jackson, ed., Durham, North Carolina, 1940).

J. J. SPENGLER, *French Predecessors of Malthus* (Durham, North Carolina, 1942).

C. E. STANGELAND, *Pre-Malthusian Doctrines of Population; a Study in the History of Economic Theory* (Studies in History, Economics, and Public Law, edited by the Faculty of Political Science of Columbia University, New York, 1904), xxi, no. 3.

J. STASSART, *Malthus et la population* (Liège, 1957).

SIR L. STEPHEN, *The English Utilitarians* (London, 1900, 3 vols.).

SIR W. W. TARN, *Hellenistic Civilisation* (London, 1927).

B. TS. URLANIS, *Rost naseleniya v Evrope* (Moscow, 1941).

T. VEBLEN, *Imperial Germany and the Industrial Revolution* (new ed., London, 1939).

A. B. WOLFE, 'The Economics of Population in Ancient Greece', *Facts and Factors in Economic History* (Cambridge, Mass., 1932), pp. 35–38.

SECTION IV

ARTICLES IN PERIODICALS ON THE HISTORY OF POPULATION THEORIES

A. ALDRIDGE, 'Franklin as Demographer', *Journal of Economic History* (May 1949), ix, no. 1, pp. 25–44.

J. BELOCH, 'Zur Bevölkerungsgeschichte des Altertums', *Jahrbücher für Nationalökonomie und Statistik* (1897), III. Folge, xiii. 321–43.

L. VON BORTKIEWICZ, 'War Aristoteles Malthusianer?', *Zeitschrift für die gesamte Staatswissenschaft* (June 1906), lxii. 383–406.

L. BRENTANO, 'Die Malthus'sche Lehre und die Bevölkerungsbewegung der letzten Dezennien', *Abhandlungen der Historischen Klasse der Königlich Bayerischen Akademie der Wissenschaften* (München, 1909), xxiv. 565–625.

E. J. BUCKATZSCH, 'The Constancy of Local Populations and Migration in England before 1800', *Population Studies* (1952), v. 62–69.

D. G. COWGILL, 'The Theory of Population Growth Cycles', *American Journal of Sociology* (Sept. 1949), lv, no. 2, pp. 163–70.

A. FLEW, 'The Structure of Malthus' Population Theory', *Australasian Journal of Philosophy* (1957), xxxv, no. 1, pp. 1–20.

O. JOLLES, 'Die Ansichten der deutschen nationalökonomischen Schriftsteller des sechzehnten und siebzehnten Jahrhunderts über Bevölkerungswesen', *Jahrbücher für Nationalökonomie und Statistik* (Neue Folge, Jena, 1886), xiii. 193–224.

A. LANDRY, 'Quelques aperçus concernant la dépopulation dans l'antiquité gréco-romaine', *Revue historique* (Jan.–Feb. 1936), clxxvii. 1–33.

S. LEVIN, 'Marx versus Malthus', *Papers of the Michigan Academy of Science, Arts, and Letters* (1936), xxii. 234–48.

J. R. MINER, 'Pierre-François Verhulst, the Discoverer of the Logistic Curve', *Human Biology* (Dec. 1933), v, no. 4, pp. 673–89.

P. Mombert, 'Die Anschauungen des siebzehnten und achtzehnten Jahrhunderts über die Abnahme der Bevölkerung', *Jahrbücher für Nationalökonomik und Statistik* (1931), III. Folge, lxxx. 481–503.

L. Robbins, 'On a Certain Ambiguity in the Conception of Stationary Equilibrium', *The Economic Journal* (June 1930), xl, no. 158, pp. 194–214.

A. Sauvy, 'Doctrine soviétique en matière de population', *Rivista italiana di demografia e statistica* (Dec. 1948), ii, no. 4, pp. 474–88.

J. Schumpeter, 'Gustav von Schmoller und die Probleme von heute', *Schmoller's Jahrbuch* (50. Jahrgang, 1926), part 1, pp. 337–88.

O. Seeck, 'Die Statistik in der alten Geschichte', *Jahrbücher für Nationalökonomie und Statistik* (1897), III. Folge, xiii. 161–76.

N. J. Silberling, 'British Prices and Business Cycles, 1779–1850', *Review of Economic Statistics* (1923), v. 219–62.

J. J. Spengler, 'Population Doctrines in the United States', *Journal of Political Economy* (Aug. 1933), xli, no. 4, pp. 433–67; (Oct. 1933), xli, no. 5, pp. 639–72.

—— 'French Population Theory since 1800', *Journal of Political Economy* (Oct. 1936), xliv, no. 5, pp. 577–611; (Dec. 1936), xliv, no. 6, pp. 743–66.

—— 'Moheau, Prophet of Depopulation', *Journal of Political Economy* (1939), xlvii, no. 5, pp. 648–77.

—— 'Malthus's Total Population Theory: a restatement and reappraisal', *Canadian Journal of Economics and Political Science* (Feb. 1945), xi, no. 1, pp. 83–110; (May 1945), xi, no. 2, pp. 234–64.

—— 'Marshall on the Population Question', *Population Studies* (March 1955), viii. 264–87; (July 1955), ix. 56–66.

J. Sutter, 'Un Démographe engagé: Arsène Dumont, 1849–1902', *Population* (Jan.-Mar. 1953), viii, no. 1, pp. 79–92.

R. F. Willetts, 'The *Neodamodeis*', *Classical Philology* (Jan.–Oct. 1954), xlix, no. 1, pp. 27 ff.

INDEX OF NAMES

INDEX OF SUBJECTS